EUTHANASIA, CLINICAL PRACTICE AND THE LAW

EUTHANASIA, CLINICAL PRACTICE AND THE LAW

Edited by

LUKE GORMALLY

Director,
The Linacre Centre for Health Care Ethics

THE LINACRE CENTRE
FOR HEALTH CARE ETHICS

LONDON 1994

Published by The Linacre Centre,
60 Grove End Road, London NW8 9NH.

First published in this format 1994

British Library Cataloguing in Publication Data
Euthanasia, Clinical Practice and the Law
I. Gormally, Luke
179.7

ISBN 0-906561-09-4 (cloth)
ISBN 0-906561-08-6 (pbk.)

Typeset by Create Publishing Services Ltd, Bath, Avon

CONTENTS

Introduction *Luke Gormally*   vii

BOOK ONE

EUTHANASIA AND CLINICAL PRACTICE: 1
TRENDS, PRINCIPLES AND ALTERNATIVES.
A Working Party Report (1982)

Detailed contents of the Report   3

BOOK TWO

EUTHANASIA AND THE LAW: 109
THE CASE AGAINST LEGALIZATION

1   Submission to the Select Committee of   111
    the House of Lords on Medical Ethics
    by the Linacre Centre for Health Care Ethics.

2   'Living Will' Legislation *John Finnis*   167

3   The BMA Report on Euthanasia and the case   177
    against legalization *Luke Gormally*

4   Some reflections on euthanasia   193
    in The Netherlands *John Keown*

5   Further reflections on euthanasia in The   219
    Netherlands in the light of The Remmelink
    Report and the van der Maas Survey *John Keown*

Contributors to Book 2   241

Index   243

Introduction

The present volume brings together work separated by more than a decade. In order to mark the distinctive character and separate origins of each of the two main parts of the volume they are titled Book 1 and Book 2.

Book 1 is a further reprint of the Centre's Working Party Report *Euthanasia and Clinical Practice: trends, principles and alternatives* which was first published in 1982. That volume was well-received by readers and reviewers, but after a subsequent reprinting has been unavailable for some time. Continuing demand for the Report has suggested the need for a further reprinting. *Euthanasia and Clinical Practice*, however, largely confines its 'attention to the ethics of euthanasia in the clinical situation, i.e. to questions, about what is the right thing to do, which arise for patients and clinicians in the context of medical care' (p.10). The question of whether euthanasia should be legalised, which was reasonably eschewed by the Centre's Working Party over a decade ago, is a much more pressing issue in contemporary political debate. It therefore seemed important to provide some extended consideration of this issue alongside the reprinted Report. Hence the contents of Book 2 of this volume. Since Book 2 brings together a substantial body of writing distinct from the contents of Book 1, a new title for the entire volume seemed justified. *Euthanasia, Clinical Practice and the Law* sufficiently marks continuity with the earlier volume (now Book 1), as well as indicating the specific emphasis of Book 2.

Despite the passage of the years, *Euthanasia and Clinical Practice* (Book 1) has retained its value in the eyes both of clinicians and of students of bioethics. But readers coming to it for the first time will need to bear in mind that the text of the Report was finalised almost 12 years ago. If the Report were being written in 1993 it would have to take account of evidence which has come to light and of a body of literature which has appeared in the intervening years. But precisely because it is the work of an interdisciplinary group which concluded its deliberations at the beginning of the last decade, the Report is necessarily unrevisable. In the reprinting of the Report no significant alterations have been made to the text.

Book 2, entitled *Euthanasia and the Law: the Case against Legalization*, brings together a number of contributions which address some of the questions raised by proposals to legalize the practice of euthanasia. The first document in this part of the volume is the Submission made on behalf of The Linacre Centre to The House of Lords' Select Committee on Medical Ethics.

The Select Committee has been invited to consider the justifiability of conduct intended to end the lives of patients, and the consequences of legalizing such conduct. The Linacre Centre's Submission addresses most of the issues identified by the Committee as falling within its terms of reference. The second item in Book 2 is a paper by John Finnis on '*Living Will*' *Legislation*. He considers legislation to give effect to advance directives, and jurisprudential advocacy of such legislation, and shows how much of what is enacted and proposed makes advance directives the vehicle for a euthanasiast agenda. My own contribution, analysing the case made against legalizing euthanasia in the important 1988 Working Party Report on *Euthanasia* prepared on behalf of the British Medical Association, concludes that there are significant defects in the case which need to be repaired if opposition to legalization is to be sustained on a sound and coherent basis. Finally, John Keown, in two contributions, provides a scholarly analysis of exactly what has been happening in Holland as a result of the way the Courts have accommodated the practice of euthanasia by doctors. A sober reading of these two chapters should help dispel widespread illusions about Dutch practice, and serve to establish exactly what is at issue in proposals to import the 'Dutch solution' to other jurisdictions.

The second part of this volume is offered as a contribution to the major debate now under way in our society about the desirability of accommodating the practice of euthanasia either by statute or by judicial decision. Those who believe some such accommodation desirable need to confront the contrary case advanced in this volume that euthanasia is incompatible with a true recognition of human dignity and is deeply corrosive of the authentic character of medical practice.

Luke Gormally
28 July 1993.

Acknowledgement
I am grateful to my colleague Dr Helen Watt for her work in compiling the index to this volume.
LG.

BOOK ONE

EUTHANASIA AND CLINICAL PRACTICE: TRENDS, PRINCIPLES AND ALTERNATIVES.

A WORKING PARTY REPORT
(1982)

Members of the Working Party (1978–1981)

Rev J Mahoney SJ MA DD *(Chairman)*
Principal, Heythrop College, University of London

Professor G E M Anscombe FBA MA
Professor of Philosophy, University of Cambridge

Miss P Ashworth MSc SRN SCM FRCN
Lecturer in Nursing, University of Manchester

Mrs M Cleary SRN QN NDN PWT
Community Nursing Sister, Liverpool Area Health Authority

Mr N Coote MA PhL STL
Secretary, Social Welfare Commission, Catholic Bishops' Conference

Dr J M Finnis LLB DPhil MA
Reader in Law, University of Oxford

Dr J Hebbert ERD OStJ MD FRCP
Consultant Physician in Geriatric Medicine, Whipps Cross Hospital

Professor P M Higgins MB FRCP FRCGP
Professor of General Practice, Guy's Hospital Medical School

Miss M M Pearce MBE SRN SCM
Chairman of Council, St Mary's Hospice, Selly Park, Birmingham

Rev B Soane PhD BSc STL ARSM
Lecturer in Moral Theology, Allen Hall, London

Dr R G Twycross MA DM FRCP
Consultant Physician, The Churchill Hospital, Oxford

Professor J E Utting MA MB BChir FFARCS
Professor of Anaesthesia, University of Liverpool

Professor R B Zachary BPharm MB FRCS FRCSI
Emeritus Professor of Paediatric Surgery, University of Sheffield

Mr A J L Gormally Lic Phil
Director, The Linacre Centre

Mr F D K Williams CBE MA
Former Director, The Linacre Centre

Sr J Milne Home SHCJ MA
Administrative Secretary, The Linacre Centre

CONTENTS OF THE REPORT

Preface   7

1 Introduction   9
1. Questions, issues and confusions in the public debate   9
2. Focus of this Report   10
3. 'Trends' towards euthanasia   10
4. What we mean by 'euthanasia'   10
5. Sources of evidence   11
6. The positive task of the Report   12

Part One   13

2 Euthanasia in clinical practice and thinking

A. *Five Specialised Fields of Care*   15

1. Care of the Newborn   15
2. Care of the Handicapped   22
3. Terminal Care   23
4. Care of the Elderly   25
5. Intensive Care   27

B. *External Influences on Clinical Practice and Thinking*   28

1. Utilitarian views of responsibility   28
2. 'Possessive individualist' conceptions of the person   29
3. Social Darwinism   30
4. Supposed implications of moral pluralism   30
5. Organised advocacy of euthanasia   30
6. Economic factors   32

Part Two   35

3 Murder and the morality of euthanasia: some philosophical considerations

Introduction   37
1. What constitutes murder   37
2. On intentionally killing the innocent   39
3. The prohibition   40
4. Why euthanasia is no exception to the prohibition   41

3

5. Proper and improper 'quality of life' judgements   43
6. Limits to moral pluralism   45
7. The possibility of murder by omission   46
8. The morality of omitting life-saving measures   47
9. The morality of killing as a side-effect of other action   48

4 The Christian Tradition

1. The gift of life   51
2. The commandment: 'Do no murder'   52
3. The conditions of our stewardship   53
4. Attitudes towards our stewardship   54
5. 'Death with dignity'   55
6. Roman Catholic teaching   55

Part Three   59

5 The rights and duties of competent patients in regard to treatment

1. The legal right to refuse treatment   61
2. The question: When ought patients to accept treatment?   61
3. The distinction between 'ordinary' and 'extraordinary' means   62
4. Considerations determining when treatment is and is
    not obligatory   63
5. Burdensomeness and patients' refusal of treatment   63
6. Which reasons for refusing treatment are suicidal?   64
7. Refusing treatment, suicide and the direction of the will:
    further analysis   65
8. Conclusion   66

6 The rights of incompetent patients and duties towards them

1. Standard of treatment   67
2. Judging the burdensomeness of treatment for the incompetent   68
3. What valid reasons are there for withholding treatment from
    the newborn?   69
4. Uniformity in treatment not to be expected   71

Part Four   73

7 Good practice: some principles

1. *Three Classes of Patient*   76

A. Patients with a lethal condition for which there are no life-saving
    treatments   76
    i) The inevitability of death
    ii) What is normally involved in saying that someone is dying?
    iii) The importance of knowing that a patient is dying
    iv) Recognising the onset of dying

    v) Treatment in the terminal phase
    vi) Relief of symptoms

B. Patients with a lethal condition for which life-saving treatment   80
exists

C. Patients with a non-lethal but incapacitating condition   81

2. *Good Team Care*   81

8 Good practice in specialised fields of care

1. Care of the Newborn   84
   a. Conditions which are lethal and for which there is no life-saving
      treatment?   85
   b. Conditions which are lethal and for which life-saving treatment
      exists   85
   c. Conditions which are not lethal in themselves but which are
      associated with severe disability   86
2. Care of the Handicapped   88
3. Terminal Care   90
4. Care of the Elderly   91
5. Intensive Care   93
   a. Dying patients   93
   b. Transplantation and the 'brain dead' patient   94

9 Conclusion   95

Glossary of some medical terms   97
Works cited   99
Note: Regina v. Arthur by *Luke Gormally*   104

PREFACE

The Report which follows is the product of three years of collaboration of a Working Party invited by the Governors of The Linacre Centre 'to consider and report on trends towards euthanasia in modern health care practices, in the light of Catholic principles and teaching'.

The Working Party first met in October 1978, and in the course of its early meetings its membership became established as indicated on page 2. In addition to various sectional meetings and regular correspondence, twenty-one plenary sessions of the Working Party were held at The Linacre Centre, the final one taking place in September 1981.

The Working Party wishes to acknowledge its indebtedness to the founding Director of The Linacre Centre, Mr. David Williams, for his experienced and energetic contributions to its activities. His sudden illness and unavoidable retirement were matter for deep regret, but his colleagues on the Working Party are gratified that he has found it possible in some measure to follow their later deliberations and so to associate himself with this final Report.

The Working Party also wishes to record its appreciation of the contribution and support provided by the present Director of the Centre and by its Administrative Secretary.

In concluding its commission and presenting this Report the Working Party confirms both the importance and the relevance of serious ethical concern on the subject of euthanasia. It also expresses the hope that its considerations on this fundamental issue of life or death will provide a positive contribution for reflection not only by members of the health care professions but also by all sectors of the community.

John Mahoney SJ,
Chairman of the Working Party

Note

After the Working Party had completed and submitted its Report, the very important and widely publicised *Arthur* case seemed to corroborate much of what is said in the Report about paediatric practice and thinking. In the circumstances, and with the agreement of the Chairman of Governors of the Linacre Centre, I have thought it appropriate to ask the Director of the Centre to supply a Note outlining the evidence for trends towards euthanasia which came to light in the course of the trial. The contents of the Note are not attributable to the Working Party itself.

J. M.
(January 1982)

1

Introduction

1. Questions, issues, and confusions in the public debate

Euthanasia is increasingly a subject of public debate and concern. There are those (notably the members of 'Exit') who strongly press for the legalisation of voluntary euthanasia. Moreover, evidence increasingly suggests that some doctors and nurses are already treating patients in ways which are designed to hasten death. Some believe these practices to be morally right even if illegal. Others believe them to be not merely illegal but morally wrong and bound to have a profoundly corrupting effect on the practice of medicine.

Some doctors who express an opinion on these matters employ dubious distinctions in defence of treatment policies. Some seem to think that what is called 'passive euthanasia' (letting a patient die) is always morally permissible, and that only 'active euthanasia' (active killing) is morally wrong. And among those who seem to think passive euthanasia quite generally acceptable are some who talk about 'letting nature take its course'. One may wonder whether any science and art of medicine could have developed if people had remained content to let nature take its course. When should nature be allowed simply to take its course? Only when it is futile to resist biological decline? Or also in circumstances in which one can alter or reverse the course of nature but has reason not to do so? But then, what reasons are morally acceptable? That a patient's life is not worthwhile, for example? Or that treatment would impose burdens of a kind that are hardly warranted by its expected benefits?

At times the phrase 'letting nature take its course' savours of euphemism. If you are sedating a patient so that he will not take food so that he will die, are you doing no more than letting nature take its course?

There are those who think such euphemism unnecessary as well as hypocritical; they wish frankly to defend active euthanasia in circumstances in which a patient is subject to considerable pain or is severely handicapped and who for either of these reasons is judged not to have (or no longer to have) a worthwhile life; these patients are sometimes said to have an unacceptable 'quality of life' or to have lives incompatible with human dignity.

There are those who think euthanasia commendable because they believe that the alternative – the traditional ethic of the sanctity of life – is too abhorrent in its implications in certain clinical situations. Belief in the

9

sanctity of life, it is said, would require clinicians to strive to prolong life to the utmost, indifferent to burdens of physical and psychological suffering.

2. Focus of this Report

In debate among the lay public, and in medical and nursing circles, there seem to be more questions than answers; and of the answers proffered, some are disturbing.

The Working Party which has produced this Report undertook to address only some of the issues currently engaging public attention in the euthanasia debate. We have confined our attention to the ethics of euthanasia in the clinical situation i.e. to questions, about what is the right thing to do, which arise for patients and clinicians in the context of medical care. We have deliberately eschewed extended discussion of the question whether euthanasia ought to be legalised. We did so in order to avoid overburdening an already complex Report and in order to keep clear our treatment of the most basic issues: how ought clinicians and patients to think and to act in situations in which euthanasia can seem an attractive option.

3. 'Trends' towards euthanasia

In Chapter 2 we seek to establish how urgent an issue euthanasia is both in the practice and thinking of clinicians. Our terms of reference were to consider 'trends' towards euthanasia in clinical practice. If a trend is considered demonstrated only when a rising graph of verifiable incidents has been produced then we must say, first, that evidence as to practice is not sufficiently public for it to be possible to produce that kind of graph; and, second, even if it had been we did not command the research resources to unearth it. So our method has had to be in part impressionistic: we have relied on the information available to clinical members of the Working Party and on such reports as are made public. But impressions about practice can receive some confirmation from evidence of clinicians' own thinking about euthanasia. We emphasise that we have for the most part concentrated on what clinicians themselves think about euthanasia rather than examining extended philosophical defences of it. Still, those clinicians who have put forward principled defences of euthanasia may indeed find their best allies amongst philosophers; and we thought it right to give serious philosophical consideration to the ethics of euthanasia in Chapter 3.

Two further points need to be made about the enquiry undertaken in Chapter 2.

4. What we mean by 'euthanasia'

First, what are we referring to when we talk of euthanasia? We settled, partly for reasons of brevity, on the following definition:

there is *euthanasia* when the death of a human being is brought about on purpose as part of the medical care being given him.

What is covered by this definition crucially depends upon the interpretation one gives to the term 'medical care'. At this stage of our inquiry it would not do to anticipate our own normative conclusions. Many justifications can be invoked for bringing about the death of the ill or handicapped; but a justification is euthanasiast, in the sense we have in mind,[1] only when it represents the death of a *patient* as a *benefit* to him, or at least as no *harm* to him (and a benefit to others). Death is made out to be a benefit on the basis of the view taken of the present or future physical or mental condition or quality of life of the patient; and in reckoning benefit to others, the quality of life of the family in particular is taken into account.

Death procured as a benefit is thought by some to be at least compatible with medical care, and by others to be a positive expression of medical care. In some justifications of involuntary euthanasia it is said that the 'unit of care' is the family, and the doctor ought to calculate what course of action will, overall, benefit the family.

That range of use of the term 'euthanasia' for which the notion of benefit is critical, stakes out the central subject-matter of our enquiry. Accordingly, our brief definition can be expanded as follows:

> in euthanasia a person's death is brought about on the ground that, because of his present or likely future mental condition and quality of life (and sometimes in consideration too of the quality of life of his family) it would be better for him (or at least no harm) if that person were dead.

5. Sources of evidence

The second matter calling for comment is the range of published material on which we have drawn. Our primary interest is in British clinical practice and in the ethical issues as they are perceived therein. Nonetheless, we have not hesitated to draw from time to time on North American publications. This may surprise readers especially when evidence is adduced from these publications in Chapter 2. For a number of reasons, however, we do not think this procedure unreasonable. Firstly, some of the American publications referred to are (wholly or partly) the work of British authors. Secondly, even when this is not the case, it is important to recognise the intellectual commerce that exists between British and North American medicine, particularly in respect of ethical issues fundamental to the practice of medicine. Thirdly (and this comment has particular relevance to Chapter 2) there is a

---

[1] 'Euthanasia', of course, can be used to refer to all forms of, and motivations for, bringing about death by medical means or medically qualified personnel. Thus broadly used it extends to killings motivated by considerations of eugenics, *Lebensraum*, etc. in which the question of benefit or harm to the person killed plays no significant part. Euthanasia of the eugenic, *Lebensraum*, etc, forms seems to us significantly different in motivation from the forms of euthanasia which principally concern us in the Report, even though it also seems to us that the *justifications* for euthanasia of the sort defined in the text above are justifications which, when analysed critically, leave no ground for excluding eugenic, etc, euthanasia.

sad paucity of British-based empirical research on those clinical practices and attitudes which particularly interest us. Such American research as exists may serve to suggest the likely shape of the picture. The reports on which we have drawn are confirmed by the personal experience of those of our members familiar with the specialities in question.

6. The positive task of the Report

Chapter 2 makes clear that euthanasia is an urgent practical and theoretical issue. We felt called upon to consider the issue as deeply as we could. Our exploration of the fundamental ethical question – philosophical and religious – will be found in Chapters 3 and 4. Their conclusion is that euthanasia is wrong.

It is not to be expected that in a pluralistic culture the insights into the nature of human existence on which the tradition of common morality depends will come readily to all readers, even to all Christian readers. But unless these insights are reappropriated and medicine honours the traditional conception of human dignity it is difficult to see what in *principle* stands in the way of a repetition of the historical betrayal of medicine that took place in Germany in the second quarter of this century.

We have not merely undertaken to explain the case *against* euthanasia, important in itself though that task is. Some views of what is required by the traditional ethic of the sanctity of life seem to us a travesty of what is truly required by that ethic. In Part Three of the Report we have sought to clarify the limits on a competent patient's obligations to undergo treatment and on the obligations of others in respect of treatment for the incompetent. In Part Four, as well as clarifying what forms of patient management may be euthanasiast, we undertake to give positive accounts of the types of care we think consistent with an authentic recognition and respect for the dignity of every patient.

Part One

2

Euthanasia in Clinical Practice and Thinking

Before discussing the morality of euthanasia we have sought to establish whether and in what ways euthanasia has become a more pressing issue for clinicians in recent years. In particular we have reviewed readily available evidence both for clinical practice in this matter and for thinking which is apt to determine practice. The present chapter reviews some evidence for both practice and thinking in five specialised fields of health care: care of the newborn, care of the handicapped, terminal care, care of the elderly, and intensive care. In the second part (B) of the chapter we identify some background influences on clinical thinking and practice.

A. Five specialised fields of care

1. Care of the Newborn

a) Practice

The situation of the newborn is distinctive in two significant ways. Firstly if there is euthanasia in childhood it necessarily is involuntary. Secondly in the neonatal period death can be readily brought about by purposeful omission since the baby cannot sustain life without ordinary nursing care, including nutrition and warmth, which others have to provide.

Commenting on striking changes in statistics for 'stillbirths' a paediatric surgeon remarked fifteen years ago that 'the immediate survival of the infant depends to a large extent on the attitude of those in attendance'.[1] A small survey published in 1967 revealed that between 1951 and 1961 recorded stillbirths of spina bifida babies varied between 10% and 40%, but that subsequent to 1962 no stillbirths were recorded. The change to some degree coincided with the introduction of new methods in the treatment of spina bifida and with a consequent optimism which then prevailed. It is not unreasonable to speculate that before 1962 'stillborn' was a label masking 'obstetrical euthanasia'[2].

Has the situation changed more recently? We think that it has. In the

[1] D M Forrest, 'Early Closure in spina bifida: results and problems' (1967) 60 *Proceedings of the Royal Society of Medicine*, 764.
[2] Freeman J M, 'To Treat or Not to Treat: Ethical Dilemmas of Treating the Infant with a Myelomeningocele' (1973) 20 *Clinical Neurosurgery*, 134–46.

following paragraphs we set out some of the evidence that euthanasia of the newborn has recently become common. And we should note straightaway that there has been another change: whereas euthanasia, if it was practised in the 1950s, was covert, euthanasia in the 1970s and early 1980s has become much more overt, something to be more or less openly advocated as an acceptable paediatric practice in relation to handicapped newborn babies. It still is not fully overt, however, since it is frequently described as 'leaving (or allowing) them to die'.

Two sorts of case can be broadly distinguished. The first is where the baby has a condition which, if not relieved, is lethal: for example, an intestinal obstruction. Duodenal atresia in a Down's syndrome baby is a type of case frequently referred to. Very few paediatricians would withhold surgery from a baby with intestinal obstruction uncomplicated by any other condition. The surgery is readily performed and generally successful. Yet a recent editorial in the *British Medical Journal*[3] rather assumes that a significant number of paediatricians would withhold surgery when the atresia occurs in a Down's syndrome baby and merely urges upon these paediatricians the desirability of sedating the baby. Two articles published in *The New England Journal of Medicine* in 1973 – one of them claiming to break 'public and professional silence on a major social taboo'[4] – each documented cases in their authors' practice of withholding treatment from Down's syndrome babies with duodenal atresia when parents refused consent for surgery[5]. In England public silence on this practice was signally broken in 1981 by civil court proceedings concerning a Down's syndrome baby with duodenal atresia; the evidence in these proceedings suggests that the withholding of surgery when parents refuse consent for surgery on the grounds that 'it would be unkind to the child to operate on her' and that death would be 'in the best interests of the child'[6], has indeed become recognised (though by no means universal) practice in these circumstances. The justification generally offered for withholding treatment in such cases is that Down's syndrome is nearly always associated with mental retardation which, at the least, is burdensome to the family and the community.

In 1975, more than 450 members of the American Academy of Paediatrics completed a questionnaire designed to survey attitudes and practice, with particular reference to cases of Down's syndrome babies with duodenal atresia[7]. 267 of the respondents were paediatric surgeons and 190 were paediatric physicians in senior positions. 24 per cent of the surgeons and 13

3 Editorial, 'Withholding treatment in infancy' (1981) *British Medical Journal* i, 925–6.
4 R S Duff, A G M Campbell, 'Moral and Ethical Dilemmas in the Special-Care Nursery', (1973) 289 *The New England Journal of Medicine*, 894.
5 The case of Baby B in A Shaw, 'Dilemmas of "Informed Consent" in Children', (1973) 289 *The New England Journal of Medicine*, 886; R S Duff, A G M Campbell, *op. cit.*, 891.
6 *In re B (a Minor)*, Law Report, *The Times* 8 August 1981, fully reported in [1981] 1 *Weekly Law Reports* 1421. The Court of Appeal in that case allowed the local authority [and doctors willing to do so] to override the parents' refusal and said that 'to terminate the life of a mongoloid child because she also has an intestinal complaint' is not 'in the interests of the child'.
7 A Shaw, J G Randolph, B Menard, 'Ethical Issues in Pediatric Surgery: A National Survey of Pediatricians and Pediatric Surgeons', (1977) 60 *Pediatrics*, 588–99. It should be noted here – as the authors of the article note – that 'the totals of over 100% for both groups indicate that several of those

per cent of the physicians said that they would seek to persuade parents not to have surgery on their baby, while 52 per cent of the surgeons and 38 per cent of the physicians said they would put all the facts before the parents and accept the parents' decision. 77 per cent of the surgeons and 50 per cent of the physicians said they would acquiesce in a parental decision to refuse consent for surgery. If faced by indecisive parents, only 17 per cent of the surgeons and 28 per cent of the physicians said they would try to persuade the parents to allow surgery, though they would not take them to court if they refused. Only some 3.5 per cent of the surgeons and 16 per cent of the physicians declared themselves willing to seek a court order directing surgery to be done if the parents refused to sign consent. There is reason to believe that in the United Kingdom a rather higher percentage of paediatric physicians than the 13 per cent of the American survey would try to influence parents against the operation. And in this country the paediatric physicians have primary clinical responsibility for the decision.

The second sort of case in which the death of the baby is sought is where the baby is suffering from one or more non-lethal conditions producing handicap. There are many conditions which, because they are serious, give rise in the lay mind to the misconception that they are lethal; for example, extrophy of the bladder, in which the baby is born not only without any covering to the bladder but with the bladder itself turned inside out. This sort of misconception is most commonly entertained of spina bifida, where it is wrongly assumed that if a child has an operation he will live and if he does not he will die. This is not true, yet it is by trading on this false assumption that a form of selection of patients for operation is often rationalised. Those who seem likely to have a considerable residual handicap are not even referred to the surgeon by the paediatric physician and parents are told that 'the child will die'. Without any operation many do not die and the open wound on the back may heal over within a few weeks or months, leaving the baby with a large swelling on the back and its disability unchanged or becoming worse on account of hydrocephalus. Since early death often does not supervene, it has become the practice of some paediatricians not only to withhold surgery but also to seek to hasten death.

One of the 1973 articles already referred to in connection with Down's syndrome reported in the following terms on 'treatment' of some spina bifida babies: 'When maximum treatment was viewed as unacceptable by families and physicians in our unit, there was a growing tendency to seek early death as a management option ...'[8] A subsequent interview with one of the authors makes it clear that what is being referred to is the emergence of killing as a standard practice.[9] A more recent contribution by the joint

who responded checked more than one of the options' (p.591). It should also be noted that one could, without inconsistency, regard some of the options as alternatives.

[8] R S Duff, A G M Campbell, op.cit., 893

[9] B Kelsey, 'Which infants should live? Who should decide? An interview with Dr Raymond Duff', (1975) 5 (2) *Hastings Center Report*, 5–8. When asked to reflect on the morality of making death a 'management option' Duff responded by observing that in some instances the distinction between killing and letting die was a 'moral quibble'. In its context this response can only be interpreted as an attempted rationale for some killing.

authors of the 1973 article reports on the basis of 'a recent study of paediatricians in the New Haven area that euthanasia was viewed quite favourably. Passive euthanasia ("letting a child die") was approved by 98 per cent. Active euthanasia (killing) was viewed favourably by 39 per cent, with mixed feelings by 28 per cent, and opposed by 33 per cent.'[10]

To say one is 'letting a child die' is certainly a euphemism for killing when one is administering sedatives to the baby so that it shall be continuously sleepy, take little or no food and die within a few weeks. In such a case it is not the condition of spina bifida that causes the death of the child but the lack of nutrition.

There is growing evidence that this form of management is common. Thus at a public meeting in 1977 a paediatrician explained the details by saying that the babies were given 60 mgs of chloral hydrate per kilogram body weight four times a day (eight times the sedative dose recommended in a modern textbook of paediatrics) starting on the day, usually the first after birth, when the decision was made not to offer a neonatal operation. The result was that after two or three days these babies became very sleepy and did not demand a feed, usually dying between two and six weeks of age[11]. In one centre 23 out of 24 babies did not have a neonatal operation and all 23 babies died, it being admitted that they were 'pushed into death'[12]. A paediatrician admitted in open meeting that when he had made the decision not to recommend operation he told his registrar to give the baby a large dose of morphine.[13] A paediatrician in a London hospital said during an open meeting in reply to a student that the babies who did not receive operation were either not fed or given only glucose and water[14]. A paediatrician invited to give his views in *The Lancet* has explained his practice in relation to such forms of congenital handicap as severe spina bifida and hydrocephalus (as well as the more severe chromosomal disorders, including Down's syndrome, multiple anomalies, bilateral anophthalmia and severe rubella syndrome). What he has to offer is 'some help in hastening the end of a life which I now have to advise the parents would otherwise be one which is not a life in any full sense'. Accordingly, in the absence of a strong expression of parental desire to rear the child, the baby is given 'careful and loving nursing, water sufficient to satisfy thirst, and increasing doses of sedation' and soon dies[15]. Two experienced consultant paediatricians have recently in separate television programmes described their practice in the management of certain handicapped babies in similar terms.[16] The unashamed fashion in

10 R S Duff, A G M Campbell, 'Moral and Ethical Dilemmas: Seven years into the debate about human ambiguity', (1980) 447 *Annals of the American Academy of Political and Social Science*, 26. Reference to American data should not be thought uninformative in respect of British practice. Professor Campbell is a British paediatrician. The joint contributions of Duff and Campbell over the past eight years amount to sustained advocacy of allowing parents and physicians the choice of euthanasia for severely handicapped children.

11 R B Zachary, 'Life with Spina Bifida', (1977) *British Medical Journal* ii, 1460–62.

12 *Ibid.*

13 *Ibid.*

14 *Ibid.*

15 Anon. 'Non-treatment of Defective Newborn Babies' (1979) *Lancet* ii, 1123–4.

16 Dr Hugh Jolly of the Charing Cross Hospital on the ATV Jaywalking programme, Sunday 22 February 1981; Dr Donald Garrow of High Wycombe General Hospital firstly on Thames Tele-

which senior members of the profession so describe their practice in public suggests confidence in a considerable measure of support from colleagues.

It is seldom admitted that the administration of hypnotic drugs to babies with spina bifida is done with the intention of causing the death of the baby and the explanation often given is that the purpose is to relieve pain. Yet the drugs most frequently used are not pain-relieving drugs, they are given in excessive doses from the first day of life before it is known whether the baby has any pain, and in any case babies seldom present any evidence of pain in the neonatal period; moreover in those babies intended to survive, if they develop pain, sedatives are not used to achieve comfort.

b) Thinking

Reasoning about the most severe forms of spina bifida often goes as follows. Without treatment the child may die, or live, but in a more miserable way than if he were treated. With treatment, he will probably live but his disease and treatment may be so great a burden to himself and his family that the family and all advisors feel the best moral choice is to kill the baby. The awesomeness of this seems exceeded only in the claim that the choice need not be faced by people who care ... Changes are necessary if patient and family centered care is to be achieved. In this regard, we have no doubt that a few choices for death are as reasonable and humane as are most choices for life.[17]

The foregoing is the considered viewpoint of two senior paediatricians, one American, the other British. Elsewhere they have explained in more general terms why they consider death may be chosen for its own sake[18] i.e. as a benefit, and why killing may in some circumstances be an obligation[19] for a clinician. It is because 'severely compromised living resulting from disease or its treatment is regarded as worse than death[20]. Certain conditions of defect or handicap amount to "wrongful life"[21]. These judgements and all they imply for treatment decisions are seen as implicit in a position which gives primacy to concern for 'the quality of life'[22]. These paediatricians believe it is possible to make quality of life judgements of a kind determining the value of a human being's existence. They think it possible to determine whether someone would be 'better off dead' and so whether death would be a benefit one should secure for a person.

A similar viewpoint is found in a series of articles which has decisively influenced selection policy in the treatment of spina bifida children.[23] These

vision's 'Afternoon Plus', 15 January 1979; subsequently on the BBC-2 'Man Alive' Programme – 'A loving thing to do', 26 February 1981.

[17] R S Duff, A G M Campbell, 'Moral and Ethical Dilemmas: Seven years into the debate about human ambiguity', (1980) 447 *Annals of the American Academy of Political and Social Science*, 26, 28.

[18] R S Duff, A G M Campbell, 'On deciding the care of severely handicapped or dying persons: with particular reference to infants' (1976) 57 *Pediatrics*, 487.

[19] R S Duff, A G M Campbell, *op. cit.*, (1976) 489.

[20] R S Duff, A G M Campbell, *op. cit.* (1976) 487; cf also R S Duff, A G M Campbell, 'Deciding the care of severely malformed or dying infants' (1979) 5 *Journal of Medical Ethics*, 65.

[21] R S Duff, A G M Campbell, *op. cit.*, (1973) 892.

[22] R S Duff, A G M Campbell, *op. cit.*, (1976) 487.

[23] The published work referred to here is by Professor John Lorber of Sheffield. A recent editorial in the *British Medical Journal* (1981) i, 926–6 on 'Withholding treatment in infancy' essentially repeats the position on selection of spina bifida babies argued by Lorber in articles published ten and nine years

articles[24] seek to establish technical criteria on the basis of which decisions for or against surgical treatment of newborn spina bifida babies should be made. But what motivates the search for the technical criteria is a particular estimate of the value of lives lived under conditions of severe handicap.

Criteria had to be found, preferably on the first day of life, which would reliably separate those infants who may die early whatever is done, *and even more importantly those who would live but were bound to suffer severe multi-system handicaps and would be unable to live an independent and dignified existence*, in spite of the best possible treatment. A line of division had to be found, so that no infant who had a chance of life with moderate handicap should be denied treatment, and that no infant should be treated who is certain to suffer from severe handicaps.[25] [italics ours]

Severe handicap is taken to be incompatible with human dignity, with a life that has worth and value.

These were babies whose initial conditions precluded any kind of existence which one could call humanely adequate or consistent with dignity, consistent with self-assurance, consistent with ability to live without extensive help from outside and who had some chance of employment, of marriage or anything like that.[26]

Babies born with certain degrees of handicap are considered to have no prospect of lives of dignity. Given what is predictable in the way of handicap and adversity, it is assumed possible to make a *comprehensive* judgement on the value of an infant's life. To have a worthwhile life it would be necessary: first that a person should not be subject to those sufferings and hardships involved in repeated operations and hospitalisation and which are said to be an inevitable consequence of multi-system defects[27], second that they should be capable of self-support in competitive employment and have the possibility of marriage; it is variously asserted or implied that these are conditions of self-respect, of happiness and of dignity.[28]

'It is the potential quality of life and the future happiness of the individual

previously. Referring to these articles, Lorber himself wrote: 'The publication of these results led to the second revolution in the management of myelomeningocele – namely an almost universal acceptance of selection which has been officially recognised as legitimate practice'; the text at this point carries a footnote reference to 'Personal communication from most paediatricians and paediatric surgeons in Britain'. J Lorber, 'Early Results of Selective Treatment of Spina Bifida Cystica' (1973) *British Medical Journal* iv, 202. Cf also the claim in J Lorber, 'Ethical Problems in the Management of Myelomeningocele and Hydrocephalus', (1975) 10 *Journal of the Royal College of Physicians*, 47–60, at 54.

24 See the list of Works Cited under Lorber at pp. 101–2.

25 J Lorber, 'The Doctor's Duty to Patients in Profoundly Handicapping Conditions' in D J Roy ed. *Medical Wisdom and Ethics in the Treatment of Severely Defective Newborn and Young Children* (Montreal: Eden Press) 1978, 20–21.

26 Dr Lorber in response to Mr Ian Kennedy, BBC Radio 3 broadcast 'The Defect' 18 October 1978.

27 J Lorber, 'Results of Treatment of Myelomeningocele. An analysis of 524 unselected cases, with special reference to possible selection for treatment' (1971) 13 *Developmental Medicine and Child Neurology*, 288; J Lorber, 'Spina Bifida Cystica. Results of Treatment of 270 Consecutive Cases with criteria for selection for the future' (1972) 47 *Archives of Disease in Childhood*, 854; J Lorber, 'Ethical Problems in the Management of Myelomeningocele and Hydrocephalus' (1975) 10 *Journal of the Royal College of Physicians*, 42; J Lorber, 'Selection – the best policy available', *Nursing Mirror* (14 Sept., 1978a), 15; J Lorber, 'The Doctor's Duty to Patients and Parents in Profoundly Handicapping Conditions', in D J Roy ed. *Medical Wisdom and Ethics in the Treatment of Severely Defective Newborn and Young Children* (1978), 17.

28 Lorber, *op. cit.*, (1971) 286; and *op. cit.*, (1972) 867.

child which should govern a decision to treat or not to treat'[29] The decision not to treat means that the child receives 'custodial management'. The open objective of such management is that the infant should die soon and painlessly[30]. It is admitted: 'There are babies we do not want to operate on because we want the babies dead, that is absolutely clear.'[31] While there are some paediatricians with this attitude to handicapped newborns who would deplore the legalisation of active euthanasia, they consider 'passive euthanasia', including the intentional bringing about of death through omission, to be morally different.[32]

In addition to an adverse quality of life judgement grounding a decision to hasten death, there are other considerations which are advanced in favour of such a decision:

− the problems created for families looking after a severely affected child[33];
− the cost to society of caring for such a child[34];
− the absorption of resources which could otherwise be devoted to the more adequate care of the moderately handicapped.

Yet these considerations would hardly of themselves be thought to justify accomplishing a child's death unless it was also believed that the child's life was disposable.

c) Conclusion

Evidence is becoming increasingly available to the general public that involuntary euthanasia of certain newborn babies is a systematic rather than

---

[29] J Lorber, op. cit., (1978b) 15–16.

[30] J Lorber, op. cit., (1973) 204. Cf equivalent declarations at J Lorber, op. cit., (1972) 854; and op. cit., (1978b) 21.

[31] J Lorber, comment in discussion at the 1975 Skytop Conference, recorded in C A Swinyard ed. Decision Making and the Defective Newborn (Springfield. Illinois: Charles C Thomas) 1978, 462.

[32] Thus Professor Lorber, whose influential writings have been examined here, believes that: 'Though it is fully logical, and in expert and conscientious hands it would be the most humane way of dealing with such a situation [viz protracted dying], legalising euthanasia would be a most dangerous weapon in the hands of the State or ignorant or unscrupulous individuals.' op. cit., (1973) 204. However, though suspecting that it may be 'inconsistent or hypocritical to oppose active euthanasia, yet support non-treatment, or what is often called passive euthanasia', he seems to go along with the view that there is some general distinction between the two. In defining our topic in Chapter 1 we indicated that purposeful killing may be by omission. For clarification of this see Chapter 3, sec. 7. Reliance on a supposed general distinction between action and omission is quite widespread in medical circles and seems to be reflected in The Handbook of Medical Ethics of the British Medical Association (London 1980) 5.19–5.20 (pp. 30–31).

[33] Professor Lorber gives an almost uniformly negative picture of what he describes as the 'disastrous effects on family life' of such babies. Typical is the following: 'A large proportion of the mothers are on tranquilising drugs and more need them. Young parents age prematurely through constant anxiety and recurrent crises. The upbringing of brothers and sisters suffers. Families break up. There are considerable financial difficulties even though treatment in Britain is free'. op. cit., (1978b) 17. Professor John Freeman has noted ('Ethics and the Decision Making Process for Defective Children' in D J Roy ed. op. cit., 35) the prejudice of which clinicians may be guilty in evaluating family stress. R B Darling Families against Society. A Study of Reaction to Children with Birth Defects (Beverly Hills – London: Sage Publications 1979) has documented for a small sample professional prejudice – including that of paediatricians – against which families have had to struggle in securing a fair deal for their handicapped children.

[34] In op. cit., (1978a) Lorber estimated 'that each badly affected child costs some £7,000 every year to the country . . . By the time a child with spina bifida has left school he will have cost some £100,000 – much more than the lifetime earnings of an average family – and yet the results are often disastrous.'

an occasional occurrence in certain paediatric units. It can be said to be systematic because it is presented as a policy option for certain kinds of condition. Infants with these conditions are selected for non-treatment and 'custodial management'; and this regularly means: for sedation with a view to starvation and death.

We do not hold that selection criteria need be employed in a euthanasiast spirit, in the sense that those not chosen for extensive surgical treatment would necessarily be sedated and starved. It is clear that there are paediatricians and paediatric surgeons who are moved to employ the criteria for other than euthanasiast reasons. But the most widely influential criteria for selection have been conceived and commended in a 'euthanasiast' spirit. They are inspired by the belief that it is possible to make comprehensive judgements on the value of human lives; and it is assumed that parents and paediatricians are in a position to judge that some infants would be better off dead and that paediatricians should treat these children in ways that ensure they die.

2. Care of the Handicapped

a) Practice

Evidence of euthanasia applied to handicapped people, whether physically or mentally handicapped or both, is hard to come by. Whereas the new born baby has a precarious hold on life and the terminally ill person will soon die anyway, so that the line between relieving suffering and euthanasia may be indistinct, it is otherwise with the handicapped person who has survived infancy. Few would risk prosecution by committing obviously illegal acts even if they considered them desirable.

b) Thinking

We refer later in this chapter (see sec. B2) to the influence of the view that a human being must possess a certain range of abilities in order to be counted as a person. One surgeon has suggested that doctors can be helped to reach decisions on whether to treat if they work with a formula which depends on quantifying natural capacity and the family and social resources available to develop that capacity. On this formula, inferior natural capacity together with marked family or social unwillingness to support the handicapped person would be interpreted as indicating non-treatment[35].

Clearly there is reason to fear that those quality of life evaluations which have an increasing place in decisions about the handicapped newborn will also come to have a place in considering treatment of older handicapped persons. There is, of course, a significant distinction between, on the one hand, advocating the death of a human being because his quality of life is so poor that he lacks dignity and human rights and the community has the right

---

[35] A Shaw, 'Defining the quality of life' (1977) 7 (5) *Hastings Center Report*, 11.

to relieve itself of the burden he represents, and, on the other hand, advocating the death of a human being because his quality of life is so poor that death is in his own interests. Advocates of the latter sort of euthanasia (the sort we have focussed upon in this Report) often deny that they are committed to advocacy of the former (eugenic or similar) sort of euthanasia. But once one accords decisive weight to the supposed worthlessness of any human life (beyond a certain degree of handicap) there seems little basis for resisting eugenic and kindred policies of euthanasia.

It is certainly proper to recall in this section the fate of many handicapped in one part of Western Europe in our century and the fact that this fate was sealed in terms similar to those which can again be heard. Nonetheless, it would be wrong to suggest that those fateful voices are at all dominant. The dominant climate of opinion in the treatment of the handicapped remains, for the present, positive: thinking is in the main directed to improving the condition and circumstances of the adult handicapped person.

3. Terminal Care

a) Practice

The situation in relation to terminally ill patients is not clear cut. It is, however, reasonable to assume that most claims by doctors to have administered euthanasia relate to those who are *in extremis*, that is, terminally ill. But, although euthanasia is probably talked and written about far more today than thirty to forty years ago, it cannot be stated with any certainty that euthanasia is administered to the terminally ill more frequently now than formerly. Since C. Killick Millard's Presidential Address to the Medical Officers of Health in 1931, there have been sporadic reports, undocumented but from reliable sources, of medical meetings at which doctors have admitted to having administered euthanasia. In a recent editorial in a leading medical journal, it was implied that there are circumstances in relation to terminally ill patients in which doctors 'are openly willing to prescribe drugs with the hastening of death as a deliberate objective'.[36]

From time to time a doctor will admit publicly to having administered euthanasia. A retired Scottish doctor claimed he had carried out between 15 and 30 'mercy-killings' during 30 years of medical practice[37]. A British psychiatrist in 1977 admitted administering what he hoped would be a lethal dose of assorted narcotics and drugs to a man with terminal cancer, and has cited the case of a medically qualified daughter who killed, at his own request, her medically qualified father who had inoperable cancer[38]. Other doctors have made similar claims. Most relate to the use of excessive amounts of morphine given deliberately to kill the patient.

The only clearly definable trend in relation to the terminally ill is, in fact,

[36] Editorial, 'Choosing When and How to Die' (1980) *Lancet* ii, 571.
[37] *The Times*, 21 Jan. 1975.
[38] C Brewer, 'Murder most inefficient' (1977) *World Medicine* (19 Oct.) 40.

with an acute respiratory infection or a myocardial infarction. Similarly with an old and frail patient who has suffered a fracture, the question arises as to whether or not to undertake a surgical operation. Apprehension of burdensome and futile treatment is the valid element in the movement (especially strong in the USA) for 'living wills'.[43] The issues raised by the likelihood that treatment will be either burdensome or futile are given extended consideration in Part Three, especially Chapter 5.

b) Thinking

Recent advances in geriatrics have been fostered by, and have in turn encouraged, a much more positive sense of the prospects for life in old age than was current forty years ago. There is not strong evidence in the published thinking of geriatricians for a negative valuation of the lives of old people even when they are much impaired.

From time to time, however, management policies are justified on grounds which are in principle 'euthanasiast'. A recent article in the *British Medical Journal*[44] contained policy proposals on withholding tube feeding from long-term geriatric patients suffering from dementia and who had been unable to take spoon-feeding. The reasons offered for these proposals in a companion article[45] seem to us dangerous in their logical implications. In the companion article the decision not to tube-feed and to allow death through dehydration is said to be justifiable on the view 'that it is better that a life of severe suffering ceases to exist. The alternative of prolonged and magnified suffering is worse than death'. While the authors reject 'active euthanasia' (because in their terms that would be a 'non-natural' way for a patient to cease to exist) they seem to think that any form of 'allowing to die' is acceptable in the case of the patients they are discussing. Unfortunately the

[43] 'Living will' is a term used in the United States to refer to a document in which a person, while still competent, requests and directs that certain measures (which may be variously specified) should not be used to preserve him if and when he becomes seriously ill (as variously defined) and incapable of consenting to or refusing treatment. Beginning with the Natural Death Act 1976 (California), a number of American States have made laws to give legal effect to such documents. Some of these laws are quite ambiguous and may amount to partial authorisation of euthanasia, even involuntary euthanasia. For example, the Arkansas statute of 1977 authorises either parent of a child, or the guardian of a mentally incompetent person, to execute a document 'on his behalf' denying him not only 'extraordinary', 'extreme' or 'radical' treatment but also all '*artificial* medical or surgical means calculated to prolong his life'; such a document is effective provided it contains 'a signed statement by two physicians that extraordinary means would have to be utilised to prolong life'. The movement to popularise and give legal effect to living wills has been particularly promoted by an organisation describing itself as 'a successor of the Euthanasia Society of America'. In England, Exit, which campaigns for euthanasia, has distributed a living will under the description 'Advance Declaration'. Broadly similar documents have been distributed by persons who have no euthanasiast intent and who are concerned only to prevent the unreasonable prolongation of dying. In every case the precise wording of the document or law must be studied closely to discern whether it has euthanasiast intent or effect.

[44] A Norberg, B Norberg, H Gippert, G Bexell, 'Ethical conflicts in long-term care of the aged: nutritional problems and the patient – care worker relationship' (1980) *British Medical Journal* i, 377–8.

[45] G Bexell, A Norberg, B Norberg, 'Ethical conflicts in long-term care of aged patients: analysis of the tube-feeding decision by means of a teleological ethical model' (1980) 7 *Ethics in Science and Medicine*, 141–5.

kind of reasons they offer for withholding feeding are such as to make death an objective (albeit chosen through inaction) to be adopted on the grounds that it is preferable to prolonged suffering. If this is to be an acceptable rationale for a form of clinical management it is difficult to see what good grounds a clinician could consistently have for excluding active euthanasia.

It is not being suggested here that proposals for withholding tube-feeding are in all circumstances unacceptable. But we do maintain that the thinking underlying the practice of some proponents is euthanasiast.

c) Conclusion

Such evidence as we have seen would not suggest there is any growing movement of opinion and practice in favour of euthanasia in geriatrics. There is no published work surveying the British scene in this respect. But two pieces of research in America[46] have failed to establish a significant relationship between the age of patients and whether the patient received life-prolonging therapy for various conditions. In one of these studies[47] surveying the treatment of patients with febrile infections in nine long-stay hospitals in an American city, it was also found that the additional factor of central nervous system impairment (e.g. stroke, aphasia, paralysis, senility, dementia, chronic or organic brain syndrome and atheroarteriosclerosis) was not significant for the non-treatment of fever. The authors were surprised by this finding, since the fevers were life-threatening and non-treatment might have ensured the death of these patients. It is difficult to be sure that a similar picture of treatment policy could be established for this country.[48]

5. Intensive Care

There is little evidence for practices amounting to euthanasia in Intensive Care Units or for thinking among clinicians in this field favouring euthanasia. To say this is to take a view about 'brain death' and especially in relation to the relatively recent practice of using heart-beating donors in transplantation. For if that practice were the killing of patients for the sake of others it would amount to euthanasia in one obvious form if not the form on which we concentrate in this Report (see Chapter 1, sec. 4, footnote). In Chapter 8, sec. 5, we record our agreement that a patient who has

---

[46] D Crane, *The Sanctity of Social Life: Physicians' Treatment of Critically Ill Patients* (New York: Russell Sage Foundation) 1975; N K Brown, J T Donovan, 'Non-Treatment of Fever in Extended Care Facilities' (1979) 300 *New England Journal of Medicine*, 1246–50.

[47] N K Brown, J Thompson, *op. cit.*, 1249.

[48] Another survey – in this case of students, house staff, and members of a university medical faculty in the United States – carried out in 1976 and compared with the data from a similar survey made in 1971 showed a decrease in support for 'death-hastening measures'. [R Noyes, P R Jockinsen., T A Travis, 'The Changing Attitudes of Physicians Toward Prolonging Life', (1977) 25 *Journal of the American Geriatrics Society*, 470–74.] The reservation and uncertainty one must have about the significance of this survey arise from the fact that its questions assume that the important moral distinction is quite simply between action and *omission*. As we hold that one can intentionally kill by omission it is not clear that the data supplied by the two surveys (1971, 1976) are evidence for a decline in support among clinicians for euthanasia.

suffered total loss of brain function is dead and so cannot be killed by use as a donor for transplant. By 'total loss of brain function' we mean that condition in which the brain has irreversibly ceased to contribute anything to ongoing bodily activities.

Since many think that medicine can be at its most meddlesome in the intensive care unit, futilely standing in the way of inevitable death (and 'death with dignity') we also comment in Chapter 8 on the proper management of dying patients in intensive care.

B. External influences on clinical thinking and practice

'External' here simply means influences which can be located in the wider culture of our society or in changing social conditions and practices in that society. So these influences are not external to the day to day lives of clinicians; but they do not have their origins in either their specialised thinking or their practice.

In identifying external influences on the practice and advocacy of euthanasia in clinical circles, attention will not be confined to voluntary euthanasia. Both practice and advocacy, as we have seen, extend to involuntary euthanasia.

1. Utilitarian views of responsibility

'Utilitarianism' as a label can be taken to refer to many things. In the present context reference is not primarily being made to a developed or elaborate form of philosophical doctrine.[49] Rather we have in mind the residue of philosophical utilitarianism as it has taken hold in the wider culture.

A distinctive teaching about euthanasia cannot be said to be an indispensable ingredient of philosophical utilitarianism. But what is distinctive to it – and also influential – is its consequentialism: the view that the moral character of action derives wholly from the consequences of action. The influence shows in the widespread inclination to frame questions of responsibility almost exclusively in terms of the question: 'What course of action will have the best outcome?' – for some more or less clearly specified group (a married couple, or a couple and their already accepted children, or the nation, or the present population of the world, or future generations).

Calculations of consequences designed to answer this question must, if they are to be made, assume that the values (attaching to the consequences) can be estimated on a common measure (i.e. it must be assumed that values are commensurable). So, for example, the value of a child's life can be calculated alongside the burdens (financial, physical and psychological) care

---

[49] To be seen, for example, in this country in the work of R M Hare and, with particular reference to medical ethics, in Jonathan Glover *Causing Death and Saving Lives* (Harmondsworth: Penguin Books), 1977.

for the child will impose if he is severely handicapped, and alongside both we may measure the value of alternative possibilities (say, for lifestyle) which will be realisable if the child is not around. The calculation may issue in the conclusion that it would be best for the majority of those concerned if the child were dead. But the calculation can proceed only if it is assumed (and it often is so unreflectingly) that the value of the child's life can be computed on some common calculus applicable to all the values adverted to. The value of the child's life can be reckoned as a positive or negative contribution to 'happiness'. This reduction of values, implicit in calculations about 'achieving the best outcome', has some currency in our society.

Utilitarianism is influential in encouraging a consequentialist conception of responsibility and in insinuating its own undefended assumption: that values can be reduced to a common measure. These are influences which accommodate minds to the reception of the arguments standardly deployed in favour of euthanasia.

2. 'Possessive individualist' conceptions of the person

Alongside a more or less vulgarised utilitarianism, which has become established in many minds, there is another philosophical conception which has gained some currency: that an infant is not, properly speaking, a person and so lacks human rights. Though the conception of 'personhood' involved here goes back to Locke[50], it has been given striking expression in its application to the ethics of medical practice only in recent decades[51]. It is maintained that a human being must possess a number of presently exercisable capacities in order to be counted as a person. Somebody lacking those abilities also lacks the rights which properly belong to persons – including the 'right to life'.

This selective view of who qualifies as possessing basic human rights is now straightforwardly asserted by secularist propagandists seeking to change the basis of our homicide laws[52].

[50] *Essay Concerning Human Understanding*, Book II, Chapter 27.

[51] Particularly by Joseph Fletcher. Fletcher, writing as an Episcopalian moral theologian, has been widely read in medical circles, particularly in North America. He itemises the following characteristics ('indicators of humanhood') which must hold good of somebody if he is to be regarded as certainly a person: he should have a minimum IQ of 40; he should be self-aware, be capable of exercising self control; he should have a sense of temporal duration, a sense of the future, a sense of the past; he should be capable of entering into relationships, be capable of concern for others, be in communication with others, be in control of his existence, be inquisitive, be capable of both adapting to and initiating change in his way of life; he should enjoy a balance of reason and emotion in his life; he should be idiosyncratic or distinctive; he should have a functioning neocortex. See Joseph Fletcher, *Humanhood: Essays in Biomedical Ethics* (Buffalo: Prometheus Books) 1979, pp. 7–19.

[52] See, for example, the comment of the President of the National Secular Society on the question 'have the newborn no rights?' 'The answer is No – not full human rights since a new-born baby is not fully a human person. They do, however, have one right – a right which they share with animals under human control: that is the right to be spared unnecessary suffering.' Letter, *The Observer* 8 February 1981. And from the same writer in The Guardian 11 August 1981: 'What makes us complete human persons is the development of human relationships: what gives us a stake in life is life-experience. A new-born baby, even a perfectly normal one, cannot therefore have a right to life ... Needless to say, new-born babies in common with all sentient animals, have a natural right to be protected from unnecessary suffering.'

29

3. Social Darwinism

One reason why these propagandists seek such change is best understood by reference to the persistent influence of Social Darwinist notions of human evolution as requiring the elimination of the 'unfit'. One member of Exit, declaring her intention to seek legislative change of a kind which would permit parents and paediatricians to allow Down's syndrome babies with duodenal atresia to die, referred to the law as a framework which should be conducive to human evolution[53].

4. Supposed implications of moral pluralism

Moral pluralism is characteristic of our society. Different groups can be characterised by the differing and incompatible conceptions they hold of what values should command human allegiance and of the nature of human responsibility. It is argued that a liberal society should allow for the un-trammelled realisation of any way of life which cannot be demonstrated to be harmful to those not party to it. Thus it is held to be neither necessary nor appropriate for our society to proscribe euthanasia. From the fact that some believe there is a 'right to die'[54] it is rather rapidly concluded that exercise of the right should be facilitated.

Legalisation of euthanasia is not our topic. But arguments about the propriety of legalising euthanasia are to be counted among the influences on clinical practice: in so far as they are thought to be persuasive they encourage doctors and nurses to do what they believe they should be free from sanction in doing.

It may be appropriate to note here (a point that should become clearer in the course of the Report) that those who think legislative changes in favour of euthanasia desirable are in effect proposing to jettison both that conception of the dignity of human life which underpins our homicide laws and a framework of laws consistently embodying that conception. Nothing can be more basic to the maintenance of a society than respect for the laws protecting human life. The legalisation of euthanasia would involve a radical change to the conception of human life underlying our homicide laws. It might be intended as a mere adjustment of law designed to accommodate various moral persuasions. But inevitably the change would introduce into the conceptions which underly these and other laws a specific view of human life, a view incompatible with that which has hitherto preserved us.

5. Organised advocacy of euthanasia

A number of tendencies already identified find a home in Exit (formerly, the Voluntary Euthanasia Society), the organisation devoted to making both an ethical and a legislative case for euthanasia.

---

[53] Mrs Peggy Lejeune, interviewed on BBC Radio 4, The World this Weekend, Sunday 9 August 1981.

[54] That is, a right to determine when and how one dies. Some proponents of the right also believe that it can be exercised on behalf of the incompetent by proxies. And so involuntary euthanasia can be represented as allowing the incompetent the exercise of their 'right to die'.

It is important in analysing the case presented by Exit to distinguish its presently declared objectives from the long-term aspirations of some of its members. Exit seeks the legalisation of voluntary euthanasia; some of its members would like to see the legalisation of involuntary euthanasia too. We shall argue (in Chapter 3) that voluntary euthanasia could be justified only if one could make a comprehensive judgement on the worthwhileness of a person's life. But if such judgements are possible then they are possible in respect of subjects who are not asking or are not in a position to ask for euthanasia. The thrust of the case for voluntary euthanasia is in the direction of involuntary euthanasia. The connection is not merely logical, however, it is also historical. But before turning to these connections it is worth examining the nature of the carefully circumscribed case that Exit currently presents to the public.

Essentially the case is that persons possess a right to determine the manner of their dying since persons are entitled to dignity and certain conditions of dying are incompatible with dignity and worth. These conditions are

- the pain and suffering which attends many deaths;
- more particularly, the extremes of suffering which may accompany certain terminal cancers; it is said that the sequelae of pain control are often undesirable;
- the pain and distress of relatives and friends.

The nub of the argument concerns dignity and worth: that lives lived under certain conditions are lives which cannot be respected, are lives which lack dignity.

If one believes (with Exit) that certain conditions as it were reduce people to a sub-human level, it then becomes appropriate to supplement the argument about loss of dignity by adverting to the fact that we do not keep alive suffering animals. The existence of hospice care (to which we shall refer later) is considered neither in principle nor practice to offer a solution. For, on the one hand, even with hospice care there will be those who prefer a 'clean death' to the dependency and indignities of physical degeneration. And, on the other hand, given the scarcity of resources, it is unlikely that hospice care can be provided for all who need and might want it.

Exit also emphasises a point with which, as will become clear, we have complete sympathy: that people in their dying should be spared futile and burdensome treatments.

It seems crucial to Exit's case that one should be able to judge that certain human beings lack dignity and worth. To kill them is to do them a benefit: it is to terminate pathetic existences; such killings are said to be merciful. If this is the core of the case for euthanasia it is difficult to see why it should not extend to involuntary euthanasia.

Neither in the past nor in the present has the movement now named Exit disassociated itself in principle from involuntary euthanasia. This is not surprising, especially given the character of its medical membership. A recent detailed historical survey of the part played by members of the medical profession in the movement for euthanasia over the past century has shown that many have been moved to participate as much by an interest in eliminating the 'unfit', and the 'useless' as by an interest in voluntary euthanasia; they have seen the latter as no more than a tactical first move to their ultimate goal[55]. In *The Last Right* Exit is careful not to state any principled objection to involuntary euthanasia and merely claims that this cannot be said to be a present objective of the Society: 'Exit does not advocate the "putting down" of deformed children and mental defectives. If there are to be any proposals to cope with this problem, they will have to be dealt with on their merits and approved or rejected by the community through their elected representatives to Parliament.' (p.4)

There are those who are sceptical about the relevance of the Nazi era to understanding the implications of the contemporary movement for euthanasia[56]. But once it is grasped that central to the argument for euthanasia in Germany in the 1920s was the concept of a 'life not worth living'[57] and how extendable that concept is (and how much it was extended) and when it is also realised that exactly the same concept is being more or less explicitly invoked at the heart of present arguments for euthanasia, then the historical lessons of the German experience can hardly be overlooked. It takes some hubris to discount them.

6. Economic factors

We have already seen that the cost of caring for handicapped children is invoked as a contributory reason for ensuring that they die. Cost-benefit analyses of the advantages of preventing the births of babies with Down's syndrome or spina bifida[58] can readily be adapted to demonstrate the advantage of preventing the continued lives of such children if they are born.

[55] See I van der Sluis, 'The Movement for Euthanasia 1875–1975' 66 *Janus* 1979:131–172. Pertinent here is the report in *The British Medical Journal* 1935 ii: 1168 on the address of the chairman of the executive committee (Mr C J Bond FRCS) to the inaugural meeting of The Voluntary Euthanasia Legalisation Society (a predecessor of Exit): Civilised man was being called upon to exercise increasing control over human development and human life, meaning control at both ends, entrance into and exit from life, but in order to exercise this control wisely there was needed a truer conception of the value of life, which consisted not in living, but in living usefully and happily. The population was an aging one, with a larger relative proportion of elderly persons – individuals who had reached a degenerative stage of life, in which cancer and other disabling diseases tended to occur. Thus the total amount of suffering and the number of useless lives must increase, and this problem required wise handling. To talk of the proposed Bill as a Bill to promote murder and the doctor working under it as a public executioner was beside the point. He added that today they were concerned only with voluntary euthanasia, but 'as public opinion develops . . . further progress on preventive lines will be possible'.

[56] See in particular the remarks of Professor Lucy Dawidowicz made at the Conference 'Biomedical Ethics and the Shadow of Nazism' and reported in (1976) 6(4) *The Hastings Center Report*, Special Supplement.

[57] See the title of the key tract by Karl Binding and Alfred Hoche: *Die Freigabe der Vernichtung 'Lebensunwerten Lebens'* (The granting of permission to destroy life that is not worth living) 2nd edn. Verlag von Felix Meiner, Leipzig, 1922. Binding, a highly reputable non-Nazi jurist, thought that there were 'not only completely worthless, but even lives with a negative value'.

[58] See S Haggard, F A Carter, 'Preventing the birth of infants with Down's syndrome: a cost-benefit analysis' (1976) *British Medical Journal* i, 753–56; S Haggard, F Carter, R G Milne, 'Screening for spina bifida cystica. A cost-benefit analysis', (1976) 30 *British Journal of Preventative and Social Medicine*, 40–53.

Reference to the cost of care as a reason for euthanasia is made in respect of other categories of patients. Over thirty years ago one British physician wrote in regard to the aged and senile:

A decision concerning the senile may have to be taken within the next twenty years. The number of old people are increasing by leaps and bounds. Pneumonia, 'the old man's friend', is now checked by antibiotics. The effects of hardship, exposure, starvation and accident are now minimised. Where is this leading us? . . . What of the drooling, helpless, disorientated old man or the doubly incontinent old woman lying log-like in bed? Is it here that the real need for euthanasia exists?[59]

No doubt this argument ends by appealing to the plight of individuals but it gains its foothold as an argument precisely by its reference to growing numbers and its implicit supposition that expenditure on the aged therefore should not or cannot be maintained at present rates.

Given the present allocation of resources in this country, in particular the reduction of support to health and social services, at least some geriatricians are finding themselves with far fewer beds and facilities than are regarded as standard provision (for the population they serve). In these circumstances some patients are inevitably neglected and the temptation arises to neglect those with a 'poor quality of life'. There is reason to think that 'quality of life' judgements, having consequences for life and death (even though, as yet, those consequences may be unintended), are thus in danger of gaining a foothold in geriatric practice.

[59] Quoted in Y Kamisar, 'Euthanasia Legislation: Some Non-Religious Objections', in A B Downing ed. *Euthanasia and the right to death*, p. 112.

Part Two

The central ethical issue raised in the trends which have been described is: are there any circumstances which would justify a person, acting in a private capacity, in intentionally killing anyone? In the two following chapters we consider philosophical and religious responses to this question.

It might seem that the best approach to determining whether euthanasia is justifiable would be by considering the ethics of suicide. Our approach here is to consider the ethics of murder. As we shall argue, the consideration which is ultimately decisive in supposed justifications of euthanasia is not that the death is voluntary but that the person to be killed is believed to be fortunate or 'better off' in being dead. It turns out that at this point the most general grounds for condemning murder can be seen to coincide with those for any condemnation of suicide. So it is useful to begin by clarifying our understanding of the nature and wrongfulness of murder, both for this reason and also because a justification of euthanasia in terms of suicide could have little or no application to various proposals and practices advocated particularly in the field of paediatrics.

Essentially our argument is that it is the recognition that man is marked off from the other animals in being also spirit that stands in the way of killing people because it is thought that they would be better off dead. In this recognition there is a sense of awe before the mystery of human life which can be described as religious, and is not peculiar to the Judaeo-Christian tradition. Chapter IV examines the moral teaching on our topic of the religious tradition to which we belong, giving special attention to Roman Catholic teaching.

3

Murder and the Morality of Euthanasia: Some Philosophical Considerations

Before considering the ethics of murder we need to consider what counts as murder. In order to understand the logic of what follows it is important to be clear that we will not *define* murder as impermissible killing. That is to say, we will identify a class of acts (which we call murder), and will then seek to explain why acts of that class are impermissible. Of course, if all such acts are impermissible, it will easily seem to some that murder is actually defined as the impermissible; but the sequence we follow should remove this mis-understanding. We recognise, too, that some people do use the term 'murder' to mean 'impermissible deliberate homicide', but that is not the way we use the term. It will happen that in order to define the class of acts we shall need to speak of intention and responsibility, and this is naturally done in terms of 'guilt ' and 'exoneration'; but the discussion does not proceed from any definition of murder as impermissible. We think, indeed, that it is. But we so understand it that there is a real question *whether* it is: whether, that is, human beings can ever be justified in incurring the guilt of murder; and the decision that they cannot is not a matter of definition.

1. What constitutes murder

Murder is a complex of disparate elements, not merely the killing of one human being by another. There is also the mental element of intent. Yet 'murder ' cannot be explained just as intentional killing: for civil authority introduces the possibility that there may be killing which is legitimate even though intentional – in struggle with violent law-breakers or, it may be, in capital punishment. The right account is one whereby murder is killing which involves a special degree and kind of responsibility for death, a responsibility which is guilt.

Responsibility itself is a shifting notion. For present purposes, it should be observed to have three levels. (1) The primary level is that at which a mere cause (for example a stroke of lightning) or contributory condition (such as the temperature of the atmosphere) is said to be responsible for something happening. (2) At a higher level, where a rational agent is involved, there is the further feature that he can be called to account. If he has caused or contributed to a human death, he may have to answer the question of guilt for that death. (3) The third level of responsibility is that of guilt itself.

When hi-jackers say that 'they will not be responsible' for deaths if they blow up a plane because their demands are not met, they mean that they will not be guilty; they are not denying level 2 responsibility, but claiming to have an exonerating answer. One who is called to account may not be guilty, even though he did cause death, because there is an exonerating answer on his behalf. The range of such answers is very wide, e.g. 'He was sleep-walking', 'he stumbled', 'he did not know he was administering poison', 'he did not intend death but something else which was quite legitimate', 'he was acting with legitimate authority', 'he had no duty to act to prevent death'. In default of an exonerating answer, the gravest sort of responsibility for a death entails that one has committed murder. It is determined by the knowledge and will with which one acts.

It should be noticed that advantage to be got by deliberately killing someone is not counted as exonerating. If anyone maintains that it can justify, then what is thereby justified will be murder itself.

We cannot offer a sharp and simple definition of murder. But there is a central part of what the term covers which can be reasonably well-defined, namely *the intentional killing of the innocent*. Whenever this is done by rulers, soldiers, terrorists or other violent men, reference is made, in reporting it, to the murder of innocent victims. This gives us a stereotype of the murderer, and constitutes the hard core of the concept.

There are, however, other intentional killings which are murder, though not all philosophers agree that this is so in the 'state of nature', i.e. where there is no government. These are: vengeful killing where the victim has wronged the killer, and planned killing by a private person in self-defence.

Intention alone, however, is not all; even where no intention to *kill* is present there may be murder. The victim may be attacked in order to hurt him badly, or to expose him to serious danger. Or the killer may not be focussing on any victim – for example he blows up a plane or he burns down a house to get insurance money, not caring whether or even that there are people inside. Such killing may be more callous and heinous than some that is intentional.[1]

---

[1] English lawyers have often used an artificial sense of 'intention' in these contexts, together with technical senses of 'malice' to help out. For in these contexts no weight is given to the distinction between intending death and foreseeing that there is a serious risk of death as a result of one's act. Yet this distinction is well understood and treated as significant when doctors give pain-killing drugs or surgeons do dangerous operations. Thus the idea that foresight entails intention is applied only in connection with serious wrongdoing of the sort that used to be called felony. It may have arisen from the obvious murderousness of such killers as the arsonist referred to in the text. But guilt requires in law guilty intent, and this was perhaps assumed to be the intent of committing the very crime charged. On this assumption, the intention to kill the victim would have to be somehow attributable; this in turn made it necessary to think foresight sufficient for the requisite intention, and so 'intention' acquired a special sense in writings of jurisprudents.

In addition there used to be the assumption that the accused understood what any rational agent in his situation would understand. This would give the rationale of counting it murder when someone dies of being savagely beaten up. But since the enactment of the Criminal Justice Act 1967, 5.8, foreseeability by a reasonable person is not to be taken as legal proof of either foresight or intention. And after 1967 the law fell into confusion: the abolition of 'felony murder' ('constructive malice') in 1957 and the enactment of 1967 together left a gap: it seemed that the equation of intention and actual foresight had to provide for the whole doctrine of murder where the killing is not intended (in the ordinary sense), and it became a moot point whether, and how, to justify a verdict of murder where death results from serious bodily harm.

It is not possible to commit murder unless *something* is done intentionally; for when death arises from mere (even gross) negligence that will rather be manslaughter. But we ought to distinguish between intending to kill and intending something else in spite of the likelihood of a death resulting.

Some moralists, as well as jurisprudents, have nevertheless equated intention and foresight of harm. So long as the equation of intention and foresight is made only in connection with gravely unlawful acts, it may seem harmless. But so to restrict it is highly illogical. Of course this equation is never actually made in such cases as high-risk surgery. But if intention and foresight of the probability of death can be equated at all, it may well be asked why not there. If the equation were made, it would certainly not be inferred that the surgeon is a murderer if his patient dies. But the alternative inference would be that the 'intention' to kill is acceptable for good purposes.

What ought to be said is (1) that intention and foresight are distinct, and (2) that the intention (i.e. the purpose) of harm or danger to the victim is not a necessary part of the mental element in murder. Even without such intent, unlawful acts can be murderous. 'Unlawful' is closer in sense to 'wrongful' than to 'illegal', and the unlawfulness of an act may reside in its endangering someone's life without excuse.

2. On intentionally killing the innocent

There are two conceptions competing for our acceptance. One, that there is an absolute prohibition on murder: this has up to now (forgetting about abortion, which has not been legally classified with murder in England) been the stance of English law, as well as being the teaching of the Judaeo-Christian tradition. The other, which appears in the Model Penal Code[2] and makes progress in many minds, would allow necessity as an exculpating (exonerating) plea in some cases of perfectly intentional killing. 'Necessity' can be understood in a very restricted or a widely extended way according to what we insist on trying to get or avoid.

Here the Judaeo-Christian teaching enters its interdict, forbidding all killing of the innocent as end or as means. We might rely on religious authority for this; but it has also generally been held that the moral law is accessible to reason.

Some think it would be within the competence of the State to authorise such killing as seems necessary for the common good. But the right of the State to use violence has such a foundation as to put that idea right out of court. For the foundation is the human need of protection against unjust

[2] See Model Penal Code, articles 2 and 3 (especially article 3, headed 'Justification and Choice of Evils', and the commentary in Tentative Draft No.8 [1958] pp. 5–10). The Code was drafted and published by the American Law Institute (Philadelphia), a private association of academic and practising lawyers, between 1952 and 1962 (definitive edition 1980). Many of the Code's provisions have been adopted in whole or part by legislatures in the US. The Director of the Institute and Chief Reporter of the Code was Herbert Wechsler. On 'necessity' and killing, see Wechsler H, Michael J, 'A Rationale of the Law of Homicide' (1937) 37 *Columbia Law Review* 701, esp. at 738–9.

attack. The fact that the attack is unjust secures the justice of supplying the need by the use and threat of violence. The need creates the first task of government, which cannot be supplied in a large society without laws and an administration of justice. Only when we have these have we civil authority. But if the civil authority itself attacks innocent people, it nullifies the basis on which its use of violence is different from that of a gangster band. This remains true even if it pleads the common good as an excuse for exterminating innocent people. Its role in promoting the common good enables it to make pertinent laws for violating which people may be punished. But that does not mean that an attack on people's lives when they are not lawbreakers but just as part of a scheme for future advantage, is within the competence of government. In acting so, the civil authority would always be nullifying the basis of its own right to command violence.

Civil authority cannot make it policy to decide on or license the killing of innocent people without losing the character of civil authority. And, whatever the appearances, the decision to take part in such killing is necessarily a private one. People rightly suppose that public authority can be invoked, and that this makes all the difference, if what is in question is e.g. police action against violent law-breakers; but whatever may be enacted by wicked legislation, the case is quite otherwise for killing innocent people and it is merely error and confusion to think the responsibility can be referred to the civil authority.

3. The prohibition

With this confusion cleared away, we have to consider the essentially private decision: to kill an innocent person because it seems a good idea that he should die. What is the basis of the prohibition? First, someone who is murdered suffers a great wrong (an injustice). Utilitarian types of morality are here compelled to talk only of the disturbing effects of murder on the living. But clearly the victim is the primary one to be wronged, and this is enough objection to murder in most cases.

If someone is wronged, he has a right which is violated. But the wrongfulness of murder seems to be the basis of the right, rather than *vice versa*, because (a) there is not a simple right to life, but rather a right not to be murdered and (b) if there were a certain right to life upon which the wrongfulness of murder was based, it would be difficult to see why it should not be waivable.

The prohibition on murder is indeed a great charter of right to all of us, but it is the prohibition that comes first and not the right.

The prohibition is so basic that it is difficult to answer the question as to why murder is intrinsically wrongful. Some think they can get an answer out of more general principles. Here we shall rather point to the character of rational argument designed to show that it is wrong to steal, or commit adultery, or that we ought to keep a rule of the road where there is traffic, or a close season for game or fish needed for food where stocks must be replenished. The arguments are of the form 'Obedience to this law is needed for human good'. The unit whose good the argument seeks is the human individual, considered generally. To kill him, then, is to destroy that being which is the point of those considerations.

Why then are there exceptions? Why may some men be made targets in war, fought in civil struggle, killed in putting them down as violent law-breakers, perhaps assassinated if they are tyrants and executed if found guilty of some crimes? The answer is that where this is so, what they receive is justice, they themselves being unjust assailants.

The meaningfulness of these considerations brings us face to face with the truth that man is spirit. He moves in the categories of innocence and answerability and desert – one of the many signs of a leap to another kind of existence from the life of the other animals. The very question 'Why may we not kill innocent people?' asks whether it may not be *justified* to do so, and this is itself a manifestation of this different life.

Here some present day philosophers produce arguments based on the concept of a person in support of killing young infants and the senile. They say that mere biologically human life does not constitute personhood, and it is only a person who has what we call human dignity and the right not to be killed. A person is defined by certain qualities and capacities. Since these are lacking in the newborn and the senile, they fall outside the ban on murder.

Such thinkers trade on the weight of the word 'person', although they define it wrongly in terms of characteristics which may come and go and which are a matter of degree.

For a person is a substantial individual being with his own identity, which he has as an individual of a particular species. In our case the species is 'human being'. Having named an individual human being we use the name with the same reference so long as it is the *same human being* we are talking about. A human being is a person because the kind to which he belongs is characterised by rational nature. Thus we have the same individual, and hence the same person, when we have the same human being. One is a person just by being of this kind, and that does indeed import a tremendous dignity. It is a mere trick to draw on the weight that this word 'person' has because of this sense – thrashed out long ago – if you then go on to explain the word so that it is rather like the word 'magnet'. A piece of iron gets magnetised and so *becomes* a magnet; later it may get demagnetised and *stops* being a magnet though it is still the same piece of iron. If indeed you explain the word 'person' as meaning someone e.g. who can talk (has self-consciousness) and lead a social life (have inter-personal relations) you may say that someone can be the same human being but no longer a person. It does not come so easy to say 'Since he can no longer do such-and-such, he no longer has rights, and it is in order to kill him'.

You cannot be killing a human being and not be killing a person.

4. Why euthanasia is no exception to the prohibition

The one kind of killing innocent people which seems to escape the argument that it is unjust, i.e. that someone is wronged, is voluntary euthanasia. So far,

41

most propaganda for euthanasia assumes it should be voluntary. Like the first justifications for induced abortion, this is only a way-station. But it impresses, because it strikes people as not wronging someone to kill him if he wills it. However, it needs pointing out that they would still think it was wronging him, but for the accompanying judgement that his condition is so irremediably wretched that it is fortunate for him 'to die'. This judgement is paramount, and that is why the stress on voluntariness tends to be spurious. Though some people are serious about it, upon the whole it is merely getting the foot in the door. The drive is in the direction of killing people when their lives are judged useless or burdensome to themselves or the world. This judgement is readily made of people whose mental capacity is gone or much diminished.

The drive to get doctors killing people and to have this accepted in medical ethics ought to be regarded as sinister even by those who regard suicide in face of terminal suffering as justified and worthy of a human being. If the ground for this opinion is the dignity of human freedom and self-determination, it is inconsonant with this to ask someone else to do so grave a thing. At this point it is often said that people who would kill themselves if they could are rendered unable to do it by physical incapacity. This is less often true than may be supposed, as it is usually possible to stop eating; though the point is not of interest to Christians, who would not be recommending suicide in any form. But the plea 'kill me: I need death but cannot kill myself' is a dubious example of self-determination. Furthermore, those called upon to assist in suicide are not thereby relieved of their responsibility to decide for themselves how to respond to the suffering human being.

Those asked for assistance are indeed being asked to judge it acceptable to treat suffering people as we treat the other animals. The impulse to 'put an animal out of its misery' may be partly an impulse of sympathy with a creature that resembles us – we feel pain at its pain. The attitude is mistakenly called mercy in the sense of loving care: mercy sustains and supports and you cannot take care of something by destroying it. But you can judge it not worth preserving, and sympathy is one of the things that can make it feel intolerable to put up with the creature's gross suffering, and may even incline one to terminate a reduced and pathetic existence.

But men, being spirit as well as flesh, are not the same as the other animals. Whatever blasphemes the spirit in man is evil, discouraging, at best trivialising, at worst denigrating life. Such is the considered recommendation of suicide and killing in face of suffering. We should not confuse this with the personal desperation which may lead to suicide. That may excite our pity. But propaganda in favour of death as a remedy is different. It is irreligious, in a sense in which the contrasting religious attitude – one of respect before the mystery of human life – is not necessarily connected only with some one particular religious system. Propaganda puts in the mouth of the potential, theoretical, suicide: 'I belong to myself, and I can set conditions on which I will consent to go on living'. Life is regarded as a good or bad hotel, which must not be too bad to be worth staying in[3]. To the man of religious feeling, the claim lacks reverence and insight. A religious attitude may be merely incipient, prompting a certain fear before the idea of ever destroying a human life, and refusing to make a 'quality of life' judgement to terminate a human being. Or it may be more developed, perceiving that men are made by God in God's likeness, to know and love God. The love of God is the direction of the will to its true end. The human heart and will are set on amenity; they may also be set on what is just[4]: that is (when it comes to dying) set in acceptance of life – which is God's gift – and of death, as it comes from him. This goes even for the most incompetently alive in whom the will is manifested mainly in the vital operations. Here there is unlikely to be any possibility of a contrast between the two orientations. But where there is intellectual consciousness there can be contrast: the human being then operates under one or the other of these conceptions of what counts ultimately for him: either amenity only, or acceptance, which is obedience in spirit, which is justice. Acceptance of life and death is what justice is in circumstances of unavoidable dying; it is accord with God's will.

Such perception of what a human being is makes one perceive human death as awesome, human life as always to be treated with a respect which is a sign and acknowledgement of what it is for.

To fight a human being to the death, to try him, condemn him to death and execute him, are grave and tragic actions. But they may be compatible with this awe and respect. To kill him (whether he is oneself or someone else) because one judges his life is wretched or not worth living, is not.

5. Proper and improper 'quality of life judgements'

There are times when anyone would be inclined to say 'I'm glad his sufferings are over. Death came as a relief to him ...'. Such expressions point, forcefully, to sheer pain. or to lack of mental capacity, or of physical capacities, or of 'potential for developing human relationships'.[5] A person's miseries, often enough, are very evident, while the good of his existence is no longer evident, being submerged from view beneath the ills of his condition. But there is a dignity which belongs to humans not in virtue of achievement

---

[3] Cf. Hume's *Dialogues Concerning Natural Religion*, Part XI.

[4] See St. Anselm, *De Casu Diaboli*, c. 12.

[5] Colloquial expressions are often used without being meant literally or 'philosophically'. Just as one may say 'life without sliced bread [or democracy] would not be worth living', so one can say, in the face of great suffering or deprivation, 'his life is no longer worth living'. The latter statement would obviously be meant more seriously than the quip about sliced bread or even than the exaggeration about democracy; but it still need not be meant to affirm what it literally states. That is to say, it need not be taken to contradict the truth that every human being's existence has a value, both in itself and in relation to others, a value which cannot in this life be known to anyone. We recognise, of course, that such a statement as 'his life is not worth living' can readily be taken as claiming to sum and balance all the values and disvalues of a person's existence, and thus as a philosophically and theologically unacceptable human judgement. But we do not think all uses of such expressions should be condemned; the important thing is that those who use them (or hear them) should not treat them as the final truth of the matter, and should not make them the basis for choices of actions (or omissions) intended to terminate or abbreviate life.

or 'good condition' but simply in virtue of the kind of beings we are: spirit as well as flesh. Because man is spirit, talk of the quality of his life is not an adequate basis for deciding to suppress his existence. The full meaning of any part of anyone's existence eludes our understanding; judgements about that meaning cannot reasonably provide the basis for a decision to move someone from existence to non-existence in this world.

We therefore reject those 'quality of life' judgements which are intended to identify death itself as a good to be pursued by the doctor, the nurses, or even the patient himself.

We do not deny that judgements which can (but need not) be called 'quality of life' judgements do enter into the process of medical decision-making. Any therapeutic recommendation is based on a consideration of likely and possible advantages and disadvantages that may accrue to the patient. The doctor makes some sort of comparison – 'weighing' is too simple a metaphor – between the benefits and the risks and burdens for the patient that will or may accrue from the specific treatment under consideration. And this comparison is inevitably made against the background of the patient's present and likely condition and prognosis. So the question being asked, implicitly, can be put thus: given his present 'quality of life', are the burdens of this (expensive or time-consuming or painful or disfiguring or undignified ...) medical treatment worth enduring, in view of (a) the probable 'quality of his life' while undergoing it and (b) the probable 'quality of his life' if and when the treatment is completed?

The same question can be asked, in the first person, by any patient or prospective patient, and at the beginning of Chapter 5 we shall analyse quite closely the ways in which different patients in similar circumstances can answer, and reasonably answer, that question in differing ways. There we shall consider, too, what answers are suicidal and so are to be excluded. For the present it is sufficient to notice the precise role of the question in trains of practical reasoning that are non-suicidal and non-euthanasiast: it focuses, and must be kept focused, on the advantages and disadvantages of specific possible treatments, given their effects, side-effects and outcome. It does not enquire about, let alone focus upon, the worthwhileness of the patient's being alive at all.

The decision resulting from the non-euthanasiast practical reflection may be that *no* possible specific treatment is now, for this patient, worthwhile. And that decision may be arrived at in the knowledge that, untreated, the patient will probably die somewhat earlier than he would if treated. And indeed that consequence of the decision may be accepted without regret, and with the feeling, expressed or unexpressed, that death will bring relief to that patient. Still, such a decision can be perfectly reasonable and morally proper. But it would be euthanasiast, and so morally improper, if it used the judgement that death would bring relief, or that the patient's life was no longer worth living, or that the patient's prospective quality of life was too poor, as the basis for a decision to regard death as the objective, or an objective, of the treatments to be decided on.

Behind justice, and the canons of right dealing which preserve us generally when they are observed, there lies that valuation of human life which we are seeking here to explain and defend. That valuation as we have said can be called 'religious': it sees in the earthly life of each individual human being, however damaged, a weight and significance such that the termination of that life can never rightly be chosen as a means of advancing overall human welfare – not even the welfare of that damaged individual himself.

Thus we conclude that the guilt of murder ought never to be incurred for any advantage to be gained or evil to be avoided.

We are not arguing here that there is a duty in justice to prevent the suicide of someone who, with full deliberation, rejects or acts against this valuation of human life. But we hold that both the duty in justice not ever to murder (the main 'right to life'), and one's own duty not to commit suicide, are based on the religious valuation we are speaking of.

6. Limits to moral pluralism

Here we have reached a limit to the practice of moral pluralism. For the sake of authenticity and integrity in people's search for moral truth, a wide moral pluralism, of practice as well as belief, is to be accepted and even constitutionally protected. But that valuation of personal freedom and authenticity itself rests (whether people realise this fact or not) upon the 'religious' sense which we have been trying to express – the sense of each individual's worth, a worth (because man is spirit) not captured by any consideration of his imperfections and poor prognosis as an organism, or of his 'contribution' to the welfare of his fellows. What we have just said is of wide significance. It is not our purpose in this Report to consider the case against legalising euthanasia;[6] our concern here is with the personal and medical ethics of the matter. But what we have just touched upon is the reason why no one is entitled (morally or legally) to ask another to do an act which expresses a rejection of the true valuation of human life, and why the community is entitled to forbid such acts as being crimes of murder or complicity in suicide. It is the reason, too, why those who do not value human life in the way we have defended do badly to fight this valuation. It is not necessary, or good, for those who do not have a religious attitude to life, and who thus are willing to kill in what they conceive to be a spirit of mercy, to seek to overthrow that attitude. For that attitude is the solid foundation for recognising that persons have *rights* to be treated *justly*.

The character of medical practice would be very radically altered, too, if quality of life judgements became a *focus* of practical reflection, rather than

---

[6] The most fundamental and helpful discussions of the case against legalising even voluntary euthanasia are, so far as we know, Yale Kamisar, 'Some Non-Religious Views against Proposed "Mercy Killing" Legislation' (1958) 42 *Minnesota Law Review* 970–1039 (another version is in A B Downing, ed., *Euthanasia and the Right to Death*, London: 1969, pp. 85–133); Germain Grisez & Joseph M Boyle, *Life and Death with Liberty and Justice* (Univ. Notre Dame P., London: 1979), pp. 149–183, 214–250. See also Hugh Trowell, *The Unfinished Debate on Euthanasia* (SCM Press, London: 1973), chs 3–6; Jonathan Gould & Lord Craigmyle, *Your Death Warrant?* (Geoffrey Chapman, London: 1971).

merely part of the background to the selection of appropriate treatment. For then opinions such as 'I'm glad his sufferings are over' or 'I hope death comes quickly to relieve him'[7] would cease to be merely the comments of someone drawing attention to the miseries from which death would bring relief. Rather, such opinions would form the basis and criterion for selection of treatment, and the proper goals of treatment would be taken to include not only life, health and comfort, but also death itself. In the context of medical practice thus conceived, 'quality of life' opinions would function as practical judgements calling for death-dealing treatment. One early sign of this transformation of medical practice would be, indeed, the new and sinister ring to that word 'treatment'.

7. The possibility of murder by omission

To complete our account of murder, we need to consider omissions. It is certainly possible to commit murder (morally speaking) by omission, as when, in order that the patient should die, a medical attendant omits e.g. to turn on an apparatus; or when people deliberately neglect to feed their child. Thus the fact that one 'did nothing' is not of itself proof that there is not the gravest responsibility for a death.[8]

In the utilitarian type of morality labelled 'consequentialism' it is supposed, first, that we always ought to act so as to produce the best possible future state of things, and hence, second, that in not doing something that one could do one is always just as responsible for the consequences as with positive action. It is even maintained that the first of these suppositions expresses what anyone has to mean who has a moral view at all[9]. This can be quickly disproved: the Socratic view that one ought to suffer wrong rather than inflict it cannot even be formulated in consequentialist terms[10]. Furthermore, the consequentialist doctrine strikes at an enormously important part of traditional morality; for since it entails that one cannot know one's duty, it gets modified into the doctrine that one must always act for the best according to one's beliefs about consequences, and thus it leads to the characteristic view that there can be no such thing as the guilt of doing evil that good may come.

Although no sane person will even try to make the constant calculations required by consequentialist theory, it is influential where it maintains that it is all one *not* to do something that would preserve or prolong a life, and to do something positive to terminate it. The examples we have just given show that this is sometimes true. But it is generally false.

First, omission is not mere non-doing. Something not done is omitted if it

---

[7] Or even 'his life is/was not worth living', in the loose colloquial sense discussed in footnote 5 (p.43).

[8] Hence we deprecate the way the term 'passive euthanasia' is commonly used. It merely serves to obscure a vital moral distinction to have it apply indifferently to (a) witholding treatment with a view to hastening death, and, for example, to (b) withholding treatment on the grounds that it is excessively burdensome in circumstances in which as a consequence the patient dies earlier than he otherwise might have done. On (b) see Chapter 5, sec. 4.

[9] See G E Moore, *Principia Ethica*, pp. 24–5.

[10] A Müller, 'Radical Subjectivity: Morality versus Utilitarianism' (1977) 19 *Ratio*, 115–132.

ought to have been done, or was needed for some enterprise in hand, or was expected etc. It is the cook who spoils the potatoes by not putting salt in the water; it is *his* omission and not that of anyone else, say the gardener.

Second, omission contrasts with positive actions in two important ways.

(1) A positive action carries the presumption that the agent incurs the responsibility of intentionally doing it; omission does not.
(2) Blame for a positive act seldom depends on how difficult not acting would have been. Blame for an omission must take account of the difficulty, inconvenience etc of the omitted act.

When something is omitted intentionally and this results in harm, the omission may have been for the sake of the harm or for some other reason. If the former is the whole story, the harm is to be laid at the door of the non-acting agent as much as if he had done something positive for the same purpose. In law, this character of his omission will probably not be considered, as it is seldom detectable. When, though intentional, the omission is not for the sake of the harm, the moral question will be what the reason was and whether it exculpates. In the absence of an exculpating explanation the harm of the result, even though it is not intended, still lies at the door of the person whose omission is responsible for it. For the harm is voluntary. And, since negligence too is voluntary, so also may be the harm produced by an *un*intended omission, if it constitutes negligence. For behaviour can be voluntary though it is not deliberate or thought about.

The principle by which such harm is voluntary was stated succinctly by St. Thomas Aquinas: it was both possible and necessary for the agent to act, and he did not[11].

'Possible' and 'necessary' have many applications. Something may be non-possible in various ways. These may even include excessive difficulty: this of course would be serious or not according to circumstances. If it is somehow – seriously – impossible, an act cannot be called ethically necessary, although it may be physically possible and necessary for a certain result. If harm can be avoided only by a wicked, i.e. ethically impossible act, then there arises no guilt (in respect of the unaverted harm) for not doing the thing. E.g. a surgeon who will not kill one person, A, to save another, B, 'lets B die' but cannot be called guilty of his death. This is not because he 'only let him die': for, if what he omitted had been ethically possible we may suppose the case to be one in which it would also have been necessary.

8. The morality of omitting life-saving measures

We must now consider a doctor who omits saving remedies, not for the sake of having the patient die, and not because they are in any way impossible. There can be various justifications. It might be that resources were needed elsewhere too. Or the consideration may be solely about the patient himself. Here it will be generally agreed that only what does not seek to harm him has

---

[11] *Summa Theologiae* Ia IIae Q6, a.3.

a rightful place. It is possible for someone with the greatest respect for life to think it does not seem a misfortune for the patient to die soon. This however is a deep matter which he cannot know; and so the only positive objection to the adoption of the means of prolonging life can be that such means would be an affliction to the patient, which he can reasonably be spared, or would be futile because, for instance, the patient is dying anyway, if that is the case.

It follows from our consideration that wrongfulness in 'letting die' will always be a consequence of a particular moral necessity of saving life. That there are such necessities is clear; but it is a mistake to think that the mere circumstance that if one did nothing some life would be lost that might have been saved imposes a necessity to do that thing. Indeed the interests served by those who argue that such non-action is equivalent to murder are not those of promoting an impossible moral concern but rather those of breaking down the objections to murder as this is commonly understood.[12]

9. The morality of killing as a side-effect of other action

It remains to say a little more of murder where the death of the victim is a side-effect. These cases constitute a penumbra or fuzzy area surrounding the central areas of murder, intentional killing. An absolute prohibition on murder, which we have in our inherited moral law, cannot be confined to intentional killing. But not all deliberate action involving risk can be prohibited. So it must be possible to have sufficient excuse for risking or accepting death as a side-effect. This is readily grasped in the case of doctors giving pain-killing drugs. The statement that this is possible is known from Catholic moral theology as the 'principle of double effect'. The phrase is needlessly mystifying: the term 'double effect' relates to 'side effects' which may be brought about in addition to the effect that is aimed at.

A side-effect is one not intended by the agent. The principle is of course not that, so long as death is not what you intend, you can cause it with a clear conscience. Nor does it imply that burning a house down to get insurance money without regard to people in it getting killed, is *less* heinous than intentionally killing the same people (for the same purpose, we may suppose). The principle of the side effect merely states a possibility: where you may not aim at someone's death, causing it does not necessarily incur guilt – it can be that there are necessities which in the circumstances are great enough, or that there are legitimate purposes in hand of such a kind, to provide a valid excuse for risking or accepting that you cause death. Without such excuse, foreseeable killing is either murder or manslaughter.

The principle seems unexceptionably instanced in examples such as we have already mentioned – dangerous surgery, closing doors to contain fire or water, having ships and aeroplanes and races. In them, we are helped by thinking of the deaths as remote or uncertain. But of course an unintended death which is a foreseeable consequence of one's action may be neither.

---

[12] See in particular J Rachels, 'Active and Passive Euthanasia' (1975) 292 *New England Journal of Medicine*, 78–80; J Glover, *Causing Death and Saving Lives*, 91–112.

Then we are confronted with cases where it strikes people that there is little difference between direct and indirect killing. Imagine a pot-holer stuck with people behind him, and water rising to drown them. And suppose two cases: in one, he can be blown up; in the other, a rock can be moved to open another escape route, but it will crush him to death.

Someone who will equally choose either course clearly prefers saving these lives to the avoidance of any intentional killing of innocent people. Such cases are often discussed with a note of absolute necessity about saving lives: a presupposition that this is unconditionally paramount. The example of the stuck pot-holer (without the choice of methods of escape) was invented to illustrate the iniquity of abortion: you would not say you could kill the pot-holer to get out – it was argued. But people did say just that, at least if the case was described so that the potholer himself was going to drown too.

But situations must often have occurred where people were in a tight corner together, and could have saved themselves by killing one of their number, and that has not struck them as a serious option at all. If that were the attitude of the people in the cave, they would be equally unwilling either to destroy their companion directly, or to move the rock and crush him. Indeed someone might ask 'Isn't that direct killing too?' But the point of not calling it direct was that it isn't being crushed that gives the escape route: that is only an unavoidable consequence of moving the rock. They might adopt this means without realising the consequence, and that possibility indicates some difference.

Here the 'doctrine of double effect' is supposed to say that they can move the rock, though they cannot blow the man up. And this is what people find intolerably artificial and unnatural. But we must ask: is that because of what is here allowed, or because of what is forbidden? The principle of the side effect is employed in relation to an absolute prohibition on seeking someone's death, as end or as means. We have expounded that prohibition. But if the objection is to what is here allowed, one ought to notice that the principle does not state or imply that they can move the rock. For it does not say what necessities excuse foreseeably causing death.

There might be people among them who, seeing the consequence, would move the rock, though they would not blow the man up because that would be choosing his death as the means of escape. This is a far from meaningless stance, for they thus show themselves as people who will absolutely reject any policy making the death of innocent people a means or end.

But, to repeat, you cannot deduce the permissibility of moving the rock from the principle of double effect. It determines nothing about that, except that it is not excluded on the score of being intentional killing. The claim that the necessity of saving the trapped people is a sufficient excuse for moving the rock may be controverted: it may be said that the immediacy and intrinsic certainty of the death of the victim excludes moving the rock. To say this is to introduce a new principle to use in judging killings which are not intended as end or means. It is a reasonable principle. Surgery for example would be thought murderous, though not done in order to kill but, say, to get an organ for someone else, if the death of the patient were expected as a pretty immediate consequence, certain from the nature of the operation.

It will be clear why the area of murder which we have called the penumbra is not sharply defined. Necessity is a highly relative term: we invoke the necessity of relieving pain when we accept the risk of giving pain-killing drugs, but where the risk is considerable we shall allow it only in cases of terminal illness. It is appropriate to recall here that it is an axiom of medical practice that even in the most extreme situations, the least drastic remedy should be employed. There are gradations and shadings when there is a comparison to be made between the importance of ends being sought and the risks to life, as also in the circumstances which affect the comparison, and there are also gradations of uncertainty and remoteness. Where agents are anyway 'up to no good' (like the arsonist) the killing they do without purposing to kill will usually fall squarely within the penumbra. Other cases will also fall there, like the hypothetical surgery above. And there are cases also which fall clearly outside it. But there will also be borderline cases. Nor need the borderline be between murder and manslaughter; it may be between murder and innocence.

4

The Christian Tradition

Christian moral teaching on euthanasia arises both from the belief that human life is a precious gift from God and from a divine command to respect and protect that gift.

1. The gift of life

The understanding of human life as a gift from God is deeply rooted in Christian tradition. When we speak of it as a 'gift' we are forced, as always when speaking of God, to strain the ordinary language of human experience in an attempt to understand a deep mystery. In particular, the creation of an individual human being differs from other gifts because there is no preexisting recipient. But the analogy has force in showing that our very existence is a sheer gift. We who receive it are completely dependent on the creating giver. We have neither any prior claim nor anything to offer in exchange as a purchase price. God's creation and sustaining of us is a gift because it is utterly free, unconstrained.

The life we are given is a great good. And as so often with gifts, it brings with it responsibilities. We honour, serve and love God by respecting, fostering and loving the goods he has created and put in our charge. The Christian sees his life as one of the 'talents' which he is to use as a steward with responsible initiative. The gifts of creation, particularly the goods of human existence, are not merely to be passively or fatalistically 'held on to'; they are to be developed, fostered and actively protected against what threatens them. That is why when medical care is necessary and available, we are morally obliged to have recourse to it, up to the point where it becomes futile, or where it would itself involve burdens that the patient need not feel obliged to undergo.

Precisely because the gift of human life is so precious in God's eyes, and should therefore be in our eyes, God protected it among his people of Israel with a strict moral commandment, which was reaffirmed by Jesus in the New Testament[1].

---

[1] Cf Matthew 25: 14–30. Cf also Romans 14:7 ('None of us lives to himself and none of us dies to himself').

2. The commandment: 'Do no murder'

The command is first found among the Ten Commandments (Decalogue)[2]. It is often translated 'Do not kill'; but this translation is too wide. The law and practice of Israel authorised the deliberate killing of human beings in such cases as punishment for murder or the defence of Israel. Another translation is 'Do no murder'. The word 'murder', however, is ambiguous in English usage. Given one sense of the term, the translation is made to seem vacuous ('Do not do the kind of killing you ought not to do'). But given an explanation such as we gave in our discussion of murder in Chapter 3, the word approximates to the range of application of the original Hebrew verb as used in the Commandment. Assuming this sense, then, 'Do no murder' is close to being a correct translation. (It may be helpful to recall here the old English usage, found from Chaucer to Macaulay, in which wilful suicide is called self-murder.)

In the Christian Church, much of the law and practice of Israel was superseded, but each of the synoptic Gospels records that Jesus reaffirmed many of the fundamental moral commands that are found in the Decalogue.[3] Indeed he did so in a way that indicates that the love of God and of our neighbour excludes what is excluded by those commands. To the question 'What shall I do to inherit eternal life?', Jesus commends the reply[4], that 'You shall love the Lord your God with all your heart ... and your neighbour as yourself'. He himself begins another reply to the very same question[5]: 'If you would enter life, keep the commandments ... "You shall not kill, you shall not ... and, You shall love your neighbour as yourself"'.

Thus the prohibition on taking innocent human life was proclaimed from the outset of Christian teaching as an unconditional requirement, proposed by God not just to a chosen people but to all. St. Paul's letter to the Romans treats these moral principles of the Decalogue as bases of God's final judgement on all men, and as principles both divinely revealed and 'written

---

[2] Exodus 20: 13; Deuteronomy 5: 17.

[3] Much of the teaching about the respect due to human life, which is expounded in the main part of this chapter, is a teaching common to Jews and Christians. In post-Biblical Judaism there is a fairly developed casuistry on medical subjects in the rabbinic responsa devoted to them. We note briefly the controlling emphases of this tradition.

Killing any innocent person, 'whether he is healthy or about to die from natural causes' is legally codified as murder. [Maimonides, *Mishneh Torah, Yad Hazakah, Roze'ah* 2:7.] Human life is held to be of infinite worth, so that any fraction of it is reckoned to be of infinite value. Hence relief from suffering is not to be secured at the cost of life itself. '... a patient on his deathbed is considered as a living person in every respect ... and it is forbidden to cause him to die quickly ... or to move him from his place (lest this hasten his death); ... and whoever closes his eyes with the onset of death is regarded as shedding blood.' [J Caro, *Shulhan Arukh. Yoreh De'ah*, 339.1 and gloss.] 'Some recent rabbinical responsa, however, are inclined to sanction the cessation of "heroic" methods to prolong a lingering life without hope of recovery. The withdrawal of treatment under such circumstances might be justified on the basis of the permission to remove from a dying person an extraneous impediment, such as "a clattering noise or salt on his tongue, delaying the departure of his soul" (J Caro, *Shulhan Arukh, Yoreh De'ah*, 339. 1, gloss).' [I Jakobovitz, art. 'Euthanasia', in *Encyclopaedia Judaica*, vol 6, p. 979.]

[4] Luke 10: 25–27.

[5] Luke 18: 18, 20; Matthew 19: 16, 18–20; cf Mark 10: 17, 19 and Luke 18: 18, 20. See also James 2: 11.

on the hearts of the Gentiles', i.e. available to the conscience of all men[6]. The moral teachers amongst the earliest Church fathers and apologists built on the Decalogue, which they included amongst the commandments of Jesus that show the Way of Life[7]. The Church of the second century met and vigourously rejected the challenge of those who argued that Christ had abrogated the Ten Commandments along with other parts of the law of Israel. In his statement of the Church's teaching, Irenaeus elaborates and amplifies Paul: the Ten Commandments are God's permanent will for mankind, fully revealed and ratified by Jesus; the moral precepts of the Decalogue correspond to the deepest and most original law of human nature[8]. When Jesus said[9] 'You have heard that it was said to the men of old, "You shall not kill, and whoever kills shall be liable to judgement", but I say to you that everyone who is angry with his brother shall be liable to judgement', he was not abrogating the commandment (as some mid-second century theologians claimed), but rather 'fulfilling, extending and affording greater scope to it'[10].

3. The conditions of our stewardship

But it might be asked: Why cannot we stewards of our life return it voluntarily to its rightful owner when the indications are that it has served its purpose and that God is recalling it to himself? Why cannot we then hasten death?

The Christian answer is that one's stewardship of one's life does not include the choice to terminate the stewardship itself. We did not ourselves participate in initiating the gift and task of that stewardship; we could not accept it on conditions chosen by us. Why God should have brought us (or anyone) into existence as 'persons created for their own sake' is deeply mysterious. So we should not be particularly surprised if we also find it mysterious that God sees meaning and value in every part – even the most miserable and reduced – of the lifespan he allots us. But that God can and does is central to the faith of Israel and to Christian faith. His ways are not our ways, and the particular workings of his purposes are inscrutable to us.[11]

The conditions of our stewardship, then, are provided by God's commandments or 'mandates'. Men and women can come (though not without the risk of uncertainty and confusion) to a knowledge of those commandments by conscientious exercise of 'natural' reason, i.e. even without the benefit of God's self-disclosure to Israel and through Jesus. In that self-disclosure there is revealed a commandment which, as explained through Scripture and the tradition of the Church, forbids us to intend to terminate our life. It has always been Christian belief that that expression of God's will holds good in all the circumstances and conditions of life.

[6] Romans 1: 29–32; 2: 5–8, 12–16; 13: 9.
[7] See *Didache* 2: 2; *Epistle of Barnabas* 4; 14; 19; 20; *Apology of Aristides* 15.
[8] Irenaeus, *Adversus Haereses* IV, 13–15.
[9] Matthew 5: 21–22.
[10] Irenaeus, *Adversus Haereses* IV, 13–15.
[11] Isaiah 40: 13; 55: 8; Romans 11: 33.

4. Attitudes towards our stewardship

Acceptance of God's gifts, on the conditions specified by God's commandments, calls for those human dispositions (which are also in God's gift) which we call 'virtues'. Christ had many things to say about them. Take, for example, 'Blessed are the meek ...' (Mt 5:5). The meekness of which Christ speaks is not the meekness (weakness) of passivity or wilful feebleness: Moses the great leader was 'the *meekest* man in the world' (Num. 12:3), and Jesus who drove the dealers out of the Temple calls on us to learn from his own meekness (Matt. 11:29). Rather, meekness is a fundamental *willingness to accept the role that truly has been allotted one*. The meekness of those who are willing to learn from Jesus is not servile. God is indeed Lord and master of life and death[12]. But Jesus reveals that 'You are *my friends* if you do what I command you. No longer do I call you servants...'[13].

We are at all times in the hands of a loving God who has given us each a life to be lived out in loving worship of him and in loving service of our neighbour, in preparation for a further life of perfect fulfilment with the God of all love and consolation. We must not therefore conclude from language which refers to the absolute claims of God's commands, and to the responsibilities and restrictions under which we exercise our stewardship of life, that our God is no more than a distant and aloof judge. The Christian revelation is not one of easy solutions or optimistic blindness to suffering; we recall the suffering and sense of dereliction of Jesus on his cross. But it is a revelation that love somehow predominates; that God is tender towards those creatures he created for their own sake; that the weak and powerless are somehow going to be privileged; and that God, despite appearances to the contrary, is a 'very present help' in all man's troubles. He is no absent God to any of his creatures but is intimately present to them. Viewed from this perspective, each person's life is not just a bleak commission from a superior being, but an enterprise to be undertaken with a friend, to be shared at every step along the way, and not least in its final stages. Here is a resource in whose existence Christians believe, but whose strength no one can fathom.

A believer, observing the sufferings of another person, may wonder whether God's presence and resource are available or helpful in those sufferings if that other is a non-believer. We must recognise the possibility of a real rejection of God's friendship and purposes, a rejection bringing desolation. But the active presence of a loving God encompasses every human being in this life, even those who are unaware of it and do not believe in it. When it is not radically rejected, that presence can sustain, and is certainly available to sustain, all human beings in their sufferings.

The ultimate source of the dignity and inviolability of the human being is God's creative love and loving purpose, which are at the depth of the mystery of every human person, and uniquely for everyone. Faith in God's loving presence, calling for trust, enriches and makes personal those con-

[12] Wisdom 16: 13; Deuteronomy 32: 39; I Samuel 2:6.
[13] John 15: 14–15.

54

clusions concerning euthanasia which earlier we spoke of only in the language of justice: euthanasia is a betrayal of that trust.

5. 'Death with dignity'

If someone speaks of 'death with dignity' or 'dying with dignity', the Christian will reflect that indeed every person in every condition of life has the dignity of one 'created for his very own sake' and called to friendship and sonship with God. He will also reflect that true dignity is not incompatible with weakness and need. In a real but superficial sense of 'dignity', some very ordinary but necessary aspects of bodily life and activity are scarcely dignified, at the best of times. The dissolution of one's bodily life in sickness and death often involves indignities of this sort, which may be needlessly multiplied and intensified by insensitive attendants, ward–round procedures and many other slights. If we go a little deeper, we find that our pride and self-esteem are threatened and aroused when we are dependent on the service, generosity and love of others; we may feel our whole situation then to be intrinsically undignified and shameful. But these are feelings to be overcome. The golden rule of doing to others as we would have them do to us is observed as much in grateful and ungrudging accepting as in generous giving. The spirit of serene acknowledgement of the reality of one's needful situation (a spirit that could be called meekness) is much more real an expression of human dignity than any struggle to maintain a fiction of independence, or any flight into death simply to preserve one's 'control over one's own destiny'.

Finally, we may reflect on the high dignity that Christianity recognises in, and affords to, human bodily life. To regard the body as a prison, or as an instrument or detachable launching rocket of the *real* person, is incompatible with the faith in which incarnation and resurrection are central. The age-old and anti-Christian temptation to body-spirit dualism has always to be resisted. The good of human life, protected by God, is the good of bodily life. One cannot justify an attack on that life, even in one's own person, by arguing that one's bodily life is useless or an encumbrance to one's *real* vocation as a person. Reverence for that bodily life is thus integral to one's most fundamental calling by God, right to the very end of one's earthly existence. As we have said above, man differs from the other animals by being spirit as well as flesh. But the human spirit, 'since it is a part of the human body, is not the whole man, and my spirit is not *me* (anima mea non est ego)'[14].

6. Roman Catholic teaching

The teaching of the Roman Catholic Church has steadily opposed euthanasia. That teaching is based on the nature of human existence as a gift from God protected by God's own command. Some of the main strands in

[14] Aquinas, *Commentary on I Corinthians*, c. 15, Lect. 2.

the Church's understanding of the respect to be accorded to the gift of life and of the wrongfulness of euthanasia are summed up in a recent address of Pope John Paul II:

... you should each cultivate within yourself a clear awareness of the very high value of human life: it is a value unique in the whole of visible creation. The Lord, in fact, created everything on earth for man; man, on the other hand – as the Second Vatican Council stressed – is 'the only creature that God wanted for its own sake' (Const. *Gaudium et Spes*, n.24).

... This is the deep content of the well-known passage of the Bible, according to which 'God created man in his own image ... male and female he created them' (Gen. 1:27); and this is also what it is desired to recall when it is affirmed that human life is sacred. Man, as a being supplied with intelligence and free will, takes his right to life directly from God, whose image he is ... Only God, therefore, can 'dispose' of this extraordinary gift of his: 'I, even I, am he, and there is no God beside me; I kill and I make alive; I wound and I heal; and there is none that can deliver out of my hand' (Deut. 32:39). Man, therefore, possesses life as a gift, of which he cannot consider himself the owner however; for this reason, he cannot feel he is the arbiter of life, whether his own or that of others. The Old Testament formulates this conclusion in one of the Ten Commandments: 'You shall not kill' (Ex. 20:13), with the clarification that follows immediately afterwards: 'Do not slay the innocent and righteous, for I will not acquit the wicked' (Ex. 23:7). Christ, in the New Testament, confirms this commandment as a condition to 'enter life' (cf Mt. 19:18); but – significantly – he follows it with the mention of the commandment that sums up every aspect of moral law, bringing it to completion, that is, the commandment of love (cf 19:19) ... [15]

The meaning and force of the commandment, as constantly taught in the Church, were summed up in the Roman Catechism (1566): the commandment does not concern the killing of animals, or accidental killing; it does not forbid killing in self-defence or a just war; it does not exclude capital punishment, and finally it would not override a special decree of God the Lord of life:

These, which we have just mentioned, are the cases not contemplated by this commandment; and with these exceptions the prohibition embraces all others, with regard to the person who kills, the person killed, and the means used to kill. As to the person who kills, the commandment recognises no exception whatever ... With regard to the person killed, the obligation of the law is no less extensive, embracing every human creature ... It also forbids suicide ... Finally, if we consider the numerous means by which murder may be committed, the law makes no exception ... [16]

Thus the Second Vatican Council could recall a very constant and firm Christian teaching on the reverence due to human life:

Whatever is opposed to life itself – such as any type of murder, genocide. abortion, euthanasia and wilful suicide; ... – all these and the like are criminal; they poison civilisation, but they harm those who carry them out more than those who suffer the injury; and they are a supreme dishonour to the Creator[17].

The Council does not say what it means by 'euthanasia'; the term had been explained less than a decade before, in two addresses by Pius XII in 1957. In the first of these, the Pope had considered the use of pain-relieving drugs and

[15] Address to Midwives, 26 January 1980; Italian original in (1980) 72 *Acta Apsotolicae Sedis*, 84–8.

[16] *Roman Catechism*, Part III, c.6. On suicide it adds: 'For no one has such power over his own life as to be morally allowed to bring death upon himself by his own decision; and thus the wording of this commandment is not "Do not kill another" but simply "Do not kill".'

[17] Constitution, *Gaudium et Spes*, para 27.

had explained how that need not amount to euthanasia even if the use of the drugs, for the sake of relieving pain, might also shorten the life of a dying person:

Every form of direct euthanasia, that is to say, the administration of a narcotic[18] in order to procure or to hasten death, is immoral because it is a claim to dispose directly of life ... One lays claim to a right of direct disposition whenever one wills the shortening of life as an end or as a means[19].

In the second address, Pius XII considered the use of techniques of artificial respiration on deeply unconscious patients who, if not already dead, would certainly die a few minutes after any cessation of the techniques:

Natural reason and Christian morals say that man (and anyone entrusted with the care of his fellow man) has the right and duty, in case of serious illness, to take the treatment necessary for the preservation of life and health ... But this duty normally obliges one only to the use of ordinary means (according to the circumstances of persons, places, epochs and culture), i.e. of means that do not impose any extraordinary burden on oneself or on someone else ...

The rights and duties of the doctor are correlative to those of the patient ... Since these forms of treatment go beyond the ordinary means, which one is bound to have recourse to, it cannot be maintained that there is an obligation to use them or, consequently, to authorise one's doctor to use them.

The rights and duties of the [patient's] family depend in general on the presumed will of the unconscious patient if he is of age and *sui juris*. As to the family's own independent duty, the only obligation in normal circumstances is to employ ordinary means. Consequently, if it were to appear that the attempt at resuscitation constitutes in truth a burden on the family such as one could not in conscience impose on them, they can legitimately insist that the doctor cease his attempts, and the doctor can legitimately comply. In this case there is no *direct disposal of the life of the patient, no euthanasia*, which would never be permissible; even when it brings about the cessation of circulation, the interruption of the attempts at resuscitation is only ever indirectly a cause of the cessation of life ...[20]

These passages from the teaching of Pius XII provide a clear indication of what the Second Vatican Council had in mind when it condemned euthanasia. Since the Council, the papal magisterium of the Church has as we have seen given further expression to that teaching and its theological bases. The *Declaration on Euthanasia* by the Sacred Congregation for the Doctrine of the Faith, dated 5 May 1980, provides a fuller treatment of the whole matter. We shall conclude by citing just two passages from that Declaration:

Human life is the basis of all goods, and is the necessary source and condition of every human activity and of all society. Most people regard life as something sacred, and hold that no one may dispose of it at will, but believers see in life something greater, namely a gift of God's love, which they are called upon to preserve and make fruitful[21].

[18] In this address, the Pope chose to use the terms 'analgesic', 'anaesthetic' and 'narcotic' virtually interchangeably.
[19] Address of 24 February 1957 to doctors and surgeons in response to questions by anaesthetists (1957) 49 *Acta Apostolicae Sedis*, 129–47; quoted extract at 146. See likewise Sacred Congregation for the Doctrine of the Faith, *Iura et Bona* (Declaration on Euthanasia) (1980) 72 *Acta Apostolicae Sedis*, 542–52, Section III.
[20] Address of 24 November 1957 to doctors, (1957) 49 *Acta Apostolicae Sedis*, 1027–33; quoted extracts at 1030–2. The final sentence concludes 'and one must here apply the principle of double effect and the principle of *voluntarium in causa*'. This is to be understood in the light of what is said in Chapter 3 above in discussing the so-called Principle of Double Effect.
[21] *Iura et Bona*, section I.

This being so, the teaching concludes, euthanasia 'is a question of the violation of the divine law, an offence against the dignity of the human person, a crime against life, and an attack on humanity'[22].

---

[22] *Iura et Bona*, section II.

Part Three

A patient who consults a doctor may be said to have three questions: what is wrong? What can be done about it? What *should* be done about it? The doctor's skill in diagnosis, his knowledge of what can be done and his judgement of what clinically should be done do not endow him with sole authority to decide what shall be done. Even though he accepts his doctor's diagnosis, a patient may still think differently from the doctor about what in the circumstances he needs or is able to accept. What is to be done remains to be settled between doctor and patient.

Relatives and guardians also have duties and rights. Good practice is something to be striven for within a web of relationships in which the exercise of responsibilities and rights does not always permit the implementation of a theoretically ideal clinical regimen. Something needs to be said, therefore, about the rights and duties of competent patients (Chapter 5), and the rights of and duties towards incompetent patients (Chapter 6), before discussing the norms of good clinical practice (Part Four).

5

Rights and Duties of Competent Patients in Regard to Treatment

1. The legal right to refuse treatment

A competent person may not be given treatment without his or her consent and is legally entitled to refuse what a doctor proposes. A doctor should not force a patient to accept medical treatment unless the patient is not of sound mind or too young to make sound judgements about himself. We need not here explore the problems that can sometimes arise in applying these principles; they are not peculiar to the situations in which euthanasia is proposed. It is clear that the doctor must respect the mature and sufficiently lucid patient's refusal of treatment even if he disapproves of that refusal, believing, in a life-threatening situation. that it is tantamount to suicide. In respecting that refusal the doctor is respecting the patient's autonomy[1]. On the other hand, because a doctor may not assist a suicide, a patient has no right to request such assistance.

2. The question: When ought patients to accept treatment?

A patient may act wrongly in refusing treatment and it is important for patients to be clear about the moral (as distinct from the legal) obligations they may have in the matter of accepting and refusing treatment. The forms in which the question of what is obligatory confronts the patient depend on his or her condition. In the context of our discussion it is useful to distinguish three broad classes from each of which there may be patients for whom euthanasia is contemplated. (When we turn in Chapter 7 to a detailed consideration of principles of clinical management of patients, we will again find it useful to distinguish between these three classes of condition).

A. Those suffering from a lethal condition for which there are no life-saving treatments

Even if a person has a lethal condition which cannot be successfully treated, the question may arise whether all possible measures to slow the onset of dying and death must be taken, or whether all possible or even all 'normal' means of sustaining life must be accepted by the patient. And there may be

---

[1] It should be pointed out here that a doctor does have a responsibility not to respect a patient's suicidal refusal of treatment if it seems reasonably clear that that wish is indicative of a depressive condition which in turn suggests that the patient is far from being able to make a 'lucid and mature' judgement.

the question whether he is bound to sustain himself by food, drink and treatments which are commonplace (e.g. some antibiotics) or which he has used before the onset of the new and lethal illness (e.g. insulin for his long-term diabetes).

B. Those suffering from a lethal condition for which there are life-saving treatments

For such a patient the question may be whether he is bound to undertake the treatment if it is costly, painful, distressing, time-consuming, damaging, leaves him with substantial defects or is even potentially lethal. Such questions, particularly the questions about risks and unwanted sequelae, are also important for his doctor.

C. Those suffering from a non-lethal condition which is painful, distressing or incapacitating (physically or mentally), and for which any improvement must remain substantially incomplete

For this kind of patient a similar range of questions arises –

i) if he comes to be subsequently afflicted by a lethal but easily remedied condition and is tempted to refuse treatment for it in order to escape from his long-term miseries;
ii) when he considers whether or not to undertake treatment that may cure one or more (but not all) of his symptoms or relieve (but incompletely) all of his symptoms.

3. The distinction between 'ordinary' and 'extraordinary' means

It has been common in Catholic teaching to refer to a distinction between 'ordinary' and 'extraordinary' means in answering questions about when a patient is obliged to accept treatment. In recent decades a number of writers have treated this distinction as synonymous with a distinction between what is obligatory and what is optional for a particular patient[2]. If it is understood in this way the distinction clearly needs to be explained by reference to the considerations which are invoked in determining whether treatment is obligatory. These considerations are outlined below.

However, there is a more familiar use of the distinction in which 'ordinary' refers to a normal and tried procedure, and 'extraordinary' refers to an unusual procedure, involving much risk, pain or heavy cost. The fact that a treatment is in this sense 'ordinary' is itself a reason for holding it to be normally obligatory, though there may be circumstances in which this reason lacks force; for example, when one considers the use of antibiotics for pneumonia in a patient in the terminal phase of another illness.

[2] Notably Paul Ramsey in *The Patient as Person* (1970). Ramsey's understanding in turn derived from his reading of Gerald Kelly S J 'The Duty of Using Artificial Means of Preserving Life', (1950) 11 *Theological Studies* 203–220, and the same author's 'The Duty to Preserve Life' (1951) 12 *Theological Studies* 550–56.

It is not necessary to be troubled by ambiguities attaching to the terms 'ordinary' and 'extraordinary'[3]. It is the underlying considerations determining when treatment is obligatory which are important.

4. Considerations determining when treatment is and is not obligatory

In general if a person is ill he is obliged to seek help (if available) to maximise his chances of recovery and to minimise the effects of chronic disability or handicap. If illness is life-threatening a person should seek to avert the threat.

There are limits, however, to the extent to which a patient is obliged to accept specific treatments to these ends. The most obvious and basic limit concerns the efficaciousness of a treatment. If there is little or no chance of a treatment succeeding in restoring health, modifying handicap or averting death a patient can rarely be obliged to undergo it. The point may seem obvious. It nonetheless needs labouring since clinicians do sometimes encourage patients to persist in *futile* treatments.

The more difficult factors to assess in judging whether treatment is obligatory concern what is traditionally called the *burdensome* character of treatment. In judging how burdensome treatment is, consideration is to be given to the degree of risk, cost and physical and psychological hardship involved relative (a) to this particular patient, his overall condition and its potential for improvement, his resources and sensibilities, and (b) to this particular doctor (or medical team), his time, effort and other obligations.

A patient is entitled (though not obliged) to refuse treatment on the ground that, considering all the above factors, it is too costly and/or physically or psychologically burdensome to him or to his dependents or to those in attendance on him, even in circumstances in which he expects the consequences of his refusal to be fatal or drastic for him.

The burden of treatment can depend, we have said, on a patient's overall condition and its potential for improvement, his resources and sensibility; as these vary from patient to patient so may and should the assessment of burden.

5. Burdensomeness and patients' refusal of treatment

There seem to be at least three lines of thought into which considerations of burdensomeness may enter and lead a patient to refuse treatment:

a) A patient might reject treatment not because he cannot envisage that it might be beneficial – he might indeed think benefits likely and in themselves attractive – but simply because he cannot bring himself to pay the price in, say, pain or mutilation that the treatment would entail. He recoils from the prospect of the burden of the treatment.

[3] To avoid ambiguities some writers suggest the terminology should be abandoned. E.g. Paul Ramsey *Ethics at the Edges of Life. Medical and Legal Intersections* 1978, p. 155; Robert Veatch, *Death, Dying and the Biological Revolution* 1976, p. 110.

b) A patient might reject treatment not so much because he recoils from the prospect of its attendant burdens, but rather because he finds the promised benefits either too improbable or disproportionately small to warrant enduring those burdens.

The first patient's line of thought is not in principle wrong; nor is that of the second. (It is, however, possible that a patient ought to judge that for the sake of some duty he owes to others he is morally obliged to put up with the burdens of a prolonged illness, degeneration and/or dying.)

c) A patient might reject treatment not precisely because that treatment would create burdens which he could specify in a way that would make it seem recognisably burdensome, but because the treatment's characteristic benefits no longer appear to *him* to be benefits. What leads him to so experience his situation is a combination of debilitation and suffering which cannot be alleviated and which in turn prevent relief from some supervening condition like pneumonia being reckoned really beneficial; as it seems, antibiotics would merely release him for lengthier endurance of his wretchedness.

Is this third line of thought suicidal? That is, must we say that such a patient's intention in rejecting treatment is that of bringing about his own death? For (it might be said) it is not the treatment which appears to be burdensome but rather his own life.

6. Which reasons for refusing treatment are suicidal?

There is certainly a clear distinction to be made between, on the one hand, rejecting life-saving treatment because one recoils from its burdensomeness – as (a) – or thinks it insufficiently beneficial relative to its costs, attendant hardship or risk – as (b) – and on the other hand rejecting treatment because one assesses one's potential future as not worth having, and so rejects treatment precisely with a view to hastening death. Rejection for the latter reason is the choice of suicide by omission. Rejection for one or other of the former two reasons is the expression of a preference for life without certain impositions or without impositions which lack compensatory benefits, even if that life be shorter than it might otherwise have been.

It seems to us, however, that an important distinction needs to be made in respect of patients suffering from terminal conditions who begin to suffer from other conditions (like pneumonia) which may hasten death. The distinction we have in mind is between the suicidal attitude of the patient who omits treatment on purpose so that death will come sooner, and the attitude of someone who omits treatment because he judges he has no obligation (and certainly has no desire) to seek to prolong his life. A patient is indeed moved to reflect on whether he has such an obligation by the thought of the burdens associated with his prior fatal condition and not because of any burdens associated with treatment for his supervening condition. But a decision to refuse life-prolonging treatment based on a reasonable judgement that one does not have an obligation to seek to prolong one's life (where death cannot be for very long delayed) does not itself embody an intention to hasten one's death.

Some may object that the distinction we have spoken of in the preceding paragraph is one that does not make a difference because the *consequence* of either attitude is foreseeably a similar hastening of death. This objection misses a point central to the argument of this Report. In Chapter 3, sec. 4 we have emphasised that justice in relation to one's own death depends on the direction of the will: towards acceptance of life and death as they may come from the hand of God. The patient who omits treatment because he judges that he does not have to prolong his life is not defeated in his intention if it happens that he survives the pneumonia; for his will is not set on the rejection of his life. But the patient who omits treatment precisely in order that death will come sooner will be defeated in his intention if he survives, for his will is set on the rejection of his life (if only by omission). The one attitude is compatible with acceptance; the other is its antithesis.

7. *Refusing treatment, suicide and the direction of the will: further analysis*

Any decision to omit treatment in order to die is suicidal and so is to be excluded. But it is quite possible for patient X to say to himself 'my life is nearly over, and is wretched in various ways, and I have no special responsibilities to others; I just *don't have* to undertake any new treatment for the sake of keeping my life going'. Such a decision need not be regarded as suicidal, even though another patient, Y, in apparently identical circumstances, might say to himself: 'I know that what they're offering me won't give me much more time or comfort; but it won't create any new burdens for me and it will keep me going a bit longer and I shouldn't spurn life while it's available to me without extraordinary burdens on myself or others'. X's 'I just don't have to . . .' need not express a rejection of life or a choice of death, and Y's 'I shouldn't spurn life . . .' is not a universal moral judgement that would commit Y to condemning X. Rather, Y's decision represents a sort of personal valuation of or commitment to life; we can describe Y's willingness to endure a longer period of wretchedness as 'noble' without having to describe as 'ignoble' X's choice not to extend his period of wretchedness.

What is important is that X's decision, like Y's, is distinguishable from the attitude and decision of Z, who says to himself 'my life is not worth living: I know I mustn't "do" anything to kill myself; but here's a way out – I'll refuse my insulin (or: my food; or: this cheap, new, painless and effective treatment)'. Z's attempt to exploit the distinction between positive action and omissions in fact amounts to the suicidal adoption of a policy of omission in order to die.

We can say of X that he rejects treatment because he lacks a reason for thinking treatment worthwhile, while Z rejects treatment because he rejects the prospect of a wretched life. This distinction is significant, we would maintain, precisely in those circumstances in which a patient is inevitably dying. If it is not the case that death is antecedently inevitable, it is doubtful that a patient can reasonably judge that he has no obligation to seek to prolong his life when he first begins to suffer from a life-threatening condition.

8. Conclusion

We seem, then, in the course of this analysis to have isolated four potentially acceptable reasons for rejecting treatment apart from considerations of excessive risk or financial cost (though the latter is one type of burden):

a) the burdens attendant on treatment impress as more than one can cope with;
b) the burdens attendant on treatment seem hardly warranted by the promised benefits;
c) treatment is not worthwhile because a dying patient has reason to think that he no longer has an obligation to seek to prolong his life;
d) treatment is straightforwardly futile i.e. inappropriate to the biological nature of one's condition, as, for example, when putatively curative treatment is offered to someone in an irreversible state of dying.

It is obvious from what has been said that there must be some difficulty in practice over distinguishing the attitude of someone – like X – who rejects treatment along the lines of (c) and someone – like Z – who rejects treatment with a suicidal intent. To the outside observer, X's and Z's situations, and their decision to refuse treatment, might appear identical. But what matters morally are their intentions and dispositions, and in this matter of refusals and omissions the 'public' character of the situation and of the treatment does not constrain us to any single characterisation of the intention or disposition of the person doing the refusing or omitting. The non-public character of the distinction between X's intention and Z's does not make the distinction either unreal or less than fundamental; whereas what is publicly observable is a distinction between two positions (X's and Y's) which are both within the field of the morally permissible: X judges rightly when he says 'I don't have to ...'

6

The Rights of Incompetent Patients and Duties Towards Them

There is a long moral and legal tradition that decisions about consent to treatment where the patient is incompetent should lie with relatives (or guardians), on the grounds that these may be presumed to have the interests of the incompetent patient at heart. Since the presumption will not always hold good, and since in any case relatives (et al.) may be unclear about what is in the interests of an incompetent patient and what is owing to him, we need to clarify the rights of the incompetent patient. What we say about the duties of relatives in respect of the incompetent is also of importance for doctors since they have a special responsibility when treating incompetents to be sure that relatives are well informed and have the patient's interests at heart. In many circumstances the doctor will have to make the decision himself because, for example, no relative is available.

It will be clear from what we have argued in Chapter 3 that it cannot be in the interests of an incompetent patient that others (e.g. parents) agree to treatment or a clinical regimen the purpose of which is to hasten that person's death. We recall the distinction we have already drawn between aiming to bring about someone's death and not aiming to prolong that person's life. Still, in the context of the modem debate we fear that an exclusive emphasis on the rights of parents in consultation with their chosen physician is all too often intended to accommodate choice of a clinical regimen designed to hasten death.[1]

1. Standard of Treatment

The basic standard in the treatment of the incompetent should be no different from that which holds for the competent i.e. they should be given

---

[1] Official professional comment (e.g. that of the British Paediatric Association; see *British Medical Journal* 22 August 1981, p.567) on the debate surrounding the recent Court of Appeal decision *In re B (a Minor)* (see Chapter 2, p.16, n.6) has relied for support on the statement about 'Severely malformed infants' in *The Handbook of Medical Ethics* of the British Medical Association (London 1980). This statement describes the doctor's duty as that of finding 'a just and humane solution for the infant and the family'. In the absence of a willingness to say what *cannot* count as a just and humane solution the requirement as stated is in danger of proving empty. This danger is heightened by the *unqualified* emphasis placed on the 'ultimate responsibility' of the parent to decide 'whether the child should be treated or not' (see section 5.10, 5.11, p.29).

There is, moreover, danger of further obfuscation through identifying what is at issue as the *child's* 'right to accept or reject treatment' (see the 'general guidance' statement issued by the BMA, in *British Medical Journal* 22 August 1981, p.567) – a right which the parents are then said to exercise on the child's behalf. The child can have no such right, since that kind of right presupposes a developed

whatever treatment is beneficial, having regard to acceptable costs in terms of expense and burden. The application of this standard in cases of the incompetent can raise difficult questions concerning what to take account of in judging whether treatment is unacceptably burdensome. As we have seen in discussing the competent patient, what counts as a burden and indeed what counts as a benefit can depend on the individual sensibility and priorities of a patient. When can we safely make judgements about these factors in the case of incompetent patients and when would we risk doing these patients injustice by hazarding such judgements?

2. Judging the burdensomeness of treatment for the incompetent.

At this point it would be useful for our purposes to distinguish three classes of incompetent patient:

 i) those who were once competent,
 ii) those who though physically mature have always been incompetent,
iii) infants and young children.

In class (i) there will be some who made a considered choice, while competent, about the medical care to be given or not given them during any later period of incompetence. If a doctor reasonably judges that that earlier considered choice has not been superseded by the passage of time, or by later indications of the patient's real wishes, or by substantial changes in the character of the treatment, he may reasonably consider himself entitled not to impose on that patient treatment thus rejected in advance, even if it may perhaps have been immorally rejected. The reason for this is that this patient's choice may here be considered to have the same force as the considered choice of a still competent patient, which even when it is apparently a choice for suicide by omission should not be overridden, since the patient's liberty and autonomy ought to be respected (see Chapter 5, sec. 1).

Judgements about the individual sensibilities of other patients in class (i), i.e. those who have not, while competent, made a considered choice of the medical care to be given them if and when incompetent, will rely on the kind of informal understanding of the patient developed by those who have not only lived close to him but also can be presumed to be well-disposed towards him. Informal understanding will similarly be the basis of judgements about the individual sensibilities of patients in class (ii). This kind of evidence should be employed with caution in arriving at judgements about the burdensome consequences for a given patient of a possible course of treatment. Here the doctor's special responsibility to assure himself of the good intentions of relatives is particularly important.

It would clearly be a mistake, however, to think that evidence of a patient's distinctive sensibility is the only sort available for arriving at

capacity which a child does not have. The child's right is the right to be treated in accordance with the general standard stated in this chapter. The problems of applying this standard in the case of very young children are examined in the chapter.

judgements about what is likely to prove burdensome. Individual sensibilities are not entirely idiosyncratic. There are reliable generalisations about what is and is not likely to prove tolerable with certain types of patient. Some of the factors cited in a now famous court case in the United States[2] against treating the patient would probably hold good for any patient of that kind. The patient in question was 67 years old and profoundly mentally retarded (with an IQ of 10 and a mental age of approximately 2 years and 8 months). He had been institutionalised all his life and was unable to communicate verbally. He was diagnosed as suffering from acute myeloblastic monocytic leukaemia, an invariably fatal disease. The only known treatment is chemotherapy which offers a 30%–50% chance of a remission lasting from 2 to 13 months. The treatment itself has serious side effects, including pain, discomfort, pronounced anaemia, bladder irritation, loss of hair, bone marrow depression, and, in rare cases, death. Apparently a majority of competent patients suffering from the condition elect to undergo chemotherapy in the hope of remission. It was argued, however, that a patient with an IQ of 10 would be unable to co-operate with the treatment and would therefore need to be physically restrained, would be disorientated by it, would find the pain unintelligible, and for these, among other reasons, ought not to be subjected to it. The reasons offered are both plausible generalisations about a patient with an IQ of 10, and also clearly relevant considerations in assessing burdensomeness, and hence pertinent to the decision to withhold treatment.

3. What valid reasons are there for withholding treatment from the newborn (class iii)?

At the end of Chapter 5 (sec. 8) we summarised our analysis of the acceptable reasons a *competent* patient may have for rejecting treatment in the following terms:

a) the burdens attendant on treatment impress as more than one can cope with;
b) the burdens attendant on treatment seem hardly warranted by the promised benefits;
c) treatment is not worthwhile because, being already dying, one has reason to think that one no longer has an obligation to seek to prolong one's life;
d) treatment is straightforwardly futile i.e. inappropriate to the biological nature of one's condition (as when would-be curative treatments are offered to someone irreversibly dying).

It will help to make clear our view of which are the morally acceptable reasons for withholding treatment from the newborn if we use the above analysis as a checklist.

It should be immediately obvious that (c) can have no place as a reason for

---

[2] *Superintendent of Belchertown State School* v. *Saikewicz* 370 N.E. 2d 417 (1977) (Supreme Judicial Court, Mass.)

withholding treatment from the newborn since it essentially involves a judgement which can be made only by a competent patient in regard to himself. The reason offered is a first-person judgement: 'I don't *have* to prolong my life'.

It should also be obvious that treatment which is in a straightforward way futile – reason (d) – *ought* to be withheld from a child (as from any other patient). But often the judgement that treatment is futile combines elements of (d) and (b); typically it will be said that significant clinical efforts or initiatives should not be made because they promise no more than minimal alleviation to a patient suffering from severe and extensive disabilities.

Two elements in such a judgement call for comment. First, it should be clear that the treatment in question does add up to a *significant* clinical effort (i.e. one which involves a deployment of personnel and resources making a substantial difference to the possible care of others). If a baby with extensive disabilities suddenly gets into difficulty with breathing, either because his tongue has fallen back or he has choked on his food, it would *not* be a significant clinical effort for a doctor or nurse to deal with the situation by, for example, aspirating the material from the back of the mouth. So one would expect them to do so.

The second element calling for comment is the judgement that the likely alleviation to be secured by treatment is 'minimal'. It would not, for example, be futile to relieve through surgery the distress caused to a child by duodenal atresia, because such relief is hardly minimal. However, it can be the case that a baby's disabilities are so extensive that the benefits of surgery would indeed be minimal and would not warrant the burden involved. But in so judging, it must be quite clear to parents and doctors that there is utter disproportion between the procedure proposed and the result to be obtained.

Finally, the judgement that the burdens attendant on treatment are more than a patient can cope with – reason (a) – has extremely limited application in the management of the newborn. Some generalisations about what would be unbearable to anyone are clearly valid. But many inferences made about what will prove unbearable to a newborn are not well founded. There certainly can be no evidence of a kind that would allow one to hypothesise about the distinctive individual sensibilities of neonates. Apart from acknowledging this it is also important to recognise that the perspective of *normal* adult experience is not an acceptable basis for making generalisations about what will be unbearable for a congenitally handicapped child. A doctor who enjoys a very active life may think of confinement to a wheelchair as a quite intolerable prospect and be quite unready to recognise that a child *could* experience it differently. A child who has never known anything different will certainly not have the same experiential starting-point as such a doctor. Residual handicaps, such as permanent colostomies, can be found bearable and become second-nature. Disability may seem far more important to the eye of the beholder than it is in the mind of the patient.

70

4. Uniformity in treatment not to be expected

In conclusion it should be said that it would be a mistake to expect universal or even general agreement, even among doctors who oppose euthanasia and accept all the principles of this Report, about what treatments are indicated for the incompetent and what treatments can be omitted (even with fatal consequences) because they are excessively burdensome or, in the context, futile. In all contexts, the consideration of risks and prospects, and of medical benefits and physical, psychological or other burdens, against the background of the patient's overall condition and prognosis, is a consideration that cannot be expected to yield a single correct answer on which all reasonable, well-informed and upright persons will agree. There are certainly some wrong answers, some wrong because euthanasiast, others wrong because they subordinate consideration of human benefits and burdens to the pursuit of feats of short-term technical mastery. But the fact that some solutions must be rejected does not imply that there is only one acceptable solution or only one acceptable treatment strategy.

Part Four

In this part of the Report we set out to identify and exemplify some basic principles for good management of typical classes of patients for whom euthanasia is seen by some clinicians as an option. Since we think no one is a suitable subject for euthanasia it is important to indicate the proper kinds of care that are or can be made available for these patients.

Chapter 7 considers care of each of the three classes of patients referred to in Chapter 5, sec. 2. There are problems of a general kind arising in each class. Something is said about how doctors and nurses can resolve these problems.

Since collaboration within the clinical team is necessary for consistent care of patients we also identify and discuss in Chapter 7 the significance of shared moral responsibility in the work of multidisciplinary clinical teams.

Then in Chapter 8 we say something about good practice in each of the five fields of care which have engaged our attention.

7

Good Practice: Some Principles

It will be clear from previous chapters that we are concerned with two general elements of clinical responsibility:

– a negative one: there should be no seeking to bring about a patient's death either by action or omission. Seeking to bring about death is, however, to be carefully distinguished from *not* seeking to prolong life;
– a positive one: what should be sought are those benefits appropriate to a patient's condition.

Medicine has a number of ends: not only restoring health and overcoming, where possible, conditions which threaten life, but also alleviating suffering and disability. Medicine has a legitimate interest in the quality of patients' lives. Hence medical care is a continuum, ranging from cure at one end to symptom control or 'comfort care' at the other. It is, therefore, never a matter of 'to treat or not to treat?' but of determining what is the most appropriate form of treatment for each individual patient.

It may, for example, become quite inappropriate to continue striving to overcome a patient's lethal condition because the patient is irretrievably dying (see section *1A* below). Or it may be inappropriate to aim to secure an improvement in function in a handicapped patient because the burden (physical or psychological) of the proposed treatment is not justified by the expected benefit (see Chapter 5 above). Now the goal that *can* be pursued in each specific case has to be settled by those who are party to the case and have some degree of responsibility. Nonetheless, it is possible to say in general terms what kinds of treatment are appropriate to differing types of condition. A doctor will have such generalities in mind in justifying his professional view of what treatment would be appropriate for a particular patient. What follows are generalisations about suitable treatment.

There are two kinds of question which doctors and nurses reading this Report might particularly wish to see answered in clinical terms:

– would it amount to euthanasia to manage a patient in such-and-such a way?
– what would be the appropriate treatment of various types of patient, given the moral principles expounded in this Report?

Clearly we cannot hope to supply answers to all the specific versions of these two questions. But we hope the answers we do give offer a sufficiently concrete picture of good practice. In what follows the two questions that concern us are not treated separately.

1. Three classes of patient.

It was found useful to distinguish in Chapter 5 between three broad classes of patient from each of which there may be patients for whom euthanasia is contemplated:

A: those suffering from a lethal condition for which there are no life-saving treatments;

B: those suffering from a lethal condition for which there are life-saving treatments;

C: those suffering from a non-lethal condition which is painful, distressing or incapacitating (physically or mentally) and for which improvement must remain substantially incomplete.

A. Patients with a lethal condition for which there are no life-saving treatments

(i) The inevitability of death

Apart from those who die suddenly and unexpectedly, everyone reaches a point where biological disintegration sets in and death is in prospect although it may be technically possible to postpone it by a few days or weeks or even months by the use of modern life-support treatments. The inevitability of death is a fact that every doctor needs to recognise as important to the practice of medicine. What is appropriate treatment for an acutely ill patient may be inappropriate for the dying.

(ii) What is normally involved in saying that someone is dying?

If we say someone is dying it is normally the case that there is an identified cause at work in that individual the operation of which is lethal and cannot be reversed so that in all probability his death will be the effect of that cause. It is, however, possible to be fairly sure that someone is dying without being sure of what he is dying from. But this does not alter the fact that the central case in standard use of the word 'dying' presupposes identification of a cause thought to be fatal.

It follows from the above that someone may be said to be dying without it being implied that death is close at hand. Hence it is useful to distinguish between 'pre-terminal' and 'terminal' phases of dying. In the terminal phase vital functions begin clearly to fade and fail. But someone may be said to be already dying (though in the pre-terminal phase) when it becomes clear that death must be accepted as the only real prospect or outcome of that person's present state.

(iii) The importance of knowing that a patient is dying

Recognition that a person is dying is important for a number of reasons. The most important of these, from the viewpoint of the clinician, is that with dying the emphasis in treatment should shift from cure and prolongation of life to comfort and improving the quality of the time that remains. It is clear that the appropriate treatment of those in the terminal phase of dying should emphasise comfort, not attempts to cure. It should be equally clear, but is often overlooked in practice, that comfort-care, not active attempts to cure, is the appropriate treatment for those who, though not in the terminal phase, are already on the way to death.

Many curative and palliative procedures, particularly in relation to cancer, are unpleasant. For example, after each 'pulse' of chemotherapy, a patient may be unwell for several days. This may mean feeling languid and losing one's appetite but, for some, it means severe nausea and vomiting and feeling physically wretched. In this situation the patient accepts that, say, for one week in three, he will be made to feel a lot worse in the hope that cure or relatively long-term palliation will be achieved. Most patients in this category also have to cope with the emotional trauma of hair loss and the use of a wig. Usually, patients are willing to accept the emotional, social and physical burdens of such treatment because of the perceived long-term benefits – improved health and longer survival. However for the person who is quite clearly not responding to treatment (tumour enlarging, blood count worsening, weight loss continuing, etc.), the burdens of treatment exceed any potential gain; a dying person is being made to feel less well without the prospect of a compensatory period of improved health.

The same is true of surgical treatment. All major operations initially cause additional suffering and increased debility, and should not be undertaken simply because of technical feasibility. Doctors are often reluctant to admit that a patient is dying, or that the anti-cancer treatment is ineffective and the patient is almost certainly going to die even if not imminently. As a result, the emphasis in care continues to assume the possibility of cure or long-term palliation to the detriment of the patient's wellbeing. He is denied the opportunity of beginning to adjust to his coming death. Moreover, because the doctor is still thinking in terms of long-term palliation, enough attention is not paid to the relief of pain and other distressing symptoms. In short, because of a failure by the doctor to accept that a patient is dying, the patient (and his family) suffers more than would otherwise be the case as a result of the continued use of burdensome treatments and the non-use or under-use of measures to relieve pain and other symptoms.

iv) Recognising the onset of dying

If certain kinds of treatment are inappropriate to the dying, it is important to recognise the onset of dying.

Consider first the more difficult case of the patient who, though evidently in the early stages of dying, has not got a clearly identifiable terminal illness. Even when uncertainty exists either about the cause and nature of the illness (as, for example, in old people) or about its course (as, for example, in severe respiratory disorders), the doctor may nevertheless reasonably conclude that death is inevitable since the clinical state of the patient shows increasing deterioration for no remediable cause that can be discovered.

A man in his late 50's had been in hospital for 8 years on account of advanced Parkinson's disease. During the last year of his life he lost weight progressively, became generally weaker and spent more time in bed. He was less able to talk clearly and needed increasing help with the basic 'activities of daily living'. During this time he had three attacks of bronchitis. The first two were treated with chest physiotherapy and antibiotics. In anticipation of a further attack, it was decided that the man was in fact dying, albeit slowly, and that the next episode of bronchitis would not be treated with physiotherapy and antibiotics but simply symptomatically on the grounds that curative treatment of the chest infection would, at this stage, be little more than 'resurrecting the man to die again a few weeks later' or 'prescribing a lingering death.' The outcome of a chest infection in these circumstances was quite likely to be the man's death and it was seen as the natural terminal event of the progressive physical deterioration.

With time, therefore, even in less well-defined situations, it is possible for the doctor to conclude reasonably that the patient is dying in the sense that hc is now irreversibly on a road to death.

Every experienced clinician knows, however, that it is extremely difficult, if not impossible, to give a precise prognosis even when there is an identifiably fatal cause at work. Witness the studies which have suggested that doctors tend to overestimate life expectancy in terminal cancer. Yet there is a minority of patients who significantly outlive their initial prognosis, usually only by months, but occasionally by years. It can be the case with others that the diagnosis of terminal cancer was incorrect (there has been a mistaken identification of a causal factor).

Since many decisions in medicine have to be based on probability (predictions of *likely* outcome) some proportion of them will be wrong, so that the possibility of unexpected recovery must not be ignored. Accordingly, except when death is likely within a few hours or days, the treatment prescribed should not bring about a substantial lessening in the potential for improvement. Should improvement unexpectedly occur, it may be sufficient to lead to a re-appraisal of the emphasis in treatment. Occasionally, this will result, for example, in specific anti-cancer treatment being offered to a patient for whom, a few weeks earlier, such treatment seemed inappropriate.

(v) Treatment in the terminal phase

When a person is within a few days of death, his interest in drinking and eating often becomes minimal. This is a situation in which it is wrong to force a patient to accept fluid and food if quite clearly he does not wish it. The lack of interest, or positive disinclination, should be seen as part of the process of 'letting go' which has death as its natural outcome. The traditional theological teaching about 'ordinary' means (see Chapter 5, sec. 3) does not in its application to this extreme situation require any steps to be taken to preserve life. To say this is *not* to make a global judgement that any extra span of life to be lived at that level would be worthless and that the patient would be better off dead; rather it is to make a judgement about particular means for a particular patient, namely that to continue these means would be the imposition on *this* patient of what had now become predominantly a burden.

(vi) Relief of symptoms

Relief of pain is a central part of medical care. To speak of the use of narcotic analgesics (morphine-like drugs) to relieve pain in the dying as 'indirect euthanasia' is to propagate confusion. If the point of giving a drug is precisely to relieve pain (or other distressing symptom), the ending or shortening of life is not one's purpose even if it is sometimes the case that a patient's life is shortened by the use of the drug, and that the probability of this effect is foreseeable; the purpose of relieving pain is frequently sufficient justification for risking or accepting death as a side-effect (see Chapter 3, sec. 8).

It is worth noting that the foreseeability of this consequence is often exaggerated. It is in practice impossible to predict that the next dose of a drug given to relieve pain, for example, will precipitate death. On the other hand, it is possible to say that a certain course of action, such as sedating an agitated, delirious patient will prevent the possibility of a spontaneous improvement in the patient's condition. The patient will probably no longer request or receive food and fluid because he is asleep for much if not all of the time and his weakened condition will become more so. This will make death inevitable and possibly (sometimes almost certainly) come sooner than would otherwise have been the case.

Patients with severe breathlessness represent another group of patients in whom it is possible to say that death may occur sooner if certain steps are taken to reduce the patient's rapid and therefore distressing pattern of respiration. However, even here (and even when making use of the respiratory slowing effect of morphine) it is not possible to say that the next dose or that this course of action will definitely shorten the patients' life. All that is certain is that *there is a risk* that this might turn out to be the case.

Contrary to popular belief, the correct use of morphine in the relief of cancer pain generally carries no greater risk of shortening life than the use of aspirin[1]. Morphine given regularly every four hours by mouth, is a very safe drug provided the patient is not dying from exhaustion as a result of weeks or months of intolerable pain associated with insomnia and poor nutrition. In fact the correct use of morphine is more likely to prolong a patient's life rather than to shorten it, because he is more rested and pain free. It is, of course, possible to use drugs that are generally safe in a dangerous (that is, more risky) way. When the dose of morphine or similar drugs is increased automatically at every administration, or, more commonly, at one or two day intervals, not because the patient remains in pain, is short of breath, or generally distressed but with the (unexpressed) intention of ensuring the patient's death as soon as possible there is clearly euthanasia, even though by instalments. (See Chapter 2, sec. A3.)

The axiom of clinical practice that, even in extreme situations, the least drastic remedy should be employed reflects medicine's respect for the traditional moral principles upheld in this Report. The following example shows how this axiom is applied in the field of terminal care. Many patients develop a number of confusional symptoms during the last few days or

---

[1] R. G. Twycross, 'Ethical and Clinical Aspects of Pain Treatment in Cancer Patients' (1982) 74 *Acta Medica Scandinavica*, 83–90.

weeks of life, notably disorientation with respect to time and, sometimes, place. Misperception of external stimuli are also fairly common and some experience visual and/or auditory hallucinations. With explanation ('Many patients experience this', 'It often happens when someone is very ill', 'It does not mean that you are losing your mind'), most patients accept these disturbances of thought with little or no distress. A few, notably those who have not adjusted to their impending death, react with increasing agitation and, sometimes, with paranoia. It is not always possible to resolve their mental suffering even by skilled psychotherapy and the careful use of psychotropic drugs. When this is the case, it is necessary to ensure that the patient sleeps for one or more periods during the day as well as at night. Reducing the length of the day in this way sometimes leads to an improvement in a patient's mental state. If the distress persists, however, it is important to recognise that the patient almost certainly has an irreversible agitated terminal delirium. In this circumstance it may be necessary to sedate the patient so that he remains asleep until death ensues a few days later. In other words, if the patient's distress is considered to be both intolerable and intractable, even in this extreme situation the least drastic remedy is to render the patient unconscious, not to kill him.

B. Patients with a lethal condition for which life-saving treatments exist

This is not a simple class of conditions, for while life-saving treatment for some of them is unlikely to leave the patient with a substantial defect, life-saving treatment for others is very likely to leave a considerable defect. In the condition known as meconium ileus in the newborn, one can remove the thick contents of the bowel and thereby avert the immediate threat to life, but one cannot cure the underlying condition of mucoviscidosis i.e. of defective glandular secretion into the bowel and the bronchi. The child is likely progressively to develop cystic fibrosis over a number of years.

No one is likely to think an immediately presenting lethal condition which can be cured without substantial defect supplies on its own a reason for euthanasia; one would expect any doctor to institute curative treatment straight away. If, however, a lethal condition is combined with an irremediable condition (lethal or not) or if life-saving treatment, though effective, would leave the patient with a substantial defect, there can arise a temptation to euthanasia by omission. The lethal condition may be exploited as a means of killing the patient; that is, the policy of omission may be deliberately adopted *in order that* he should die, or die sooner. Such a decision may be thought of as made for the sake of the patient, it being judged that he will be better off dead. Or it may be made, or also made, for the sake of others, or for 'society', this life being judged as now meaningless and not worthwhile. We understand as 'euthanasiast', and reject, any policy of seeking the death of the patient, whichever of these reasons is operative.

On the other hand, we must recall again the distinction between aiming at the patient's death and not aiming at a prolongation of his life. (See Chapter

3, sec. 8; Chapter 5, sec. 6.) There is no doubt that if a lethal condition for which life-saving treatment exists (say condition P) is found in conjunction with a lethal condition for which no such treatment exists (say condition Q), and it is the case that Q will bring the patient to a death within weeks regardless of any treatment for P, there is no duty to seek treatment for P. Such treatment would be futile.

In a situation in which a lethal condition can be successfully treated without residual defects, and in the absence of other uncontrollable lethal conditions, the doctor – especially the doctor who is resolved not to practise euthanasia – is faced with an opposite temptation. He may be tempted to forget that a doctor has no responsibility to give a mature person treatment which that person is unwilling to accept, even when that refusal may result in his earlier death. We have already commented on the limits of a doctor's duty in this matter when discussing the rights and duties of competent patients (see Chapter 5, sec. 1.).

C. Patients with a non-lethal but incapacitating condition

We have in mind here all those conditions that more or less severely impair a patient's quality of life. In Chapter 3, sec. 5, we explain the fundamentally important distinction between on the one hand withholding treatment because one does not regard a patient as having a worthwhile life (and we rejected the view that such global assessments of 'quality of life' are either possible or appropriate), and on the other hand withholding treatment because the treatment is of too little benefit relative to the risks or burdens involved, (or even, in the case of a dying competent patient, because it is not worthwhile since the patient's condition is too poor for the proposed treatment to secure what would be experienced as an improvement; see Chapter 5, secs. 5, 6). In regard, however, to the incompetent (as noted in Chapter 6, sec. 3) great care must be observed in judging whether a treatment will be sufficiently beneficial to warrant attendant or consequent burdens; in particular one must take care not to be prejudiced against the possibility of benefiting a given patient.

The tendency to make global quality of life judgements a basis for 'treatment', and the temptation to make euthanasia the goal of that treatment, are most prominent in the care of the newborn. So it is in the section of Chapter 8 devoted to care of the newborn (sec. 1) that readers will find a positive exemplification in clinical terms of what is implied by the moral principles central to this Report.

2. Good team care

More than one kind of expertise is required for the care of the patients considered in this Report. It is common nowadays that those with different types of knowledge and skill consciously co-ordinate their contributions in the context of a clinical team. It is clearly in the interests of patients that this co-ordination should take place.

The concept of the 'multidisciplinary clinical team' first emerged in psychiatry. It is, now well established in care of the elderly – with physicians (geriatricians), nursing staff, occupational therapists, psychotherapists and social workers all working together. It is equally necessary for good terminal care of the kind envisaged in this Report. Though the concept of a multidisciplinary clinical team is perhaps less commonplace in paediatrics, intensive care and care of the handicapped, some degree of co-ordinated implementation of an agreed treatment policy by doctors, nurses and therapists is essential in these fields.

Where persons are jointly carrying out treatment they share responsibility for that treatment. The fact that care is rarely other than a shared responsibility is of considerable significance in the context of this Report. In order to bring out this significance something needs to be said in general terms about the conditions of effective teamwork. They can be stated in the following summary way:

- members of the team should agree about the aims of treatment;
- there should be a clear understanding of the main potential contribution of each member;
- there should be respect for the professional competence and integrity of each member;
- there should be clear leadership by senior medical or, where appropriate, nursing staff;
- the opportunity should exist for questioning the treatment being given or proposed;
- it should be recognised that there will, from time to time, be disagreements as to what is the most appropriate form of treatment;
- it should be recognised that where disagreement or doubt exists then if a team is to operate as such the decision of the doctor in charge must be accepted (or, in more strictly nursing matters, the decision of the senior nurse).[2]

It will be clear from this list of conditions that the team leader has both a central and a delicate role to play, particularly in cases where all team members are to be involved in a regimen in which it is proposed to withhold treatment, and questions may arise about the purpose of doing so. It will also be clear that the list of conditions of teamwork does not cover the question when a member of a team should, on moral grounds, withdraw from collaboration. In relation to the moral constraints on teamwork we confine ourselves here to considering the role of the leader. That role is subject to a fundamental moral constraint.

In Chapter 3 (sec. 6) we observed that there are important limits to moral pluralism and that defence of a pluralism so extensive as to embrace private killing on the grounds that some human beings would be better off dead is incoherent: for the defence of pluralism must appeal to a valuation of human

[2] This brief characterisation of teamwork relies quite closely on Ivor Batchelor and Jean McFarlane, *Multidisciplinary Clinical Teams* (King's Fund Project Paper RC12, London 1980).

life which cannot be held consistently with such killing. Accordingly we argue that simple justice in the treatment of fellow human beings must constrain a team leader whatever his or her personal inclinations in the matter of euthanasia. If a whole team is inclined to concur and cooperate in practices which amount to euthanasia, then the arguments of Chapter 3 are addressed to them all. It is unlikely, however, that a team leader who judges euthanasia to be desirable will at the outset secure the ready concurrence of all members of a team. If, however, he were to succeed, in face of some dissent, in making euthanasia a 'management' option in team care, it could only be with one or a number of the following consequences:

- refusal to respect the professional integrity of other members of the team; in this kind of case the persons dissenting may fairly claim to be upholding precisely those values which have inspired the health care professions and been central to their traditional ethic;
- the effective exclusion of dissenters from those areas of care in which such a policy option is systematic[3];
- the corruption of attitude and disposition which overtakes those who acquiesce or co-operate in practices incompatible with reverence for human life: since this reverence has been central to the ethics of clinical practice the loss of it in practitioners will corrupt that practice.

The respect that a team leader should show for professional colleagues ought to preclude his pressing a policy of euthanasia.

Good leadership and good teamwork are not technical accomplishments which might be exhibited in the pursuit of just any objectives. People's minds and hearts need to be engaged by purposes consistent with human dignity. A good team leader will facilitate collaboration in the realisation of such purposes. In striving to do this the leader will be sensitive to the need to avoid whatever is calculated to undermine human dignity.

[3] There is reason to believe that exclusion of the kind we have in mind has occurred in the field of obstetrics and gynaecology. For one personal testimony see R. Walley, 'A Question of Conscience', (1976) *British Medical Journal* i, 1456–58.

8

Good Practice in Specialised Fields of Care

In this penultimate chapter we look at the implications for good practice, in five specialised fields, of the principles examined in this Report. The specialities are those reviewed in Chapter 2; specialities in which one might anticipate some practice of euthanasia since it is not difficult to see how the temptation might arise to view some patients as not having or no longer having worthwhile lives. It seems clear that in paediatrics at least clinicians very often take this view of their patients and believe themselves justified in killing some babies either on the ground that they are benefiting the child, or on the ground that they are securing the best state of affairs for the family or society.

We do not believe it is possible to make comprehensive judgements on the value of any human life or to quantify that value on some calculus of contributions to human welfare. Our support for the reverence due to every human life demands, in the context of this Report, detailed comment on the clinical care we take to be consonant with our stance.

(1) Care of the Newborn

The newborn are necessarily incompetent patients. The general standard to be observed in the treatment of the incompetent was stated in Chapter 6: that they should be given whatever treatment is beneficial, having regard to acceptable costs in terms of expense and burden. The criteria for acceptable costs should not be different from those applied in the treatment of the competent.

We also observed that in assessing likely burdens it is not possible to hypothesise about the individual sensibility of a baby and that it is particularly misleading to view the prospects for such a patient, especially if handicapped, from the standpoint of adult normality.

In general if a specific treatment is to be withheld from a baby it should be because it is clear that there is an utter disproportion between the burdens caused by the treatment and the anticipated result. It may not be clear at the time of starting treatment how much benefit can be secured for the child and what the attendant burdens or residual disabilities might be. If the response to treatment is not good, and it is thought to be excessively burdensome to the child, that the chances of success are extremely limited, and the foreseeable relief would in any case be slight, there will come a time when the doctor has to decide whether to continue this particular line of treatment. He will be influenced by:

a) the degree of relief from suffering and improvement in the condition to be expected from successful treatment;
b) the chances of achieving that success;
c) the burden to the patient in doing so.

a) Conditions which are lethal and for which there is no life-saving treatment

If a baby is dying from one of these conditions, or is irretrievably on the way to a rapid death within a matter of days or a week or two, the child will be given ordinary nursing care and symptoms will be treated as they arise. If, for example, a baby has sustained some intra-cranial damage, possibly from haemorrhage, there may be muscular spasms or fits which require treatment by sedatives; similarly in the rare examples where a baby presents visible signs of pain, drugs may be given which are specifically pain-relieving. However, it is important to draw a distinction between this type of symptomatic treatment and a sedative regimen intended to bring about the early death of the child by dehydration and starvation. Even during this very short span of life, if the baby were to show symptoms of choking it would be reasonable to take simple steps to stop this – for example, obstructive material in the air-way may be sucked out, since choking would cause the baby distress. However, it would not be justifiable to impose upon a baby a major operative procedure in the hope that the baby might survive a few days longer; for example, some babies are known to have an extremely short life span due to chromosomal abnormalities, possibly a week or two; occasionally it will happen that one of these babies might have in addition oesophageal atresia, a condition in which no food can pass to the stomach and which is likely to be fatal in one to three weeks if not treated. There is no point in undertaking the difficult operative procedure for oesophageal atresia if, in fact, it is unlikely to extend the baby's life significantly.

b) Conditions which are lethal and for which life-saving treatment exists

In the uncomplicated condition where there are not likely to be any residual disabilities or defects, no one has any doubt about the importance of advising treatment. However, some lethal conditions which can be treated may be accompanied by other serious disabilities and the question arises whether these disabilities can be so severe as to be a contra-indication to saving the baby's life by operation. One example, referred to earlier, is the condition of meconium ileus, in which there is obstruction of the bowel of a new-born baby by extremely thick contents. It is possible to operate on the bowel with perhaps a 70% chance of success. However, the obstruction of the bowel is part of the more widespread disease in which it is not only the glands in the intestine which are abnormal – resulting in thick intestinal contents – but also the glands of the respiratory tract, resulting in repeated attacks of pneumonia, so that in past years very few children so affected reached their twenties. The outlook for these chest complications is now considerably better and in between the attacks the children can be involved in ordinary family life. In cases of this sort we would not think there is any justification for withholding operation in the new-born period because of the likelihood of frequent bouts of pneumonia. With some of these babies operation may not be necessary since the intestinal obstruction can be relieved sometimes by special enemas.

Another important condition in which the justification for immediate operation has been questioned is obstruction of the duodenum, the part of the bowel just beyond the stomach. About one third of the babies with this condition also have Down's syndrome (mongolism). In addition to the unusual appearance of the face, these children are nearly always mentally retarded, mostly to a moderate degree but in a small proportion of cases very severely. It must have happened many times that operation to relieve the intestinal obstruction is withheld in order that the child should die, simply because there is a likelihood of moderate or severe mental retardation. It is easy to see that such babies may well be a considerable additional burden on the families and also on the community, but there is no case for claiming any advantage *to the baby* in withholding operation so that he might die. It should not be forgotten that a baby with intestinal obstruction has distressing symptoms of repeated vomiting. If not relieved the vomiting will persist for perhaps two to four weeks, with increasing hunger and thirst until the baby dies.

As well as giving the baby a chance of surviving one should also make sure that he has the opportunity to develop his capacities to the maximum. These children certainly are able to appreciate a proportion of the values of this life, and are often happy. Moreover, in recent years it has been found that although their level of attainment tends to diverge more and more from the normal with growth, this divergence may be considerably reduced or modified by appropriate stimulation.

c) Conditions which are not lethal in themselves, but are associated with severe disability

The most widely known example of this type of condition is open spina bifida, in which there is swelling on the back at birth with the nerves of the spinal cord lying exposed on the surface. The alternative methods of management of this condition are generally described as operation or allowing the baby to die, yet a brief consideration of the purpose of operation will reveal that this antithesis is unsound.

We must consider several different grades of severity.

i) There are a small number of babies in whom death is likely to occur in a matter of days or a week or two, babies in whom there is severe hydrocephalus complicated by haemorrhage into the ventricles or babies with spina bifida and also severe congenital heart disease. An immediate operation on the swelling on the back of the baby would have no influence at all on whether the baby lived or died, and could not be justified. Such babies should be given ordinary nursing care and any symptoms given appropriate treatment.

ii) Babies in whom there is little evidence that they are likely to die in a matter of days or a week or two, but in whom the swelling on the back is extremely large or associated with a considerable bony deformity of the spine. Any attempt to operate on the back and close the defect in the skin probably has little chance of success. Wound breakdown may occur and the resulting infection could well be worse than if the open wound were left and simply covered by appropriate sterile dressings.

iii) The third group of cases is those babies who do not seem to be in imminent danger of death and in whom the surgeon thinks there is a good chance of operation on the back leading to sound healing of the wound. Amongst these babies will be some who have been seen to be kicking their legs after birth. Almost all paediatricians and surgeons would agree that there is an urgent need for operation on the back to cover the exposed nerves with the purpose of preserving good function in the lower limbs.

At the opposite extreme, there are other babies in whom no movement of the lower limbs has been seen at all since birth. Operation on the back will have no influence at all on the function of the legs, and it is possible to manage these babies by putting simple protective dressings on the back, as was the practice 30 years ago. In many children the skin grew over the open wound, but it was a considerable burden to mothers to care for this swelling on the back as well as looking after the handicapped baby. Although such conservative treatment is an acceptable method of management, the presence of this large swelling on the baby's back is an additional and unnecessary burden on the mother, since the swelling can be removed in the new-born period just as easily as at one or two years of age.

Between these two extremes of activity and inactivity in the lower limbs at birth, there are some babies who will show evidence of activity in the muscles which flex the hips and extend the knees. There are some paediatricians and surgeons who believe that there is a case for operating on these babies in the hope of preserving this activity, so that when the baby grows up there will be more active muscles which the orthopaedic surgeon can use in improving function. On the other hand there are those who would not recommend operation because they believe that conservative treatment does not, in fact, lead to loss of function of active muscles, and consequently for these babies conservative treatment (that is to say simple dressing of the wound) is a perfectly legitimate option.

It is good practice in the care of spina bifida babies, whether they have had a neonatal operation or not, to ensure that as the baby grows he receives the care and attention that any other baby would be expected to receive. The responsible physician would ensure that the baby receives appropriate treatment for problems related to the kidneys and bladder, for any excessive accumulation of fluid within the brain (hydrocephalus) and also for any problems of the legs, with which an orthopaedic surgeon will be able to help.

It is clear that immediate surgery for open spina bifida in new-born babies is not concerned with saving the baby's life, but for the most part with preserving and improving function. If it is the case nowadays that babies operated on are more likely to live than those not operated on, this is not precisely because of the operation. Operation is, itself, evidence of a commitment to improve the child's quality of life, a commitment that also ensures normal standards of medical and nursing care for the child. It is mainly because some children enjoy that good, general care (to which any baby is entitled) that they live. Many who die do so because they are systematically and deliberately deprived of that care.

(2) Care of the Handicapped

The term 'handicap' is applied to people with a wide range of conditions, from those with full mental capacity but almost no physical independence e.g. the quadriplegic who can only move the head, or even less than that, to those with considerable mobility and strength, but who lack the mental ability to co-ordinate and control this for their benefit. There are also those who are almost totally immobile as well as giving little human response to others. Good practice must be considered in relation both to such chronic conditions and also to supervening acute illness.

As regards chronic conditions it is useful to have in mind more precise definitions of the problems of those who cannot function in everyday life as most people can: *impairment* – a defect in the normal structure or function of the body; *disability* – the loss of the functional ability and activity which results from impairment; and *handicap* – the disadvantages the individual suffers because he cannot function normally and carry out the normal activities of daily living[1]. These distinctions are important because it may be impossible to do anything to remedy the impaired state, but quite possible to change the degree of disability and/or handicap. There are a number of people[2] who have lived with severe disability and yet have gained and given to others a great deal in their lives. Treatment must therefore be directed to maximising the impaired person's capacity to live rather than just survive. Careful assessment of abilities and disabilities must be made in order to provide help when required and to enhance independence where possible, if necessary with mechanical aids.

In the planning of care and treatment nurses and others having day-to-day care of handicapped people have an important contribution to make. It does not seem to be the degree of mental or physical impairment which matters

[1] World Health Organisation, *International Classification of Impairments, Disabilities, and Handicaps* (Geneva: WHO) 1980, p.11.
[2] See, for example, J Earekson, *Joni* (London – Glasgow: Pickering & Inglis) 1976; D Clarke Wilson, *Hilary. The Brave World of Hilary Pole* (London– Sydney: Hodder & Stoughton) 1972.

most, but what use is made of what remains, the development of potential, and in particular potential for relationships with others. Perhaps more than physical distress it seems to be hopelessness or a sense of worthlessness which produces a demand for euthanasia. Hopelessness is particularly likely to affect the families of children (or adults) with mental as well as physical impairment. Often much can be done by hospital or district nurses, health visitors, or other services to provide the practical and psychological support that is so much needed by families caring for a severely disabled person, if they are to avoid feelings of helplessness, hopelessness and continuous exhaustion. The amount and quality of support provided for the family may play a considerable part in determining not only the quality of the disabled person's life, but also whether there are thoughts (expressed or unexpressed) of euthanasia.

In illness the principles of treatment for a pathological condition in a handicapped person must be the same as for any other persons. In particular, it is important to establish without prejudice whether treatment offers benefits which are not rendered insignificant by attendant burdens. Often survival is not dependent just on intervention or non-intervention by doctors, but also on the action or non-action of other health-care workers and possibly the family too. If a severely handicapped person has a chest infection then antibiotics may make less difference to survival than changing the patient's position, clearing the chest of secretions by various means, or devoting extra time and effort to feeding. It is as possible to bring about death by omitting these things as by giving a lethal dose of a drug. It is the people who spend long periods performing such activities, rather than doctors who see the patient quite briefly, who are likely to experience the acutest dilemmas over the worthwhileness of their efforts, especially if they find them distressing to the patient. Hence decisions about appropriate care and treatment may well need to include consultations with all the professional health-care staff involved as well as the patient (if possible) and the family.

Some treatment may inevitably cause extra suffering to some whose limited intelligence does not allow them to understand either the treatment or the need for it. Or the benefits to be expected from a particular course of action may be limited by mental or physical impairment, and thus some treatment, though usually appropriate for a particular pathological condition, may be inappropriate for an individual with that condition. In the case of some patients it may be inappropriate to go so far as to administer artificially (e.g. by intragastric tube or intravenously) the basic life sustaining elements of food and drink which one should always offer.

If euthanasia is to be excluded for any human being, strenuous efforts should be made to ensure that those who have to care for a handicapped person should, however great the impairment, be encouraged and supported in securing as full a life as possible for that person.

(3) Terminal Care

A terminal illness may be defined as a progressive incurable disease in which the prognosis (life expectancy) is relatively limited. In relation to cancer, it can be thought of as the period after specific anti-cancer treatment has been stopped. The emphasis in care moves from both prolongation of life *and* comfort to just comfort, that is, the relief of symptoms. Commonly, there is a period of transition rather than an abrupt change of direction in management. In practice, a terminal illness may last from a few weeks to several months and, on occasions, to one or two years. Survival beyond 6–9 months is, however, unusual. The term 'terminal care' is perhaps best reserved for the care given in the terminal phase of a terminal illness – the time when a patient is more obviously deteriorating physically and, generally, is requiring an increasing amount of support from family or friends, and the caring professions.

The dying cancer patient exemplifies many of the problems and dilemmas that doctors and nurses face in terminal care. About two-thirds of patients with far-advanced cancer experience severe pain; one third suffer with shortness of breath, and many are troubled by a variety of alimentary symptoms.

It is sometimes claimed (see Chapter 2, sec. B5) that the sequelae of pain control are themselves often undesirable. Hospice doctors dispute this, though they emphasise the need for careful monitoring of treatment in order to prevent complications such as nausea, vomiting and constipation. That hospice care can be dramatically effective in this respect is shown by the following extract from a patient's letter to a TV producer following a programme on euthanasia:

'My cancer was diagnosed in November 1979 and my health deteriorated rapidly thereafter. By January of this year I was bedbound by pain and weakness, having been able to drink only water for six weeks. My wife had been told by our family doctor that I "would die a painful death within three months". I felt desperate, isolated and frightened and at that time I truly wished that euthanasia could have been administered. I now know that only my death is inevitable and since coming under the care of the Macmillan Service my pain has been relieved completely, my ability to enjoy life restored and my fears of an agonising end allayed. As you can see, I'm still alive today. My weight and strength have increased since treatment made it possible to eat normally and I feel that I'm living a full life, worth living. My wife and I have come to accept that I'm dying and we can now discuss it openly between ourselves and with the staff of the Macmillan Service, which does much to ease our anxieties. My experiences have served to convince me that euthanasia, even if voluntary, is fundamentally wrong and I'm now staunchly against it on religious, moral, intellectual and spiritual grounds. My wife's views have changed similarly. I'm no longer in such misery that her love for me would make her want me to be dead. And after I've gone she will not have to fear the burden of guilt which would have been upon her had she wished for my early death'.[3]

Good terminal care extends far beyond the relief of pain and of other symptoms. It includes supporting the patient during the adjustment to increasing physical disability and through periods of 'anticipatory mourning' for the loss of family and friends, and of one's hopes for the future. It

[3] S Cohen, in *Macmillan Service, 5th Report* (London: St Joseph's Hospice) 1980, p.5.

also includes supporting the family as they adjust to the fact that their loved one is dying.

Much mental suffering is caused by 'depersonalisation' of the dying patient. The tendency to withdraw from a dying person is natural but must be resisted. This may happen even at home but happens more easily in a busy hospital ward. The patient, dying in the corner bed largely ignored, not participating in the usual traffic of discussion, investigation and treatment, concludes that he is no longer of any consequence. Resentment and bitterness may increase his suffering and worsen his condition.

The first requirement of good terminal care is that the dying patient should be treated as a person. Frequent visits by the doctor(s) responsible for care must be maintained. In addition, the patient should be brought into the discussion of his problems as other patients are. Secondly, treatment that serves simply to prolong the process and distress of dying must be avoided. The primary aim is no longer to extend life but to make the life that remains as comfortable and as meaningful as possible. Treatments that are appropriate for acutely ill patients may be completely inappropriate for the dying. Cardiac resuscitation, artificial respiration, intravenous infusions, nasogastric tubes and antibiotics are all primarily for use in acute (or acute-on-chronic) illnesses in order to assist the patient through a period of crisis towards recovery. Their use, without careful consideration of the intended purpose of that use, in the care of those approaching death is poor medical care. On the other hand particular types of treatment should not be classified rigidly as measures for cure, palliation or comfort. Treatments such as radiotherapy, chemotherapy, and even surgical procedures can contribute to any one of these purposes and, in specific instances, their use to alleviate will be appropriate even though cure is not possible.

(4) Care of the Elderly

Much of what has been written elsewhere in this chapter about the dying patient or the patient on the way to death is also applicable to the care of the elderly. There is however a general sense that for the old death is an expected event; with increasing age death comes nearer, in most people health deteriorates after the age of 75 and problems multiply; the old and particularly the very old are at risk at any time.

Until comparatively recently old people were often housed in institutions to wait for death. Detailed assessment of the problems of the elderly and active rehabilitation and energetic management are recent developments in medicine. The modern geriatric unit seeks to keep people active, mobile and enjoying as much independence as is compatible with good care; as far as possible patients are managed in their homes.

Some of those concerned with the care of the elderly may assess too optimistically the benefits of active treatment in individual cases; some without experience of what modern geriatric care can achieve may underrate the capacity of the elderly to survive and recover. Age alone should not determine what the doctor ought or ought not to do. The physical and mental capacity of elderly people varies greatly; some are in a better state at 85 than others at 65. Those who have reached an advanced age have demonstrated an unusual capacity for survival and their expectation of a reasonable life may be little less than that of others ten years younger.

Thus no general rule of management based on age alone is possible. The whole of the circumstances must be taken into account in individual cases. It may be right, in exceptional circumstances, to deploy a wide range of medical interventions. Surgical operations should not be ruled out if the benefit seems worth having; it is a poor sort of kindness to keep people in bed on pain-relieving drugs if relatively straightforward surgery can both relieve pain and even restore some measure of mobility. For those with cancer, for example, treatment with radiotherapy and cytotoxic drugs are as little likely to be of value in achieving cure at this age as at any other, but may be of use in alleviating symptoms or in averting a serious risk, for example, of ulceration and consequent haemorrhages that would distress the patient.

The clinician has to be realistic about the benefits to be expected from his treatment. He should bear in mind not only that death is inevitable and near but also that certain concomitants of old age make his task more complicated. Old people react unfavourably to certain drugs, are more likely to suffer from multiple problems and have more difficulty in following a regime because of forgetfulness, diminished vision or hearing or poor locomotive control. Failing mental faculties present particular difficulties, diminishing the patient's ability to co-operate with treatment or express his wishes and affecting the range of possible interventions. In these circumstances however the doctor must not too readily conclude that all is lost. He must be alert to detect depression masquerading as dementia, for the former may be remediable. Moreover the natural history of certain disease processes is different in the elderly. Cancer, for example, may be less serious than in younger people and less relentlessly progressive.

The decision to give or not give specific treatment therefore depends on an assessment of the whole of the circumstances of the patient bearing in mind that the elderly could be said to be on the way to death. When the patient is able and willing to express his own wishes they should be respected. The doctor must exercise gentleness in persuading patients of the course he thinks they should pursue; he must give information, listen and assess what his patient says in the light of his behaviour; what people say may be less informative than what they do – those who express a desire to die may for example manifest, by their eagerness to eat, a contrary view.

While it would be wrong not to offer treatment that has a good chance of benefiting the patient, it is equally wrong to force treatment on someone whose hold on life is loosening. There is little difficulty in making such a decision if the patient is clearly dying. It is less easy not to intervene when the patient has not yet reached that stage. When the patient's grip on life seems to be weakening, and particularly if there is no clear reason for the steady downhill course, it is hard to know just when to cease to try. The process of fading away is a natural one and the old must be allowed to let go of life. Loss of interest, loss of appetite, loss of desire even to drink may be a sign that that stage has been reached. It may then be justifiable not to add to the patient's burdens or to prolong the process of dying by treating conditions that are an expected part of that process such as basal pneumonia. It may also be justifiable not to distress him or her by forcing them to take nourishment or fluids.

In no field of medicine is it more important for the doctor to know his patient; management is eased if he has a long acquaintance with him and has his confidence. Nowhere is there a greater need for fine clinical judgement, nowhere less place for rules of thumb. The greatest need is that the old should be cared for in a place where death is not a shameful affair.

(5) Intensive Care

Most patients entering intensive care units get better, and of the remainder some die rapidly, despite being subject to the most sophisticated available treatment. From time to time, however, it happens that patients originally accepted for treatment in the belief that they would recover are subsequently shown to be in a hopeless condition i.e. to be dying in a lingering fashion. There is also a distinct group who have suffered so-called 'brain-death'.

Each of these last two categories of patient raises problems. In the case of those dying a lingering death, questions arise about what is good practice in the treatment of these patients. In the case of those diagnosed as 'brain dead', some of whom are treated as cadaveric donors for transplantation purposes, the question arises as to whether they are truly dead. Though we diverge in our views on the reasons which lead to this conclusion, the members of the Working Party are agreed that someone with *total* and irreversible loss of brain function is dead. Given our agreement that such 'patients' are truly dead we comment briefly on the practice of transplantation from 'brain dead' donors.

a) Dying patients

If patients whose prognosis has become hopeless are being treated, for example, with artificial pulmonary ventilation, such treatment is merely further prolonging the process of dying. Usually, in fact, the treatment that is slowing the progress towards death is complex, and involves varied and continuously changing procedures and devices over and above the artificial pulmonary ventilation. As time goes on, additional forms of therapy become necessary to meet new contingencies; for example, a patient originally accepted for treatment of severe peritonitis may develop kidney failure, tendencies to bleed and so on.

93

When the patient's physical condition has become hopeless it is often appropriate, depending on the type of case, either to withdraw some of the treatment already instituted or, without stopping existing treatment, to cease instituting treatments for new disorders as they arise. Thus, depending on the case, it may be right, for example, to discontinue an infusion of cardiac stimulants, or to allow, say, renal failure, supervening on an already hopeless condition, to take its course without treating it.

It may also be right to discontinue artificial pulmonary ventilation. It should be clear from our discussion of general principles that switching off a pulmonary ventilator when the patient is still alive is not always morally wrong. When a patient's condition is hopeless, the use of the machine is futile since it can only be described as merely prolonging the process of dying. This decision is, of course, a very grave one and should only be taken after adequate consultation.

When the machine is switched off, an attempt is made to re-establish the patient's spontaneous breathing. If this attempt is unsuccessful, ventilator treatment is not resumed and the patient is allowed to die. The illness, whatever it may be, has taken its course, and the patient has succumbed to it.

The obvious relationship between 'turning off' and the patient's death may give the impression of a deliberate act of taking life. It is incumbent therefore, on the physician sensitively to ensure that those concerned understand the nature of the problem and the principles behind its solution: the purpose is to terminate, not the life of the patient, but only a futile and onerous procedure. If the patient were, unexpectedly, to start breathing for himself, no steps would be taken to bring about his death.

b) Transplantation and the 'brain dead' donor

In agreeing that total loss of brain function is an adequate basis for declaring someone dead we also accept that it is possible to diagnose such total loss of brain function. This diagnosis is a medical matter and it is very important that it should be based on certain knowledge. We have not undertaken as a committee to reach an agreed view on which tests are adequate for this diagnosis, since this seems to us to be a matter to be settled by those with the required expertise. The general public, however, is rightly concerned with the degree of certainty required before the diagnosis is made.

When brain death has been satisfactorily diagnosed and organ transplantation is contemplated it is usual to stop artificial ventilation of the lungs and wait till the heart has stopped before organs are removed. It can be, and has been, argued that organs such as the kidney may be removed from the brain dead patient before the ventilator is stopped ('the heart-beating donor') as the patient is already truly dead, even though there is still a circulation. There is no moral objection to this procedure, if it can be shown beyond all doubt that brain death has taken place.

94

9

Conclusion

In concluding our Report we do not attempt to summarise it but rather to emphasise some of the salient points arising from it which are particularly relevant to contemporary discussions.

1. We have identified a feature crucial to justifications of euthanasia, voluntary as well as involuntary: the claim that the condition of the person to be killed is so lacking in worth that to die is either a benefit for him or (when the intended beneficiaries are others) at least no loss.

2. Against this claim we have argued that nobody can pass comprehensive judgements on the value of another human being's life. Men are not like the other animals: they are spirit as well as flesh. Their lives are sustained by the power of God and at his will and, being spirit, a man can either consent to or rebel against that will. The contest between good and evil in a man's life is a mystery not open to human judgement. So the value of any part of that life cannot be known by others.

   This valuation of human life is clearly religious. Though it is profoundly illumined by the revelation summed up in Christ, some religious sense of the mystery of human life is quite accessible to anyone. A basically religious valuation of human life underpins our homicide laws and has hitherto preserved us.

3. What presume to be comprehensive judgements on the worthwhileness of human lives are being invoked with increasing explicitness in order to justify management of patients amounting to euthanasia. Evidence for this is strongest in the field of paediatrics.

4. Euthanasia in paediatrics is principally by omission: by omission of life-saving operations (as with Down's syndrome babies born with duodenal atresia) or by omission of feeding (as with spina bifida babies). These children are judged not to have worthwhile lives and precisely for that reason their deaths are sought after. What is happening under the description 'benign neglect' (or 'custodial management') is the evil of murder. To admit the justification some clinicians and some parents invoke for neglect would strike radically at the foundation of respect for human life in our society.

5. Opposition to intentional killing of the innocent (whether by action or omission) does not commit one to never omitting treatment, even when it is life-saving. There is an important distinction between aiming to bring about someone's death and not aiming to prolong that person's life.

There can be good reasons for ceasing to strive to prolong a person's life. It is mere caricature to say that those who uphold the sanctity of life require that one should always preserve and prolong life as far as possible.

6. We have sought to identify those sorts of omission (or refusal) of treatment which are justifiable for a competent patient. In short these are omissions in circumstances in which

   - the burdens attendant on treatment are more than a patient can be expected to bear;
   - the burdens attendant on treatment are too great to be warranted by the expected benefits of treatment;
   - life-saving treatment, in the case of a dying patient, does not seem worthwhile since the patient has reason to think he no longer has any obligation to seek to prolong his life; or
   - treatment would be manifestly futile.

   Judgements about burdens are to a significant degree dependent on the disposition and sensibility of the individual patient.

7. The same basic standard in the provision of treatment should apply in cases of the incompetent as applies in cases of the competent: they should be given whatever treatment is beneficial, having regard to acceptable costs in terms of expense and burden.

8. In estimating what treatment might be unacceptably burdensome to or not worthwhile for the incompetent one must proceed with caution and with a desire to give whatever may be owing in justice to these patients. The question about worthwhileness should never be a question about the worthwhileness of the patient's life but only about the worthwhileness of the treatment (though in judging that one must clearly take account of the patient's condition).

   Judgement of the burdensomeness of treatment in cases of the incompetent can rely variously on

   - the earlier considered choice of a once competent patient;
   - in the case of a patient who has always been incompetent: reliable testimony to his individual dispositions from those who have lived close to him.

9. In the case of the newborn it is not possible to make distinctive judgements on the individual dispositions of a child and it is important to beware of the dangers of interpreting their prospective life-experience or disability from the perspective of adult normality. Omission of treatment on the grounds that it is too burdensome requires sober judgement that the burden (*consequent upon* treatment) is significantly excessive relative to the objective benefit to the child. In making this judgement the continued existence of the child is not itself to be counted as a burden.

10. We have sought to indicate in some detail what typically is required by way of good practice in the care of those patients for whom some think

euthanasia a preferable option. What we have written should be read as accounts of the *kind* of practice we take to be consistent with an authentic recognition of the dignity of every patient. The fact that some 'solutions' to the problems of care must be rejected does not imply that there is only one acceptable solution or only one acceptable treatment strategy for a given problem.

11. We hope that the indications we have given of the directions good practice can take will lead many to realise that there are positive alternatives to euthanasia; alternatives which as individuals we should want to support and for which as a society we urgently need to provide resources. For what is at stake is the dignity of man.

Glossary of some Medical Terms used in the Report

analgesic: a substance which modifies the perception of pain or the reaction to pain without causing loss of consciousness.

aphasia: inability to express oneself properly through speech, or loss of comprehension of language.

arteriosclerosis/atherosclerosis: narrowing of the medium and large arteries, with ulceration and formation of blood clots, leading to progressive damage of the tissues served by the diseased arteries.

basal pneumonia: infection, initially in the base of the lungs, secondary to the pooling of secretions, in a debilitated person no longer able to expectorate.

bilateral anophthalmia: congenital absence of both eyes.

bromide: hypnotic drug (q.v.).

chemotheraphy: literally a general term for the treatment of disease by means of chemical substances or drugs. Now usually limited to the treatment of cancer by chemical substances.

chloral, chloral hydrate: hypnotic drug (q.v.).

chronic brain syndrome: impairment of brain function, generally irreversible, and of insidious onset; formerly called 'dementia'.

colostomy: a surgical operation designed to provide a substitute for the natural opening of the rectum: a portion of the large intestine (colon) is brought through the muscle onto the skin of the abdomen; its opening acts as an artificial anus. A bag is worn to cover the opening and collect faeces.

cytotoxic drugs: drugs that suppress reproduction of cells. Among other uses, are employed to suppress the rapidly growing cells of certain types of cancer (see: chemotherapy).

Down's syndrome: a congenital defect of physical and mental development. The children have 47 instead of the normal 46 chromosomes. Physical characteristics include flattish, round face and a fold of skin over the inner corner of the eye, resulting in alleged similarity of appearance to Mongolians (hence 'mongol'). More significant is the existence of mental retardation, varying from severe to mild. If effort is concentrated early in the life of the child it is possible to improve mental ability to some degree.

duodenal atresia: the duodenum is the portion of the small intestine immediately beyond the stomach; if the channel running through it fails to open completely during development, that is duodenal atresia and no food can then pass to the rest of the intestine.

extrophy of the bladder: condition at birth in which the abdominal wall has failed to close in its lowest part and the bladder protrudes through it; the bladder itself remains open, so that its inside red lining can be seen.

hydrocephalus: condition in which cerebro-spinal fluid is being produced in excess of the baby's ability to reabsorb it into the blood-stream so that it accumulates in the ventricles of the brain. Occurs frequently with myelomeningocele, the most serious form of spina bifida (q.v.). Unless controlled by surgery i.e. by the insertion of a valve draining off excess fluid (usually into the vascular system), it will cause in the majority of cases rapid headgrowth, increased pressure on the brain and consequent damage to it. In some cases it can be controlled by drugs, and sometimes it arrests spontaneously.

hypnotic drugs: drugs used to induce sleep. They act by depressing brain function. They are not primarily for controlling pain, and so would not be used if sleeplessness was caused by pain. Some hypnotics when used in smaller dose are effective daytime sedatives.

meconium ileus: intestinal obstruction due to the contents of the intestine at birth (meconium = greenish black faeces of the newborn) being abnormally thick and viscid. It is due to defective production of mucus by the glands of the intestine and is almost always associated with a similar abnormality of the glands in the bronchi of the lungs. The total picture is often called mucoviscidosis (q.v.).

morphine: the main active principle of opium, highly effective in suppressing pain. Large doses depress the whole brain and especially the centres controlling respiration and circulation and can therefore in overdosage be fatal. Also useful as a cough sedative.

mucoviscidosis: otherwise known as cystic fibrosis. It is an hereditary defect of the glands of the bronchi, the pancreas and the intestine and also of the sweat glands – in fact sweat is often used to confirm its presence. Since the first pathological abnormality to be discovered was formation of abnormal fibrous tissue (fibrosis) and cysts in the pancreas, the name cystic fibrosis has been used when meconium ileus (q.v.) was absent. Among symptoms are severe digestive disorders, breathing difficulties and lung infections caused by thick mucus obstructing air-flow to the outer parts of the lungs. Nowadays it is possible to control the symptoms and many of those suffering from the condition can be helped to live to adult life.

myeloblastic monocytic leukaemia: a form of acute leukaemia i.e. a disorder of the bone marrow in which large numbers of abnormal white blood cells are produced with a corresponding reduction in the production of red cells and platelets, so that a patient becomes anaemic, and the blood does not clot properly.

myocardial infarction: death of part of the heart muscle, due to shortage of blood supply to it. The shortage may be due to a blood clot (coronary thrombosis) or to a severe narrowing of the artery.

narcotic: a morphine (q.v.) or codine related analgesic (q.v.).

oesophageal atresia: the oesophagus or gullet leads from the back of the throat to the stomach. If that channel is obstructed by imperfect development there is oesophageal atresia. No food or drink can enter the stomach.

organic brain syndrome: phrase referring to a group of psychiatric disorders caused by or associated with brain damage or impairment of brain function.

palliative care: used in this Report to mean the modification of the pathological process by treatment in order to delay the inevitable consequences of that process.

psychotropic drug: drugs used to modify or alter mood and experience.

rubella syndrome: the range of defective developments that may occur in a child if the mother contracts German measles early in pregnancy. When this occurs some 40% of babies are affected and among serious defects are deafness, blindness and disorders of the heart, lungs, nervous system and other organs.

spina bifida: in this Report the reference is to 'spina bifida cystica' in its more common and serious form, myelomeningocele. All forms of spina bifida result from the fact that the bones of the spinal column (vertebrae) have failed to fuse in some part of its length. There is a visible 'cystic sac' when the membrane (meninges) covering the spinal cord protrudes through the gap in the vertebrae. When the spinal cord itself also protrudes through the cystic sac there is myelomeningocele. In this condition a child suffers some degree of paralysis to legs, bladder or bowels. The severity of the handicap depends on the position of the defect and on the number of vertebrae involved. The greater number of children suffering from myelomeningocele will develop hydrochephalus (q.v.).

Works Cited

American Law Institute, *Model Penal Code*. Tentative Draft No. 8 (Philadelphia) 1958; definitive edition, 1980.

Anon., 'Non-treatment of Defective Newborn Babies' (1979) *Lancet* ii, 1123–4.

Anselm, St., *De Casu Diaboli* in *S. Anselmi Opera Omnia* vol. 1, ed. F S Schmitt (Edinburgh: Nelson) 1946.

Apology of Aristides on behalf of the Christians ed. from a Syriac Ms. with introduction and translation by J Rendel Harris in *Texts and Studies. Contributions to Biblical and Patristic Literature* vol. 1, ed. J Armitage Robinson (Cambridge: University Press) 1891.

Aquinas, St. Thomas, *Commentary on I Corinthians* in *S. Thomae Aquinatis Super Epistolas S. Pauli lectura* vol. 1, ed. R Cai (Turin: Marietti) 1953.

Aquinas, St. Thomas, *Summa Theologiae*. Latin text and English translation in 60 vols. under the general editorship of T Gilby (London: Eyre &

Spottiswoode; New York: McGraw-Hill) 1963–76. Vol. 17, *Psychology of Human Acts (1a 2ae. 6–17)* ed. T Gilby, 1970.

Batchelor I, McFarlane J, *Multidisciplinary Clinical Teams*, King's Fund Project Paper RC12 (London: King's Fund) 1980.

Bexell G, Norberg A, Norberg B, 'Ethical conflicts in long-term care of aged patients: analysis of the tube-feeding decision by means of a teleological ethical model' (1980) 7 *Ethics in Science and Medicine*, 141–5.

Binding K, Hoche A, *Die Freigabe der Vernichtung 'Lebensunwerten Lebens'* 2nd. edn. (Leipzig: Verlag von Felix Meiner) 1922.

Bond C J, Address to the inaugural meeting of The Voluntary Euthanasia Legalisation Society. Report in (1935) *British Medical Journal* ii, 1168.

Brewer C, 'Murder most inefficient' (1977) *World Medicine* (19 Oct.) 39–40.

Brewer C, '"Insufficient Evidence" – or a Subtle Shift in Policy on Euthanasia?' (1979) *World Medicine* (13 Jan.) 28–31.

British Medical Association, *Handbook of Medical Ethics* (London: BMA) 1980.

Brown N K, Thompson D J, 'Non-Treatment of Fever in Extended Care Facilities' (1979) 300 *New England Journal of Medicine*, 1246–50.

Cohen S, in *Macmillan Service, 5th Report* (London: St. Joseph's Hospice) 1980.

Crane D, *The Sanctity of Social Life: Physicians' Treatment of Critically Ill Patients* (New York: Russell Sage Foundation) 1975.

Darling R B, *Families against Society. A study of Reaction to Children with Birth Defects* (London: Sage Publications) 1979.

Dawidowicz L, Contribution to the Conference on 'Biomedical Ethics and the Shadow of Nazism' (1976) 6(4) *Hastings Center Report* (Special Supplement).

Didache in *Ancient Christian Writers* vol. 6, translated and annotated by J A Kleist (Cork: Mercier Press) 1948, pp. 15–25.

Downing A B, ed. *Euthanasia and the Right to Death* (London: Peter Owen) 1969.

Duff R S, Campbell A G M, 'Moral and Ethical Dilemmas in the Special-Care Nursery' (1973) 289 *New England Journal of Medicine*, 890–94.

Duff R S, Campbell A G M, 'On deciding the care of severely handicapped or dying persons: with particular reference to infants' (1976) 57 *Pediatrics*, 487–93.

Duff R S, Campbell A G M, 'Deciding the care of severely malformed or dying infants' (1979) 5 *Journal of Medical Ethics*, 65–7.

Duff R S, Campbell A G M, 'Moral and Ethical Dilemmas: Seven years into the debate about human ambiguity' (1980) 447 *Annals of the American Academy of Political and Social Science*, 19–28.

Earekson J, *Joni* (London & Glasgow: Pickering & Inglis) 1976.

Editorial, 'Choosing When and How to Die' (1980) *Lancet* ii, 571.

Editorial, 'Withholding Treatment in Infancy' (1981) *British Medical Journal* i, 925–6.

Epistle of Barnabas in *Ancient Christian Writers* vol. 6, translated and annotated by J A Kleist (Cork: Mercier Press) 1948, pp. 37–65.

Fletcher J, *Humanhood: Essays in Biomedical Ethics* (Buffalo: Prometheus Books) 1979.

Forrest D M, 'Early closure in spina bifida: results and problems' (1967) 60 *Proceedings of the Royal Society of Medicine*, 763–7.

Freeman J M, 'To Treat or Not to Treat: Ethical Dilemmas of Treating the Infant with a Myelomeningocele' (1973) 20 *Clinical Neurosurgery*, 134–46.

Freeman J, 'Ethics and the Decision Making Process for Defective Children' in **Roy D J** (1978), 25–38.

Glover J, *Causing Death and Saving Lives* (Harmondsworth: Penguin) 1977.

Gould J, Lord Craigmyle, *Your Death Warrant?* (London: Geoffrey Chapman) 1971.

Grisez G, Boyle J M, *Life and Death with Liberty and Justice* (London: University of Notre Dame Press) 1979.

Haggard S, Carter F A, 'Preventing the birth of infants with Down's Syndrome: a cost-benefit analysis' (1976) *British Medical Journal* i, 753–56.

Haggard S, Carter F, Milne R G, 'Screening for spina bifida cystica. A cost-benefit analysis' (1976) 30 *British Journal of Preventive and Social Medicine*, 40–53.

Hume D, *Dialogues Concerning Natural Religion* in David Hume, *The Natural History of Religion* ed. A Wayne Colvy, and *Dialogues Concerning Natural Religion* ed. J V Price (Oxford: Clarendon Press) 1976.

Irenaeus, St., *Adversus Haereses*. English translation in *Five Books of S. Irenaeus Against Heresies* translated by John Keble (Oxford and London) 1872.

Jakobovitz I, art. 'Euthanasia' in *Encyclopedia Judaica* vol. 6 (Jerusalem: Keter Publishing House) 1971.

John Paul II, Pope (1980) 72 *Acta Apostolicae Sedis*, 84–88.

Kamisar Y, 'Some Non-Religious Views against Proposed "Mercy Killing" Legislation' (1958) 42 *Minnesota Law Review*, 970–1039; in abridged version in **Downing A B** (1969), 85–133.

Kelly G, 'The Duty of Using Artificial Means of Preserving Life' (1950) 11 *Theological Studies*, 203–220.

Kelly G, 'The Duty to Preserve Life' (1951) 12 *Theological Studies*, 550–56.

Kelsey B, 'Which infants should die? Who should decide? An interview with Dr. Raymond S Duff' (1975) 5(2) *Hastings Center Report*, 5–8.

Locke J, *An Essay Concerning Human Understanding*, ed. P H Nidditch in The Clarendon Edition of the Works of John Locke (Oxford: University Press) 1975.

Lorber J, 'Results of Treatment of Myelomeningocele. An analysis of 524 unselected cases, with special reference to possible selection for treatment' (1971) 13 *Developmental Medicine and Child Neurology*, 279–303.

Lorber J, 'Spina Bifida Cystica. Results of Treatment of 270 Consecutive Cases with Criteria for Selection for the Future' (1972) 47 *Archives of Disease in Childhood*, 854–73.

Lorber J, 'Early Results of Selective Treatment of Spina Bifida Cystica' (1973) *British Medical Journal* iv, 201–204.

Lorber J, 'Ethical Problems in the Management of Myelomeningocele and Hydrocephalus' (1975) 10 *Journal of the Royal College of Physicians*, 47–60.

Lorber J, Contributions to discussion in **Swinyard C A** (1978), 111–20; 231–58; 304–11; 344–56; 446–64; 562–86; 598–617.

Lorber J, 'Ethical Concepts in the Treatment of Myelomeningocele' in **Swinyard C A** (1978), 59–67.

Lorber J, 'The Doctor's Duty to Patients and Parents in Profoundly Handicapping Conditions' in **Roy D J** (1978), 9–23.

Lorber J, 'Selection – the best policy available' (1978) *Nursing Mirror* (14 Sept.), 14–17.

Moore G E, *Principia Ethica* (Cambridge: University Press) 1903.

Müller A, 'Radical Subjectivity: Morality versus Utilitarianism' (1977) 19 *Ratio*, 115–132.

Norberg A, Norberg B, Gippert H, Bexell G, 'Ethical conflicts in long-term care of the aged: nutritional problems and the patient-care worker relationship' (1980) *British Medical Journal* i, 377–8.

Noyes R, Jockinsen P R, Travis T A, 'The Changing Attitudes of Physicians Toward Prolonging Life' (1977) 25 *Journal of the American Geriatrics Society*, 470–74.

Parkes C M, 'Home or Hospital? Terminal Care as seen by Surviving Spouses' (1978) 28 *Journal of the Royal College of General Practitioners*, 19–30.

Pius XII, Pope (1957) 49 *Acta Apostolicae Sedis*, 129–47.

Pius XII, Pope (1957) 49 *Acta Apostolicae Sedis*, 1027–33.

Rachels J, 'Active and Passive Euthanasia' (1975) 292 *New England Journal of Medicine*, 78–80.

Ramsey P, *The Patient as Person. Explorations in Medical Ethics* (New Haven & London: Yale University Press) 1970.

Ramsey P, *Ethics at the Edges of Life. Medical and Legal Intersections* (New Haven & London: Yale University Press) 1978.

Roman Catechism. Short title for: *Catechismus ex decreto Concilii Tridentini ad Parachos Pii V Pontificis Max. et deinde Clementis XIII issu editus.* Among English translations: *Catechism of the Council of Trent for Parish Priests* translated into English with Notes by J A McHugh and C J Callan (New York: Wagner; London: Herder) 1934.

Roy D J, ed., *Medical Wisdom and Ethics in the Treatment of Severely Defective Newborn and Young Children* (Montreal: Eden Press) 1978.

Sacred Congregation for the Doctrine of the Faith, 'Iura et Bona' (Declaration on Euthanasia) 72 *Acta Apostolicae Sedis*, 542–52.

Shaw A, 'Dilemmas of "Informed Consent" in Children' (1973) 289 *New England Journal of Medicine*, 885–90.

Shaw A, 'Defining the Quality of life' (1977) 7(5) *Hastings Center Report*, 11.

Shaw A, Randolph J G, Menard B, 'Ethical Issues in Pediatric Surgery: A

National Survey of Pediatricians and Pediatric Surgeons' (1977) 60 *Pediatrics*, 588–99.

Sluis I van der, 'The Movement for Euthanasia 1875–1975' (1979) 66 *Janus*, 131–172.

Swinyard C A, ed., *Decision Making and the Defective Newborn. Proceedings of a Conference on Spina Bifida and Ethics* (Springfield, Illinois: Charles C Thomas) 1978.

The Last Right. The Need for Voluntary Euthanasia (London: Exit) n.d.

Trowell H, *The Unfinished Debate on Euthanasia*, (London: SCM Press) 1973.

Twycross R G, 'Hospice Care – redressing the balance in medicine' (1980) 73 *Journal of the Royal Society of Medicine*, 475–81.

Twycross R G, 'Ethical and Clinical Aspects of Pain Treatment in Cancer Patients' (1982) 74 *Acta Medica Scandinavica*, 83–90.

Vatican Council II, *Lumen Gentium* (Dogmatic Constitution on the Church). English translation in *The Documents of Vatican II*, ed. by Abbott W M (London–Dublin: Geoffrey Chapman) 1966, pp. 14–96.

Veatch R, *Death, Dying and the Biological Revolution* (New Haven & London: Yale University Press) 1976.

Walley R, 'A Question of Conscience' (1976) *British Medical Journal* i, 1456–58.

Wechsler H, Michael J, 'A Rationale of the Law of Homicide' (1937) 37 *Columbia Law Review*, 701–61; 1261–1325.

Wilson D C, *Hilary. The Brave World of Hilary Pole* (London–Sydney: Hodder & Stoughton) 1972.

World Health Organisation, *International Classification of Impairments and Handicaps* (Geneva: WHO) 1980.

Zachary R B, 'Life with Spina Bifida' (1977) *British Medical Journal* ii, 1460–62.

Note: Regina v Arthur
Luke Gormally

Introduction

Some four hours after John Pearson was born in Derby City Hospital on Saturday 28 June 1980, Dr. Leonard Arthur learned from consultation with his parents that they did not want their baby to survive because he was handicapped with Down's syndrome. Dr. Arthur ordered that the baby be given 'nursing care only' (51C).[1] There was no evidence that at the time of making this decision Dr. Arthur had reason to believe that John Pearson was suffering from anything other than the Down's syndrome, the consequences of which could not be modified by any medical treatment in the earliest period of a child's life. Furthermore the severity of the syndrome cannot be diagnosed for several months (perhaps two years) after birth [79E; see also *In re B. (a Minor)* [1981] 1 *Weekly Law Reports* 1421 at 1423 G-H, 1424H].

'Nursing care only'[2] was an instruction understood by those to whom it was given to involve the following:
- the child should be removed to a side-ward where the nurses were to 'cherish him and remain in the ward until he died' (35C);
- the paediatrician was not to be called in the event of the child's condition worsening (34G); the only known visit of a doctor to John Pearson after he was placed on 'nursing care only' was from a senior house officer who asked to be told when the child died so that specimens could be taken from him (34A); it was not thought necessary to keep 'proper case records' (11B; cf. 31G);
- the child was to be kept comfortable and fed with water (34G);
- he would be sedated. Dr. Arthur prescribed dihydrocodeine (DF 118) for this purpose to be administered by the nurses as they thought necessary, but not to exceed 5 mgs. every four hours (51 D–E). The function of DF 118 in this context was described by Dr. Arthur (when the police first interviewed him) as that of stopping the child seeking sustenance (47G). Subsequently he claimed that 'the purpose of the drug's administration would be solely to reduce any suffering on the part of the baby' (51 E–F). In fact the baby seems to have suffered a good deal in his short life (see the references to 'laboured breathing', struggles for breath and vomiting, 32–4 passim). A little more than 69 hours after his birth John Pearson died.

Forensic evidence suggested that John Pearson's death might have been caused by a congenital heart condition and/or by broncho-pneumonia

---

[1] All statements about *Regina v Arthur* are based upon the transcript of the Judge's summing-up prepared by the Official Court Reporters, and all statements attributed to witnesses are quoted from this transcript. References in brackets are to the transcript.

[2] The phrase traditionally connotes the provision of that care and sustenance which a mother would give to a normal healthy baby (excluding, that is, only special therapeutic measures). But in many paediatric units it has been re-defined in the sense outlined in the text.

incipiently present at birth. For that reason an original charge of murder was altered to a charge of attempted murder. In Leicester Crown Court on 5 November 1981 Dr. Arthur was acquitted.

The testimony of defence witnesses at the trial provided additional evidence for the trends towards euthanasia which Chapter 2 of the Report had found to exist in paediatric practice and thinking. What follows is confined to drawing attention to some of that evidence.

Euthanasia in paediatric practice and thinking

The picture of 'nursing care only'[3] assembled above from what emerged at the trial is probably the most detailed available to the general public. It is not peculiar to the paediatric unit in Derby City Hospital. For the defence witnesses affirmed that what was described was accepted paediatric practice (see statements of Professor A G M Campbell at 54F and 57D–E; of Dr. Dunn at 66B, 69B, 70H–71 A; of Sir Douglas Black at 81G; of Dr. Bluett at 85D). Given this testimony some of the observations made by defence witnesses about the nature of a 'nursing care only' regimen are of great interest.

1) *The regimen is adopted with the intention that the child should die.* Thus Professor Campbell speaking of his own management of Down's syndrome babies:

   'The problem of deciding the question whether the baby should survive has arisen in my career some seven or eight times. In some of them the decision was made to keep the baby alive. I have put a baby on "nursing care only" on four or five occasions *with the intention it should not survive*. These were cases of Down's coupled with duodenal atresia.' (59A–B) [Emphasis added]

   The President of the Royal College of Physicians, Sir Douglas Black, had the following to say:

   'Where there is an uncomplicated Down's case and the parents did not want the child to live, the child requires normal, healthy care, but I think there are circumstances where it would be ethical *to put it upon a course of management that would end in its death*. If the parents expressed the wish repeatedly and there is no prospect of the child being adopted I would take all factors into account. I would possibly not act as Dr. Arthur did, but I would be far from condemning what he did. I say it is ethical that a child suffering from Down's and with a parental wish that it should not survive, it is ethical to *terminate life*, providing other considerations are taken into account, such as the status and ability of the parents to cope in a way that the child could otherwise have had a happy life.' (79F–80A) [Emphasis added]

2) Though it is acknowledged that the child's death is intended in adopting a 'nursing care only' regimen, it was nonetheless claimed by defence witnesses that this is ethically acceptable since death is not caused by a *positive act* but rather *allowed* to come about. Professor Campbell offered

---

[3] This use of the phrase 'nursing care only' corresponds to the similar 'specialised' use of the phrase 'custodial management' noted at p.22 of the Report.

the following testimony:

'There is an important distinction between allowing a baby to die and taking an action which will accelerate or cause death[4] ... There is an important grey area in between. It is important not only to doctors but also to parents. To most paediatricians and to most parents that I have discussed this with we hope we break no law that makes sense. There is an important difference between allowing a child to die and taking action to kill it. Withholding food is, I think, a negative, not a positive act. It is not a positive step to cause the child's death. The doctor indeed has a duty to order feeding, but if he orders food to be withheld, and he does it with the knowledge and wish of the parents, then that is permissible.' (59G–60B)

Sir Douglas Black likewise relied on a distinction supposedly holding between acts on the one hand and omissions on the other:

'I distinguish between allowing to die and killing. It is a distinction that is somewhat difficult to defend in logic, but I agree it is good medical practice not to take positive steps to end life.' (78D–E)

Two implausible contentions seem to underlie this line of thought: (i) that it is not possible to commit murder by omission, a claim which Chapter 3 of the Report shows is morally unacceptable (cf. pp. 46–48) and which has been elsewhere shown to be legally unacceptable[5]; (ii) instituting a nursing care regimen is not *doing* anything which brings about death.

3) The reasons for aiming at the child's death by instituting 'nursing care only':

- (a) *Parental rejection of the baby*; evidently the most decisive consideration in the minds of defence witnesses. Thus Sir Douglas Black maintained: 'With a *healthy* mongol *and the mother not wishing the child to survive* he [viz the paediatrician] can do what was done in this case as a matter of medical ethics. And that consequence is that it would end in the baby's death.' (81A–B) [Emphasis added] Comparable statements on the decisiveness of parental rejection were made by Professor Campbell, reported at 53C, 57D, 58E, 60B; by Dr. Dunn at 67B, 69D, 72G–H; additionally by Sir Douglas Black at 78A and 79F–H; and by Dr. Bluett at 86B.

  (Most remarkably the judge at a number of points presented to the jury the defence claim that a *conjoint* decision by doctor and parents to 'allow' a child to die was not 'arbitrary', without warning that doctors and parents have no *joint* power of life and death. See 23B, 23H, 64H, 70G.)

- (b) *A child with severe irreversible handicap has not got a 'worthwhile life'*. That final phrase was not used by defence witnesses but the

---

[4] Contrast this with Professor Campbell's support elsewhere for *active* killing of certain patients, as in R S Duff, A G M Campbell, 'On Deciding the Care of Severely Handicapped and Dying Persons: With Particular Reference to Infants' (1976) 57 *Pediatrics*, 492: 'we believe that choices for death, whether by active or passive means, should be permitted'.

[5] See *Regina v. Arthur. A verdict on the Judge's summing-up in the trial of Dr. Leonard Arthur, November 1981* (Published by Life, 7 Parade, Leamington Spa); Ian Kennedy 'Reflections on the Arthur trial' *New Society* 7 January 1982, 13–15.

thought seems to be required in order to make sense of the decisions they were prepared to defend. Dr. Bluett came close to expressing it: 'The quality of the handicap has a great deal to do with the approach. The paediatrician knows what life is going to be like for that baby. If you know life is awful, or going to be awful, one may counsel the mother that the baby should not live.' (83D–E) That fairly exhibits the kind of comprehensive judgement on the value of a child's life that the Report argues it is not open to us to make.

– (c) *The baby's right to life is conditional not merely on acceptance by the family, but also on the family's ability to cope:* 'With a baby born with severe irreversible handicap it is a matter of weighing up the severity of the handicap and the effect on its life and on its family. This is the basis for the decision which has to be made.' (Professor Campbell at 55F–G)

– (d) *The alternative to life in a family – life in an institution – is [by implication] regarded as a life not worth living.* At the end of the first of his two reviews of Down's syndrome Mr. Justice Farquharson said:

'... in nearly every case if the parents want the child the doctor will give them every encouragement to have it and keep it. But if not the likelihood of the child ever being taken into another family, either by adoption or fostering, is very remote and the most likely course is that it will be placed in some form of institution. So it is not just a simple question of saying: it is a mongol child; it will have to be put down. It is a case, say the defence, in putting this case before you, of where the most careful and agonising consideration has to be given as to what should be done in the best interests of the child.' [16C–E]

Neither here, nor when quoting Professor Campbell (58D) and Sir Douglas Black (at 79G) to similar effect, did the Judge comment on this line of thought.

107

BOOK TWO

EUTHANASIA AND THE LAW: THE CASE AGAINST LEGALIZATION
(1993)

1

SUBMISSION TO THE SELECT COMMITTEE OF THE HOUSE OF LORDS ON MEDICAL ETHICS

by

THE LINACRE CENTRE
FOR HEALTH CARE ETHICS
June 1993

CONTENTS

0. Introduction

PART ONE

1. Sanctity of Life and Autonomy

1.1 *Justice and the Sanctity of Life*
    1.1.1 The Sanctity of Life
    1.1.2 Sanctity of Life, Human Dignity and Justice
    1.1.3 Contemporary denials that human worth and dignity belong to all human beings.
        1.1.3(i) A characteristic explanation of the unequal value of human lives.
        1.1.3(ii) Warnock and Dworkin.
    1.1.4 The Basis of Human Dignity and Justice.
    1.1.5 Dualism and the false valuation of human life.
    1.1.6 Justice and the Sanctity of Life Ethic Recovered.

1.2 *Justice and Killing*
    1.2.1 Killing for reasons incompatible with recognition of human dignity.
    1.2.2 Euthanasia: killing incompatible with recognition of human dignity.

1.3 *Autonomy and Killing*
    1.3.1 Autonomy and a 'Right' to Personal Autonomy.
    1.3.2 Autonomy and the Justification of Voluntary Euthanasia.
    1.3.3 Autonomy and the Justification of Non-Voluntary Euthanasia.

1.4 *Sanctity of Life and Autonomy: Conclusion*

2. The Duties of Doctors: Duties of Treatment and Duties of Care

2.1 *The Purpose of Medicine and Duties of Treatment*
2.2 *Limits on Duties of Treatment*
    2.2.1 Patient Consent and Duties of Treatment
    2.2.2 Duties of Treatment and Suicide
    2.2.3 General Grounds for Limiting Treatment
        (i) Inefficacious Treatment
        (ii) Excessively burdensome treatment

2.2.4 Duties of Treatment to the Incompetent
2.3 *Doctors' duties of ordinary care towards hospitalised patients*
2.3.1 Feeding the PVS patient

3. Withdrawing Treatment and Intentional Killing

4. The Role of Advance Directives and Proxy Decision Makers
4.1 *Advance Directives*
4.1.1 The unilateral emphasis on autonomy
4.1.2 Advance declarations and the burdensomeness of treatment
4.1.3 Advance directives and the refusal of ordinary care
4.1.4 Advance directives and the doctor-patient relationship

4.2 *The Proxy Decision-Maker*

PART TWO

5. The Courts and 'Responsible Medical Opinion'

6. Proposals to Change the Law

6.1 *Proposals which should not be adopted.*
6.1.1 Medical Treatment (Advance Directives) Bill
6.1.2 Termination of Medical Treatment Bill
6.2 *Proposals which should be adopted*
6.2.1 The *Bland* ruling on lawful intention to terminate life should be overturned
6.2.2 Unacceptable kinds of advance directive should be deprived of all legal effect

PART THREE

7. The Hospice Movement and Advances in Palliative Care

8. The Dutch Experience
8.1 *The Law*
8.2 *Medical Guidelines*
8.3 *Euthanasia in Practice*

Concluding Observations

Introduction

This Submission has been prepared on behalf of The Linacre Centre for Health Care Ethics[1], a national Catholic bioethics centre established in 1977 by the Roman Catholic Archbishops of England and Wales, who are its Trustees. The Centre has a record of academic research and publication in the field of health care ethics,[2] and an involvement in teaching and in consultancy work both for the Church, nationally and internationally, and for other bodies.

It is not the aim of this submission to make a documented presentation of the teaching of the Roman Catholic Church on the topics which concern the Select Committee.[3] A simple statement of position is unlikely greatly to aid the Committee in its deliberations. The Centre has always sought to make intelligible to non-Catholics and non-Christians the Church's moral teaching in its bearings on the practice of medicine. Much of that teaching belongs to what has been called the tradition of *common morality*, whose central tenets belong to the moral patrimony of civilized societies.

Accordingly, the present submission is devoted to a broad exposition of that framework of moral understanding which has long shaped the

[1] The document has been prepared on behalf of the Centre by Luke Gormally, its Director, by Professor John Finnis FBA, Professor of Law and Legal Philosophy in The University of Oxford and Vice-Chairman of The Board of Governors of the Centre, and by Dr John Keown, Lecturer in Law in The University of Cambridge and a Governor of the Centre. Extensive use has been made in the preparation of the document of material which also appears in the following published writings:

John Finnis, 'Bland: Crossing the Rubicon?' *Law Quarterly Review* 109 (July 1993) pp.329–37.

John Finnis, 'Living Will Legislation' in Luke Gormally (ed) *Euthanasia, Clinical Practice and the Law* London: The Linacre Centre, 1994 pp.167–176.

Luke Gormally, 'A Response [to Roy Fox, Palliative care and aggressive therapy]' in R J Elford (ed) *Medical Ethics and Elderly People* Edinburgh: Churchill Livingstone, 1987, pp.177–198.

Luke Gormally, 'Introduction' (pp.1–10) and 'The Living Will: the ethical framework of a recent Report' (pp.53–69) in Luke Gormally (ed) *The Dependent Elderly. Autonomy, Justice and Quality of Care* Cambridge: Cambridge University Press, 1992.

Luke Gormally, 'Definitions of Personhood and Implications for the Care of PVS Patients', *Catholic Medical Quarterly* 44/4 (May 1993), pp.7–12.

Luke Gormally, 'Against Voluntary Euthanasia' in Raanan Gillon (ed) *Principles of Health Care Ethics* Chichester: John Wiley, 1993 [forthcoming].

I J Keown, 'The Law and Practice of Euthanasia in The Netherlands', *Law Quarterly Review* 108 (1992), pp.51–78.

[2] Noteworthy here is the Centre's Working Party Report, *Euthanasia and Clinical Practice: trends, principles and alternatives* first published in 1982. (See Book 1 of this volume.)

[3] Some documentation may be found in *Euthanasia and Clinical Practice*, especially chapter 4, 'The Christian Tradition', and in an earlier publication by the Centre: [Luke Gormally] *Ordinary and extraordinary means of prolonging life* (Linacre Centre Paper 3) London: The Linacre Centre, 1979.

traditional ethic of medical practice. Offering such an exposition seemed the most useful exercise we could undertake in relation to the deliberations of the Select Committee. For it is unlikely that the members of the Committee will find themselves disagreeing only about relatively derivative issues. Decisive disagreements are more likely to focus on the most fundamental issues: the value of human life, the moral significance of intention, the ethics of killing, the claims of autonomy, the purpose of medicine and its relation to duties of treatment and duties of care. Fundamental topics such as these are what the present submission seeks to illuminate, in a way accessible to those who do not share the religious faith of its authors.

Part One of this submission (Sections 1–4) is a sustained exposition which seeks to clear away some of those systematic misunderstandings of traditional moral principles which have obstructed a clear grasp of their continuing relevance to the practice of medicine and their implications for legislation and public policy. Without an accurate understanding of these principles it is not possible to appreciate what a traditional ethic requires of medical practice. Central to that ethic has been the prohibition on intentionally killing patients, a prohibition respect for which has been a necessary foundation of the trust between doctor and patient which is so essential an ingredient of the therapeutic relationship.

Systematic misunderstandings of traditional moral principles, and false inferences from them, are nowadays offered to justify jettisoning a traditional ethic of medicine in the interests of having doctors kill patients. In some cases this change is supposed to be in the interests of patients. But often enough the change seems to be promoted in response to the concerns of those who want patients killed because they are perceived to be an unwelcome burden either to families or to the Health Service.

In **Part Two** of this Submission (Sections 5–6) the proper role of the Courts in interpreting the law is discussed along with general and specific proposals for change in the law.

In **Part Three** (Sections 7–8) the Submission comments on (a) the changed character of the apologetic for legalizing euthanasia which has in part come about in response to the success of the Hospice Movement, and (b) the lessons to be learned from the permissive practice of euthanasia in Holland.[4]

Lord Justice Hoffmann rightly remarked in *Airedale NHS Trust v Bland*[5]: 'This is not an area in which any difference can be allowed to exist between what is legal and what is morally right.' There cannot be a true determination of what is morally right and legally appropriate if competing moral viewpoints on so fundamental a matter as killing are treated as having equivalent claims, and, in consequence, proposals for legislative change are designed as a pragmatic compromise between these viewpoints.

The moral issues which confront the Select Committee are not radically new in character, though they may have been given new forms by advances

---

[4] The organization of topics in this submission follows the listing of topics in section 2 of the Special Report of The Select Committee (9 March 1993).

[5] [1993] 2 *Weekly Law Reports* 316 at 350.

in medical technology and clinical practice. Questions about when to withhold or withdraw treatment and whether it can ever be right for doctors to kill patients are questions with a long history. A carefully considered and elaborated set of answers to them has for centuries supported a humane practice of medicine, of which a shining example in our own age has been the development of palliative care in the Hospice Movement. Those carefully considered answers and their relevance to contemporary variations on old challenges deserve the attentive consideration and endorsement of the Select Committee. It is in the hope of promoting those ends that this Submission is respectfully offered.

PART ONE

1. Sanctity of Life and Autonomy

Central to the concerns of the Select Committee are the questions: What may justify decisions and courses of conduct intended to bring about a person's death?[1] and: Can such decisions and conduct be justified by either the wishes or the best interests of the person to be killed? These questions are nowadays apt to give rise to talk of a conflict between respect for the sanctity of human life and respect for autonomy (self-determination). Accordingly, it seems appropriate to begin with a consideration of the significance and grounding of these moral requirements and of their precise implications for certain central issues in medical practice.

1.1 Justice and the Sanctity of Life

1.1.1 The Sanctity of Life

In the Christian tradition the idea of the sanctity of life was employed exclusively of *human* life, to assert its inviolability, i.e. the entitlement of any human being to protection from unjust attack. So employed the idea connotes the specific grounds for such inviolability, namely that human life possesses an intrinsic dignity and value because created by God in his own image (Genesis 1:26) for the distinctive destiny of sharing in God's own life. A significant body of theological reflection on this revealed doctrine analysed the meaning of the image of God (imago Dei) in terms of the distinctive *capacity for rational existence* inherent in man's nature. It is in the nature of human beings to possess the capacity to develop both the ability to understand what is truly good and the ability to be moved by the desire for what is good. The authentic development of these abilities can lead us into a life of self-giving love which mirrors the very life of God: being made in the image (imago) of God, we are able to acquire his likeness (similitudo), an achievement which is the proper fulfilment of a human life.

Traditional understanding of the sanctity of human life, set in its original theological context, may be summarised in three points:

---

[1] We shall call such decisions and courses of conduct 'intentional killing', and the phrases 'intentional killing' and 'intentionally kills' are to be understood throughout as having that precise sense (and not just as a way of signifying all non-accidental killing). Like several of the Law Lords in *Bland*, we use 'course of conduct' to include both 'positive actions' and deliberate 'omissions'.

118

(1) The notion of the sanctity of life explained why certain reasons for killing human beings were inadmissible precisely because incompatible with the distinctive dignity human beings possess. Allowing for certain justifications of killing which were thought compatible with recognition of human dignity,[2] the core of the principle of the sanctity of human life was formulated in the requirement that one ought never intentionally to kill the innocent (that is, one ought never to adopt any course of action or omission intended to terminate the life of an innocent human being).

(2) The distinctive dignity of human beings belongs to them in virtue of a radical capacity inherent in their nature. Since it belongs to them in virtue of their *nature* it belongs to all human beings equally.

(3) The rational abilities that human beings characteristically develop (in virtue of the radical natural capacity for such development) may be exercised in ways which are consistent or inconsistent with the fulfilment which is proper to human beings. To choose and to act in ways which are inconsistent with our proper fulfilment is to choose and to act at variance with the *point* of the radical capacity in virtue of which we possess dignity. But to act in ways at variance with human dignity is not to lose human dignity: for there remains the ability to repent of bad choices and to give a right direction to a hitherto disordered life.

1.1.2 Sanctity of Life, Human Dignity and Justice

In modern Western societies the theological understanding of human dignity has been transformed into secularised doctrines of the equal dignity of all citizens, doctrines which are the basis of what is sometimes called the 'politics of universalism', which insists on the *equal* basic rights and entitlements of citizens. Secularised doctrines of human dignity need to provide (a) some account of what underpins the claim that human beings possess dignity, and (b) some account of what is required if choice and action are to be consistent with human dignity. In what follows some of the accounts which are on offer in our society will be assessed with particular reference to

---

[2] It was not thought incompatible with human dignity to execute a criminal found guilty of a capital crime insofar as what he received was considered *deserved punishment*; for the assumption behind the view that someone deserves death is that he knowingly chose to do what he did and so is answerable for it. The belief that human beings are answerable for what they do and can be found to deserve punishment implies a high conception of human dignity; we are not left to be pushed hither and thither by uncontrollable impulse and fate.

Similarly, the intentional killing of unjust aggressors in warfare has been justified on the grounds that they are answerable for actual (or threatened) violent and grave harm to the common good of a society.

Both justifications – of capital punishment and of the killing of unjust aggressors in warfare – yielded a common formula stating the basic norm in regard to killing: one ought never intentionally to kill the innocent, i.e. those not guilty of crime which it is one's task to punish or of unjustified violence which it is one's office to resist. This is what is identified in the main text as the core of the principle of the sanctity of life.

Failure to recognise the precise character of this principle led Lord Goff in *Airedale NHS Trust v Bland* to say that it is not absolute: [1993] 2 *WLR* at 367. Lord Goff's explanations for this observation seem to have in mind two quite distinct 'principles': (i) 'It is unlawful to kill (take another man's life)'; (ii) 'Human life should be preserved if at all possible, by any available means, regardless of circumstances'. Neither is the principle of the sanctity of life as traditionally understood.

the adequacy of the answers they offer to the question of when killing is justified. A correct answer to this question is clearly fundamental to an understanding of justice in society, and to the criminal law, since protection from being unjustifiably killed is a precondition of enjoying whatever rights an individual may have.

1.1.3 Contemporary denials that human worth and dignity belong to all human beings.

The traditional belief in equal human dignity, both in its religious and secularised versions, is denied by a number of influential voices in our society. The understandings they offer of the basis for attributions of human dignity entail that dignity does not belong to all human beings. Broadly speaking, possession of human dignity is said by these thinkers to depend on two requirements: (a) on a human being having developed presently exercisable psychological abilities for understanding, choice and rational communication; and (b) on a human being actually exercising such abilities in the enjoyment of an acceptable quality of life. The precise relevance of the first requirement is variously explained.

1.1.3(i) A characteristic explanation of the unequal value of human lives.

A number of thinkers begin from the assertion that human beings are not equal in possessing basic dignity (and the value such dignity imports); they regard belief in the equal and distinctive dignity of human beings as a manifestation of an irrational prejudice (sometimes labelled 'speciesism'[3]). Rather, they say, a human life has value only in so far as the person whose life it is is in a position to value things and projects and activities and does value them. This means that if one does not possess the developed mental abilities to make it possible for things to seem valuable to one then there is no account one can give of one's life having value. Human beings who do not possess the mental capacities to make things matter *to them* do not *in themselves* matter.

On this account a human being can *give* worth and dignity to his life in so far as he is able to maintain a sense of things and projects being worthwhile and valuable. The corollary of this account of what it is for a human life to have value is that those lacking the mental abilities to confer value on their own lives must depend on others to attach value to their lives. This means, for example, that if those one would normally expect to value the life of an unborn child (the child's parents) or the life of a senile parent (his or her children) do not themselves account that life valuable, then not only is there unlikely to be a social basis for treating that life as valuable, but there is no account to be given of its value.

---

[3] Notably by Peter Singer. Singer's position is taken as a starting-point by Grant Gillett in developing his account of the value of human life. See Grant Gillett, *Reasonable Care*, Bristol: The Bristol Press 1989, p.14.

1.1.3(ii) Warnock and Dworkin

The requirement that a human being possess presently exercisable abilities in order to possess dignity or distinctive value underlies the distinction Mary Warnock makes between 'simply being alive' and 'the specifically human consciousness of having a life to lead'. Only those enjoying such consciousness, and having the abilities responsibly to lead their lives, possess a distinctive value; and it is only the possession of that consciousness which explains the gravity of killing certain human beings. For humans with some idea of having lives of their own to live, for which they are responsible, 'dying, or being killed, is a different matter from the mere cessation of life'. Those, on the other hand, who are 'simply alive', who have merely 'biological life', cannot have lives with distinctive significance, value or dignity.[4]

Despite immediate appearances, a similar distinction and a similar conclusion are also basic to Ronald Dworkin's more complex reflections on human worth and dignity and his explanation of why there should be extensive liberty for medicalised killing of innocent human beings. Professor Dworkin claims that almost all citizens have a shared ideal of wishing to honour the conviction that human life is sacred. He himself speaks of human life being intrinsically valuable and sacred, and formally rejects the view that nothing is valuable unless someone wants it or needs it to get what he wants.[5] But he also considers that one reasonable 'interpretation' of this value and sacredness of human life is the 'liberal' view that 'life's inherent value ... depends on the intrinsic importance of human creative investment' in it; that is, on what people 'make of their own lives', so that the life which is sacred and inviolable is not 'biological life' but the 'human life ... created ... by personal choice, training, commitment and decision'.[6] So Dworkin's own (liberal) view is that a person suffering from Alzheimer's dementia

---

4 Mary Warnock, *The Uses of Philosophy* (chapter 2: 'Man's Duties to his Own Species') Oxford: Blackwell Publishers 1992, at pp.22–23. Baroness Warnock holds that we can be justified in killing human beings either *for their own sake* [about such justifications see 1.2.2, 1.3.2 and 1.3.3 of the main text] if we believe their lives are likely to be full of suffering and to deteriorate in misery, or *for the sake of others*, when those to be killed do not understand themselves to have lives for which they are responsible and when they are likely to impose what are perceived to be unacceptable burdens. The latter contention is straightforwardly an apologia for killing for the sake of convenience. Discussing the situation in which there is nothing about the prospective quality of life of the unborn child which might be invoked to justify abortion, Warnock considers the situation in which it is simply the case
  'that the mother does not want it [the child] to be born ... Are we here justified in preferring to consider the quality of *her* life rather than that of the foetus? ... in the case of social abortion, it is the suffering of the mother if this child is born that is the decisive factor. And this ... is consistent with the non-adoption of the principle of equal value to all lives.' (*ibid.*, pp.34–35)
The general argument that we may justifiably kill those presently unable to think of themselves as responsible for their lives if and when they are perceived as diminishing the quality of life of others is a radical attack on the *moral* fabric of human solidarity and justice. Neither solidarity nor justice can be maintained by reliance on sentiments of affection uninformed by recognition of duties of care to those who in the course of nature (because of immaturity and decline) are necessarily dependent and without a sense of responsibility for their own lives. The lives of many of us have depended at some stage on others recognising duties of care towards us, a recognition overriding any strong inclination to abandon care for us.
5 Ronald Dworkin, *Life's Dominion* London: Harper Collins 1993, p.69.
6 Dworkin, *op.cit.*, pp.157, 93; Dworkin, 'When can a doctor kill?' *The Times* (London) 27 April 1993. So, for example: 'Recognising the sanctity of life ... means ... not frustrating investments in life that

'is no longer capable of the acts or attachments that can give it [life] value. Value cannot be poured into a life from the outside; it must be generated by the person whose life it is, and this is no longer possible for him.'[7]

On Dworkin's view, while some locate the 'transcendentally important source of ... sacred value' in 'biological life', others (like himself) think the source of that value lies in the exercisable abilities, especially for rational control of one's life, in virtue of which people can give the shape and significance they wish to their lives.

It is clear, then, that Dworkin's talk about the 'shared ideal of sanctity of life' is *practically* empty.[8] The ideal can guide no one's deliberations until it is given content by 'interpretation'; the interpretations which ground competing claims about right conduct and just law are *contradictory*; and Dworkin's conclusions coincide with the position favoured by Warnock. The contest which he professed to expel with his talk of consensus about life's sacredness returns with undeniable vigour in the struggle between the thesis (which he dubs 'conservative' but which in many periods and cultures has been recognised as radical and transforming) that human life has dignity even in the most undeveloped human beings or in those severely disabled by disease or decrepitude, and the thesis (which he approvingly dubs 'liberal') which accords to the relatively powerful lethal dominion over the relatively weak. This is a struggle in which the law simply cannot be neutral without abdicating its claim to uphold basic justice, the state's most fundamental duty to protect the lives of innocent citizens against deliberate extinction at the hands of others.

One does not have to rely on religious premises to see that the understand-

---

have already been made. For that reason liberal opinion cares more about the lives that people are now leading, lives in earnest, than about the possibility of other lives to come'; and the context shows that the lives which Dworkin here treats as mere 'possibilities' are the actual lives of healthy unborn children. See *Life's Dominion*, 99.

[7] *Life's Dominion*, p.230.

[8] The claim that the idea of the sanctity of life is shared even by those who favour the most liberal regimes of abortion and euthanasia has three functions in Dworkin's argument.

(1) It gives him a premise for his claim (see e.g. *Life's Dominion*, pp.164–5) that for purposes of U.S. constitutional law all questions about abortion and euthanasia are 'religious', so that choices to 'kill' the unborn or to commit or assist in suicide or to carry out euthanasiast killing cannot be prohibited without violating the 'free exercise of religion' guaranteed by the First Amendment to the U.S. Constitution.

(2) It enables him to clothe the aspirations and choices of healthy adults (e.g. healthy pregnant women, and by implication the relatives of the demented) with the aura and the borrowed dignity of a sanctity heretofore reserved for the divinely bestowed being and status of the human subject who is always equal in dignity to his potential killer. The 'sanctity' appropriated by Dworkin is now remarketed as a self-assertive sanctity, bereft of awe, gratitude or humility, and parcelled out so as to ascribe to human beings a radical *inequality* of dignity. Consciously seeking argumentation 'likely to succeed in the political forum' (*ibid.*, p.29), Dworkin strives to deprive the common morality underlying our law about protection of life of its very vocabulary, press-ganging it into the service of the campaign to overthrow that law, a campaign more frankly and lucidly waged by others in the name of self-determination or autonomy.

(3) It enables him to launch a claim to be the moderate who reconciles two warring positions, while all the time he is siding definitively with the practical conclusions of one of those positions, pervasively misdescribing what the other position holds, and retailing unmeasured denunciations of what it promotes, e.g. nursing care of PVS patients ('the ultimate insult') or laws against assisting suicide or against voluntary euthanasia ('a devastating odious form of tyranny': p.217).

ing of human worth advocated by Baroness Warnock and Professor Dworkin, precisely because it is a direct attack on the principle of the basic equality-in-dignity of human beings, is radically subversive of justice. A secularised doctrine of human dignity needs to be consistent with our fundamental intuitions about justice.

1.1.4 The Basis of Human Dignity and Justice

What are the implications for justice of the kind of understanding of the worth and dignity of human life proposed by Warnock and Dworkin and similar thinkers who would like to see a radical revision of our homicide laws? Common to their positions is the requirement (explicit or implicit) that human beings possess *presently exercisable abilities* in order to be counted subjects of justice, and specifically to be counted among those entitled not to be killed intentionally without just reason. For such exercisable abilities are necessary if one is to find value in objects or projects, or to entertain some idea of having a life of one's own for which one is responsible (Warnock), or if one is to be well placed 'to make something' of one's life, thus having a 'life in earnest' whose 'sacredness' might count for something in any competition with the 'investments' which someone else has made in his own life (Dworkin).

The rational abilities necessary to these activities are various, and come in varying degrees in human beings. If actual possession of such abilities is a necessary condition of the claim to be treated justly, questions will have to be faced about precisely *which* abilities must be possessed, and how developed they must be before one enjoys this claim to be treated justly. And these questions could be answered only by *choosing* which to count as the relevant abilities and precisely how developed they must be to count. But any such line-drawing exercise is necessarily arbitrary. A distinction between A and B, where A and B fall on either side of a line determining some minimal level of proximate capacity for the exercise of an ability, will not admit of reasoned defence when what is at issue is whether A and B are subjects of justice. If A qualifies for just treatment, B will fail to qualify even though there is very little difference in the degree to which he possesses the relevant abilities.[9]

Arbitrary choices may be reasonable and unavoidable in determining some entitlements (such as the requirement that one must have been a member of a club for three years in order to enjoy certain benefits). But if one's understanding of human worth and dignity commits one to being arbitrary about who are to be treated justly (i.e. about who are the very *subjects* of justice) it is clear that one lacks what is recognisable as a

---

[9] Note that this is not a slippery slope argument, i.e. an argument from the alleged unacceptable consequences (logical or social) of an attempted discrimination between what is to be regarded as morally (or legally) acceptable and what unacceptable. [Some slippery slope arguments are cogent, others not: see Douglas Walton, *Slippery Slope Arguments* Clarendon Library of Logic and Philosophy, Oxford University Press, 1992] The argument here, however, is that the proposed discrimination under consideration is inherently unreasonable. It is no answer to this point to say that a distinction between the status in law of A and B can be made legally *effective*, by writing it into law and making it difficult to revise and by effectively policing its application so that departures from it are made difficult.

framework of justice. For it is incompatible with our fundamental intuitions about justice that we should determine who are the subjects of justice by arbitrary choice. The need for a non-arbitrary understanding of who are the subjects of justice requires us to *assume* that *just treatment is owing to all human beings in virtue of their humanity*.

This indispensable assumption is also intrinsically reasonable. It is true that the distinctive dignity and value of human life are *manifested* in those specific exercises of developed rational abilities in which we achieve some share in such human goods as truth, beauty, justice, friendship and integrity. But the necessary rational abilities are acquired in virtue of an underlying or radical capacity, *given with our nature as human beings*, for developing precisely such abilities. Yet it should be clear that the dynamic development of this radical natural capacity[10] is not directed to the acquisition of rational abilities for them to be exercised in just any fashion. Our abilities to know and choose are not properly exercised by, for example, believing falsehood or choosing to act unjustly, any more than our abilities to see and to walk are properly exercised in double-vision and tripping over obstacles. The nature in virtue of which we come to acquire rational abilities has its proper fulfilment, then, in exercises of rational abilities in which we recognise worth and dignity. But if it is characteristic of the nature of human beings to acquire abilities which are properly exercised in ways which are inherently valuable, then it is reasonable to hold that there is an inherent value or dignity in the nature we share in common, and seriously unreasonable (and radically subversive of justice) to judge that the lives of some human beings lack inherent value because those human beings lack certain presently exercisable psychological abilities.

1.1.5 Dualism and the false valuation of human life

It is clear enough from the brief descriptions offered above that Warnock's and Dworkin's accounts of which human lives possess worth rest on contrasting what they term the condition of 'simply being alive' or possessing mere 'biological life' with the condition involved in 'having a life' (on which worth depends). Discussing obligations to patients in a persistent vegetative state in his essay 'The Right to Death' Dworkin writes:

'... nothing in the idea that life has intrinsic importance ... can justify a policy of keeping permanently comatose people alive. The worth of their lives – the character of the lives they have led – cannot be improved just by keeping the bodies they used to inhabit technically alive.'[11]

---

[10] The radical dynamic capacity for rational life which normally results in the development of rational abilities may, of course, be *impeded* by failures of organic development, most importantly by failures of brain development. But whatever is conceived with the basic constitution necessary for human development should be recognised as possessing the radical capacity characteristic of human nature. Organic failures, either in development or decline, are failures in respect of the organic *vehicles* necessary for the exercise of rational abilities. But such failures in the life of a human being are not a reason for saying someone is not a human being, with the basic dignity which belongs to human beings.

[11] 'The Right to Death', *The New York Review of Books*, 31 January, 1991, pp.14–17, at p.17c.

Here we have a contrast between, on the one hand, a personal life (a life which a person has consciously led, to which value attaches), and, on the other, the ongoing biological life of a body which for some stretch of its existence may be inhabited by a person ('may be', because according to some of these thinkers some human bodies may never have truly 'personal' inhabitants).

This dualism left clear traces in the judgements in *Airedale NHS Trust v Bland*, in which a distinction was made between Tony Bland himself and his body; e.g. 'his spirit has left him and all that remains is the shell of his body' (Brown P); 'his body is alive, but he has no life . . . He is alive but has no life at all' (Hoffmann LJ, consciously echoing Dworkin).

A dualism 'which thinks of the body as if it were some kind of habitation for and instrument of the real person, is defended by few philosophers . . . It renders inexplicable the unity in complexity which one experiences in everything one consciously does. It speaks as if there were two things . . .: a non-bodily person and a non-personal living body. But neither of these can one recognise as oneself. One's living body is intrinsic, not merely instrumental, to one's personal life. Each of us has a human life (not a vegetable life plus an animal life plus a personal life); when it is flourishing that life includes all one's vital functions including speech, deliberation and choice; when gravely impaired it lacks some of those functions without ceasing to be the life of the person so impaired.'[12]

Living human beings are organisms. On a non-dualistic view the unified life of the human organism is throughout *human*. There is not some separable organic substrate, the life of which is 'purely biological', and to which some personal subject, whose life is uniquely manifested in psychological activities, may be attached. The life that is exhibited in thinking is the *very same life* that is manifested in respiration and heartbeat. To cease to be able to think is to lose an ability, not to lose one's life.[13]

The rejection of (anthropological) dualism is important to recovering an appreciation of the inherent dignity of every human life. There is a fundamental conflict between the position of those who acknowledge a value and dignity in human beings *given with their humanity* and the position of those who think that value and dignity belong to a life *only* in so far as a person is in control of his life and can give it a valued meaning. The latter position is not reasonable. It fails to acknowledge the value of the radical natural *capacity*

---

[12] J M Finnis, 'Bland: Crossing the Rubicon?' (1993) 109 *Law Quarterly Review* 329–37. See more fully *idem*, 'On the "Value of Human Life" and "The Right to Death": Reflections on *Cruzan* and Dworkin' 17 *Southern Illinois University Law Journal* 1 at 9–11.

[13] The movement to have irreversible destruction of the neocortex taken as the criterion of death rests on a dualism of biological life/personal life. This movement has clearly influenced official BMA positions (see especially paras. 32 and 34 of the 1988 BMA Working Party Report on *Euthanasia*). In the diagnosis of human death there is no alternative to employing criteria analogous to the criteria we employ in diagnosing death in other kinds of animals. Living human beings, like other animal organisms, die when they irreversibly lose the capacity for the integrated organic functioning characteristic of organisms. In the days before artificial ventilation, cessation of heart and lung function was an unambiguous indicator of the loss of the capacity for integrated organic functioning. If there is validity in taking 'brain stem death' as an indicator of death, it can only be because a functioning brain stem is a necessary condition of integrated organic functioning.

to develop abilities to find meaning in life, and the dignity of the nature in which that radical capacity inheres. And it fails to acknowledge that the developed abilities find their fulfilment not in just any way of life which one can be said to be in control of but in a way of life in which one submits, for example, to the claims of truth and justice. And one is not in control of what counts as true and just. To attach value and dignity exclusively to autonomous control is to have blinded oneself to the true source of the basic value and dignity in a human life.

It is of considerable importance to note one implication of the inseparability of recognising someone's human dignity and recognising his status as a subject of justice. Since denial of the former entails denial of the latter, our practical reasoning should never involve us in judgements which amount to the denial of the inherent worth or dignity of a human being. The basic human dignity of the other is an *ineliminable* consideration when we deliberate about how we should treat him.

1.1.6 Justice and the Sanctity of Life Ethic Recovered

1.1.4 and 1.1.5 have argued for the necessity and reasonableness of attributing a fundamental worth and dignity to *every* living human being if we are to have a defensible understanding of justice. In so doing we have recovered from contemporary criticism, without benefit of religious premises, the basic truth about human worth and dignity which shapes the content of a sanctity of life ethic.

1.2 Justice and Killing

1.2.1 Killing for reasons incompatible with recognition of human dignity

Anyone who causes the death of another human being with intent to do so (i.e. who intentionally kills by 'act' or omission) acts on the basis that there is some reason for thinking that the person killed should have died. Quite generally what one does intentionally is identified by reference to one's *chosen purpose* in acting (under that description which makes clear its perceived desirability) and the *means* which are chosen (under that description which makes clear their perceived relevance to the achievement of one's purpose). Both of these must feature in any adequate statement of why one is acting, i.e. in any adequate statement of one's *reasons* for doing precisely what one is doing.

It is clear that one can intentionally bring about someone's death **by an omission which is intended to bring about death**: one can want someone dead and one can bring it about that he dies precisely by choosing to omit to do what one *could* (and otherwise would) have done to keep him alive. When what one omits with such an intention to terminate life is not merely something one could have done but something one had a *duty* to do, then the law has rightly regarded such intentional omissions bringing about death as

126

murder.[14] There is no morally significant *general* distinction to be made between killing and letting die, and any attempt to rely on such a distinction is intellectually perilous.[15] One may let a patient die for perfectly sound reasons (see 2.2 below), but one may also 'let a patient die' for unacceptable reasons, including the absolutely unacceptable reason that one wants (however reluctantly) to hasten his death.

Both omissions contrary to duty which intentionally bring about someone's death and actions which intentionally cause death raise two questions which the person responsible should answer:

– Why was it that X should die?
– What entitled you to bring about the death?

Distinguishing between acceptable and unacceptable answers to the first question is the most fundamental task in determining what is justifiable killing.

Since it is in virtue of the worth and dignity which attaches to our humanity that we establish to *whom* justice is owing, recognition of that dignity is the precondition of human beings treating each other properly. That being so, any purported justification of killing must at the very least be *consistent* with recognising the dignity of every human being. What is *absolutely* excluded, therefore, is bringing about another's death for *reasons* incompatible with recognising the dignity of the person killed.

As we have already remarked, at the beginning of this subsection, the relevant reasons are identified in the description of one's intended course of action which identifies the perceived desirability of one's goal/purpose and the perceived relevance to one's goal of one's chosen means.

This general account of which causations of death are absolutely excluded by recognition of the basic worth and dignity of every human life (viz. those *intentional* causations decided upon for reasons incompatible with the recognition of human dignity) makes intelligible the *moral* significance of the distinction between intentional (intended) and (merely) foreseen causation of death. When death is merely foreseen, one's causing it does not feature among the reasons one has for acting, and so is not chosen whether as end or as means (and thus is not intended). Many worthwhile activities, entirely consistent with recognition of human dignity, would be made impossible if all foreseeable causation of death were forbidden (examples would be: high-risk surgery, the giving of opiates for pain control in doses likely to hasten death, high-risk sports).

It is clear that one of the motives of those who seek to show that there is no morally significant difference between intention and foresight is to make a

[14] R. v. Gibbins and Proctor (1918) 13 *Criminal Appeal Reports* 134.
[15] The Working Party of the British Medical Association which produced the 1988 Report on *Euthanasia* relies heavily on the distinction at crucial points throughout that document. (See below pp. 184–185.) Since the Report represents official BMA policy, this reliance on the distinction, together with unclarity about the scope of intention, influences the September 1992 *Discussion Paper on Treatment of Patients in Persistent Vegetative State* produced by the Medical Ethics Committee of the BMA. Even more regrettably, the Law Lords in *Bland*, following the lead of the doctors, also rely on the distinction, though clearly aware that it is untenable: see 6.2.1 below.

prohibition of the intentional causation of death seem as unreasonable as an absolute prohibition of foreseen causation of death would evidently be. It should now be clear why an absolute prohibition can justifiably cover at least some intentional causations of death, namely all those the reasons for which are incompatible with recognising the basic dignity of the persons to be killed. To allow such killings would be to grant that human beings may be treated as though their dignity were irrelevant to how one chose to act towards them.

1.2.2 Euthanasia: killing incompatible with recognition of human dignity

In this section it will be argued that the core reason a person proposing to carry out euthanasia would have to identify, to make intelligible what he sees to be the desirability of causing death, is a reason for action incompatible with recognising the dignity of the person to be killed.

It ought to be evident that the killing of a person for advantage or convenience is inconsistent with recognition of that person's dignity, for the person killed is certainly not treated as of equal dignity with those advantaged by his death. Much advocacy of non-voluntary euthanasia is motivated by the thought that it is advantageous to others, in relieving them of the burdens of care for the handicapped and senile.

Purported justifications for voluntary euthanasia, however, as also for much non-voluntary euthanasia, speak of it as a *benefit* or a *good* for the patient. If the reason for saying that death is desirable *qua* benefit to the patient is to be consistent with recognising the basic worth and dignity of the patient's life, then it cannot rest on tacitly assuming (or seeking to show) that no positive value attaches to that life. That assumption *would* be made if the reason for saying that death would benefit the patient were that it would terminate a condition of negative value, depriving the patient of nothing of positive value. Justifications of that type, if they have any place at all for recognising a value attaching to our humanity (and many do not), in effect treat it as a *commensurable* and therefore *eliminable* value in calculating the overall 'worth' of a life. But to treat the basic human dignity of some human beings as an eliminable value is to proceed by denying to those human beings their status as subjects of justice.

All standard justifications of voluntary euthanasia, in so far as they represent it as a benefit to the patient killed, do so in a way which is inconsistent with recognition of the basic dignity of every human being. Here are four standard patterns of justification:

(1) One justification[16] represents human existence as no more than the possibility of enjoying goods. A human life is a benefit in so far as it comes up to a standard of normality in the goods available in it. But if it sinks below that standard and is overtaken by evils it is overall an evil.[17] Deliberately to end a life in that condition (if the patient asks to have it ended) is to benefit the patient.

---

[16] Philippa Foot, 'Euthanasia', in her *Virtues and Vices*, Oxford: Basil Blackwell, 1978, pp.33–61, at p.34.
[17] *Ibid.*, p.43.

Clearly this justification of voluntary euthanasia as a beneficial choice begins from the premise that our mere existence has no worth or value as such. So the justification is not consistent with recognising the dignity of every human being.

(2) Sometimes an attempted justification of voluntary euthanasia will concede that human life has value, but then argue that this value can be eliminated by the realities of suffering.[18] But if one treats the value attaching to our humanity as eliminable by countervailing disvalues one denies that basic dignity belongs to every human being whatever his or her condition.

(3) Some justifications of voluntary euthanasia start from the premise that human lives do not essentially possess a basic dignity and value. What gives a life value, it is claimed, is the ability of the person whose life it is to find value in projects, activities and relationships. Without a felt, *subjective* sense of worth and value a life lacks value. If a person is competent he is the only possible authority on whether he enjoys a subjective sense of value. If he soberly says he doesn't, his life lacks value. And those who lack presently exercisable abilities for finding value in their lives in consequence lack lives of value.

A justification of euthanasia which relies on the assumption that human lives do not *essentially* possess value straightforwardly denies the basic dignity of every human being.

(4) Some proponents of voluntary euthanasia speak of recognising the dignity of the person to be killed while asserting that continued life is not in the interests of that person. But this is mystificatory rhetoric. If one says that someone's continued existence is not in the interests of that person one means that person would be better off dead, that the non-existence of that bodily person is of less disvalue than continued bodily existence. This could be true only if continued existence is reckoned to have a negative value, for death itself can hardly be thought to have positive value. So this form of justification is inconsistent with recognition of the basic dignity of every human being.

1.3 Autonomy and Killing

It will be said that the above argument against euthanasia, both voluntary and non-voluntary, is narrow-minded in basing itself exclusively on a doctrine of equal human dignity. It will be argued that at least in respect of voluntary euthanasia there is a case to be answered in its favour based on a right to personal autonomy. As already noted, there is much talk of 'conflicting moral principles of the sanctity of life and the right to personal autonomy'[19], and of the need to balance their differing claims. A reasoned

---

[18] James Rachels, 'Euthanasia' in T. Regan (ed) *Matters of Life and Death*, New York: Random House, 1980, pp.28–66, at p.46.

[19] See para.2 of the Special Report (9 March 1993) from the Select Committee of The House of Lords on Medical Ethics, echoing observations in the judgements in *Bland*.

assessment of such talk must depend on what kind of claims in the name of autonomy are well-grounded, and more particularly on whether 'a right to personal autonomy' ever reasonably overrides what is required by recognition of human dignity. Something, therefore, needs to be said in general terms about autonomy and a 'right to personal autonomy', and about its relation to the normative constraints on killing imposed by recognition of human dignity.

1.3.1 Autonomy and a 'Right' to Personal Autonomy

The words 'autonomy' and 'autonomous' are used in respect of a capacity, a condition and a right.

To be autonomous, as the word implies, is to be self-governed or self-directed or self-determining in the conduct of one's life; that is the condition. 'Autonomy' is used of the capacity to be self-directed in the conduct of one's life. 'Respect for autonomy' involves respect at least for this capacity. 'A right to autonomy' must be a right to at least *some* exercise of the capacity for self-direction in one's life. But what exercise of that capacity? The answer we give to that question must surely depend on the understanding we have of the value of autonomy.

Some semi-popular talk about autonomy and the right to have one's autonomy respected seems to suggest that what people value is doing what they want (in the sense of acting on the wants, wishes and desires they *happen* to have) as distinct from having to do what someone else wants.

But it seems fairly clear that the ability to do what one *happens* to want to do is not sufficient for self-government in the conduct of one's life. Someone whose condition is one of wanton self-indulgence does what he happens to want to do. What is valued in the capacity for self-government is at the very least our ability to evaluate our desires and to act selectively in accordance with our evaluations.

But will action in accordance with *any* kind of evaluation count as an exercise of autonomy? Our answer to this question will depend on what we think the point of self-government or self-direction is.

The capacity for self-government is properly exercised and developed with a view to the flourishing or well-being of the person who possesses it, and of the communities to which that person properly belongs in friendship and justice. If so exercised it is indeed an aspect of that flourishing. In what way is it an aspect?

Human happiness or well-being is not left to be wholly a matter of luck, or of grace which does not require willing cooperation; what we make of ourselves (our character) makes an important difference to whether or not we flourish as human beings. And our characters are decisively shaped by our chosen actions: these do not merely bring about effects external to us, they also serve to form our dispositions. A person's exercise of choice will in this way inescapably make for well-being or misery in his life.

So there is a clear case for valuing human choice, and hence for valuing the exercise of autonomy, precisely in so far as it serves to form in us those dispositions which are conducive to human flourishing.

People differ in their views on how wide an exercise of the capacity for self-direction should be respected. One very important factor in determining those differing views is whether or not one believes there is human knowledge of moral truths, that is, knowledge of the objective requirements we need to meet if we are to flourish as human beings.

If there is such knowledge, then it is clear why we should value the exercise of choice in conformity with that knowledge: for evidently that would be an exercise of autonomy which makes for human flourishing. But it would not be obvious why we should value exercises of autonomy at variance with the objective requirements of human flourishing.

Still, if there is to be choice one has to allow not just for the possibility but also for the reality of erroneous choices. So, necessarily, respect for autonomy must leave scope for *some* erroneous choices. But it does not follow that any and every exercise of choice is to be respected. We need to bear in mind why this capacity is to be valued; and if our choices seriously undermine in us the capacity to flourish as human beings, and a *fortiori* if they aim to damage aspects of this capacity in others, there is no reason of moral principle why those choices should be respected.

1.3.2 Autonomy and the Justification of Voluntary Euthanasia

Can a right to autonomy be invoked to justify voluntary euthanasia? It is important to recognise how limited a role in justification the actual request to be killed can play. Certainly the mere fact of a request in itself provides little reason for a doctor to kill a patient. Can we envisage a doctor thinking it justifiable to kill a patient just because the patient has asked to be killed? Hardly. Indeed, we can envisage many circumstances in which doctors who are not opposed in principle to euthanasia would refuse requests; as when they think the request is prompted by an erroneous view of the prognosis, or by some relievable depression, or by circumstances which can be readily changed. Any doctor who feels that a given patient still has a worthwhile life to live will not accede to a request for euthanasia from that patient. *By contrast, it is precisely the judgement that a patient no longer has a worthwhile life which will seem to justify euthanasia.* The role of this judgement in justifying euthanasia is not altered by the different grounds a doctor may have for arriving at it. Sometimes it will seem true on the basis of evidence which the doctor can independently take stock of: pain, degeneration, depression, wretched circumstances. At other times the judgement will be clinched in the doctor's mind only by what the patient asserts: that his life is no longer worth living.

A doctor, minded to think that at bottom a human life can have value only if the person whose life it is consciously finds value in it, may well accept, in the presence of some corroborative evidence, a patient's judgement that his life has irrevocably lost value and dignity. But that fact about the doctor's background reasoning is not a ground for thinking that the doctor is not himself responsible for the judgement that this patient no longer has a worthwhile life. For it is *this* judgement which will make it appear to *him* that a choice to bring about the patient's death is a beneficent choice.

Notwithstanding, then, that the killing which carries out voluntary euthanasia is requested, the justification of that killing rests centrally on the contention that the patient no longer has a worthwhile life. *But precisely that contention is inconsistent with recognising the continuing worth and dignity of the patient's life.*

In any apparent conflict between, on the one hand, the requirement that we do not deny equal human dignity and respect for the sanctity of human life and, on the other, the putative claims of respect for autonomy, the principle of the sanctity of human life must always trump those claims. For recognition of equal human dignity is fundamental to recognition of all human beings as subjects of justice.

There is no authentic conflict between rightly respecting the sanctity of human life and rightly respecting autonomy. The exercise of human autonomy in giving shape, direction and character to a human life is not a source of value and dignity which is properly at *odds* with the fundamental source of human worth and dignity in human nature itself. For, as we saw (1.1.4), what makes it reasonable to recognise human nature as the source of our basic worth and dignity as human beings is the fact that our nature in its development is intrinsically directed to human fulfilment and human good. And what best makes sense of the ideal of respect for autonomy is the role played by free choice in the achievement of that fulfilment to which our nature is directed; for self-determining choice is integral to that achievement. But if the moral significance of autonomy is to be understood in that way, then the value of autonomy is derivative from, and reflective of, that which gives value to our humanity. So it should be clear that the claims of autonomy cannot properly extend to choices which are inconsistent with recognising the basic worth and dignity of every human being.

1.3.3 Autonomy and the Justification of Non-Voluntary Euthanasia

It is sometimes said[20] that debility, degeneration and dependency experienced by those who have become permanently incompetent, or the undignified way in which (sometimes unavoidably) they are treated, are inconsistent with the meaning and character they had given to their lives while competent. It is then claimed, or insinuated, that this meaning and character have been the exclusive source of dignity in the lives of many such people so that their present condition should be recognised as completely depriving them of dignity. For this reason, therefore, it would be beneficent to put an end to their lives.

Sufficient has already been said to show that such a line of reasoning provides no defensible ground for euthanasia of the incompetent who were

[20] For example by Ronald Dworkin, 'The Right to Death' at pp.15–16; *Life's Dominion*, ch.7.

formerly competent. As many of those nurses and others who care for such persons know, and testify to by their dispositions and acts of solidarity, communion or friendship with them, these people, though sadly weakened or wounded and scarcely or no longer able to exercise their autonomy, remain the very same persons they always were. Their state is in a sense undignified, but it is *not an indignity* (of the kind inflicted upon people by demeaning actions). Right down to their deaths they continue to share in the radical equality-in-dignity of all human beings.

1.4 Sanctity of Life and Autonomy: Conclusion

The teaching of Christian tradition about the sanctity of life can be recast in secular terms as a doctrine of equal basic worth and dignity. This doctrine has to be assumed if there is to be a non-arbitrary understanding of who are the subjects of justice, but the intrinsic reasonableness of the assumption can be defended.

Since we must hold all human beings to possess an ineliminable worth and dignity if they are to be recognised as subjects of justice, any justification for killing incompatible with recognising that worth and dignity is inadmissible.

Justifications of voluntary and non-voluntary euthanasia as beneficent rely *essentially* on the judgement that, overall, the present life of the person to be killed is of negative value (not worthwhile). But such a judgement is incompatible with recognising the ineliminable worth and dignity of the person to be killed. Hence intentional killing (by act or omission) for euthanasiast reasons falls under the absolute prohibition of intentional killing of the innocent (itself the core requirement of respect for the sanctity of life).

2. The Duties of Doctors: Duties of Treatment and Duties of Care

2.1 The Purpose of Medicine and Duties of Treatment

Doctors are skilled practitioners of the art of medicine. The generic skills of diagnosis, prognosis and treatment draw on a basis of scientific knowledge, itself based on research.

It is of the first importance in seeking to define the duties of doctors in respect of treatment to be clear about the purpose of medicine. The purpose of medicine is the restoration and maintenance of health (or of some approximation to health) or the palliation of symptoms. Traditionally, health has been understood as that condition of the body in virtue of which it functions well as an organic whole, so that the individual both enjoys physical vitality in itself and is well-placed to achieve some of the other goods intrinsic to human well-being.[1] Health is valued as inseparably an intrinsic and an instrumental good. The palliation of symptoms (when cure is not achievable) aims precisely to control those impediments to participation in other human goods which arise from organic malfunctioning; in other words, given that not even an approximation to health can be achieved, one aims to secure as *tolerable* a state of the organism as possible so that conscious living (with family and friends and others) may continue. Thus, palliative medicine, in deploying techniques of pain control, is focussed, just like other forms of medicine, on the organic component of our aptitude to share in other human goods.[2]

The prolongation of life has not traditionally been understood as an independent goal of medicine, without reference to the good of health. It has been considered a justifiable aim only in so far as a patient has had some continuing capacity for organic well-functioning sufficient to allow him to share in some of the goods of human life (e.g. contemplation, the exercise of choice, communication, or – and these are particularly relevant to babies – some form of play, the affection of others, the enjoyment of one's own vitality).

The recognition that prolongation of life has not been considered as *per se* an objective of medical practice should help to dispose of a radical misunderstanding of the requirements of respect for the sanctity of life which has been encouraged in recent years by those who wish to subvert the core requirement (that one ought never to kill the innocent intentionally). The

---

[1] A clear exposition of this understanding may be found, for instance, in Leon R Kass, M. D., *Toward A More Natural Science. Biology and Human Affairs* (New York: The Free Press 1985), especially Chapter 6: 'The End of Medicine and the Pursuit of Health', pp.157–186.

[2] This is what symptom control is *aiming for*, except in the extreme situation – now, in principle, rare – in which acute pain is so intractable that the patient has to be rendered unconscious. What justifies doing that, given the rationale for palliative medicine offered in the text? It is the belief that for *this* patient *conscious* participation in other human goods has been rendered impossible by overwhelming pain so that there is nothing further to be achieved by maintaining a state of consciousness which is nothing other than consciousness of pain. But that understanding of the patient's situation does not amount to judging that the very existence of this patient is without value.

misunderstanding has been to the effect that those who claim that a life has worth or value must mean that one should seek to prolong that life.[3]

Section 1 has shown that recognition of human dignity would require that a doctor should never intentionally kill a patient. The fundamental worth and dignity of every human life has its source in the human nature each of us shares precisely in existing as a human being. A proposal to kill a patient is a proposal to put an end to that person's existence. But such a proposal cannot be justified for a reason compatible with recognising the worth and dignity of his very existence.

It is in the nature of human beings that they die. There is nothing that we have come to know in recent years which suggests that medicine should revise its traditional goals and seek to defy the inevitability of death. A doctor's decision not to seek to prolong a patient's life need not find its justification in reasons entailing any denial of the fundamental worth or dignity of that patient's life. There may be sound reasons for such a decision, compatible with respect for the fundamental dignity of the patient; these reasons are discussed in the next section.

It follows from the nature of the purpose which the institution of medicine exists to serve that the central duty of a doctor to an ill patient is that of competently employing those medical skills relevant either to aiding and abetting whatever capacity the patient may have for a return to health or to palliating those symptoms arising from disease or disability which impede a patient's remaining capacity to live well.

2.2 Limits on Duties of Treatment

2.2.1 Patient Consent and Duties of Treatment

Two statements by Pope Pius XII may usefully introduce the topic of patient consent in relation to a doctor's duties of treatment. In 1952 he said:

'First of all, one must suppose that the doctor, as a private person, cannot take any measure or try any intervention without the consent of the patient. The doctor has only that power over the patient which the latter gives him, be it explicitly, or implicitly and tacitly. The patient for his part cannot confer rights which he does not possess'[4]

And in 1957 he made the same point in connection with restating the traditional norms on 'ordinary and extraordinary treatment':

'The rights and duties of the doctor are correlative to those of the patient. The doctor, in fact, has no separate or independent right where the patient is concerned. In general he can take action only if the patient explicitly or implicitly, directly or indirectly, gives him permission.'[5]

These statements reflect a centuries-long tradition of theological thinking on

---

[3] The misunderstanding features prominently in the writings of Helga Kuhse and Peter Singer. Its influence on the writings of Mary Warnock is also evident.

[4] Pope Pius XII, Address to the First International Congress of Histopathology, September 13, 1952. *Acta Apostolicae Sedis* 44 (1952), pp.779–89.

[5] Pope Pius XII, Address to Gregor Mendel Genetic Institute, November 24, 1957; *Acta Apostolicae Sedis 49 (1957)*, pp.1027–1033.

the doctor-patient relationship, which offers no support for the unbridled paternalism which is sometimes said to have been accommodated by a traditional ethic of medical practice.

It is important to understand the underlying reasons for the place given to patient consent in the traditional thinking articulated by Pope Pius XII.

Medicine is a body of practices which are given their unity by the varied relations they have to the good of health. But the good of health as it is instantiated in the lives of individuals is an aspect of their personal well-being. Precisely as a personal good each person's health is primarily his responsibility. Once a person has reached that stage of physical development at which he is also able to exercise responsible choice, health is effectively promoted only through the choices and commitments of the person himself. For some the choices at a certain stage of their lives need be no more than moderation and good sense in regard to what they eat and drink; for others the required choices are much more exacting.

The view that there is an intimate connection between health and personal responsibility implies that health cannot be viewed as a commodity which one can acquire by going to a doctor's surgery or to hospital. Health is effectively promoted only when a person takes responsibility for his health. The doctor's responsibility to aid and abet the restoration of health can best be discharged if the basic responsibility of the patient is recognised and respected. This means that the doctor must, within limits, respect the competent patient's choice.

There is a second important reason for insisting on respect for the competent patient's choice. Because health is a personal good it may be more or less intensively realised in one's life. The degree to which it is achieved depends in part upon the place other commitments occupy in one's life and the demands they make on one. What persons devote themselves to is a matter of choice influenced by aptitude, opportunity, inclination and inspiration. Sometimes it is a consequence of a serious and worthy choice of a way of life that health is impaired and one loses the opportunity to recover it. A doctor lacks the competence and so the authority to tell us to abandon the shaping commitments of our lives.

Because health is a personal good, an aspect of the flourishing of persons, it is wrong to neglect health problems simply because of laziness, it is wrong to damage health through self-indulgence, and it is wrong because of cowardice to avoid seeking the treatment one needs. While such behaviour is morally unreasonable, it is rarely the case that a uniform course of action is alone morally reasonable: the place one can give to fostering or restoring the good of health in one's own life will depend upon the responsibilities which arise from one's other basic commitments. So for this reason, too, the choice of the patient must be respected.

Nothing in this way of explaining the significance and importance of patient consent suggests that the rationale for its true significance is the right of patients to construct (and deconstruct) their lives as they will, providing

136

only that they do not damage the legitimate interests of non-consenting parties.

The second line of argument for the importance of patient consent suggests that a doctor has a duty to provide therapeutic or palliative treatment of a kind compatible with the reasonable commitments a person has undertaken, even if the 'compatible' treatment is not, in the doctor's view, the ideal therapy for the patient's condition. That kind of compromise is necessary and reasonable.

But there are patient wishes a doctor cannot justifiably accommodate. One such wish is the demand for euthanasia: the case against accommodating it has been fully explained in Section 1. At this point it would be appropriate to add consideration of the request for aid in suicide.

2.2.2 Duties of Treatment and Suicide

A request for euthanasia is not, of course, a request for assistance in suicide. A request for euthanasia from a patient to a doctor is a request that the doctor kill the patient. Suicide is the carrying out of a choice directly to kill oneself. One can carry out such a choice either by a positive course of action, e.g. by taking a lethal substance, or by deliberately omitting life sustaining treatment or care (precisely in order to end one's life).

Just as willingness to carry out euthanasiast killing rests on a false valuation of the life of another, so willingness to commit deliberately chosen suicide rests on a false valuation of one's own life (to the effect that it is no longer worthwhile). Since that valuation is incompatible with respect for one's own fundamental dignity, it is morally impermissible to aid a person to carry out an act of suicide.[6]

It is clear what this conclusion excludes when suicide is to be accomplished by an act such as taking a lethal dose of a drug: it excludes providing the necessary quantity of the drug with the intention of enabling the person to commit suicide.

When a competent person proposes to commit suicide by refusing necessary life-prolonging treatment (e.g. insulin for diabetes) or by refusing basic care (e.g. being fed) one does not collaborate by failing to override his proposal. The alternative to respecting the requirement of consent is to take

---

[6] The Voluntary Euthanasia Society falsely imply that the decriminalization of suicide in 1961 involved recognition of 'the right of individuals to determine when their own life was insupportable' [*The Last Right. The Need for Voluntary Euthanasia* revised edition, London: The VES, 1989, p.4] Suicide was decriminalized because it was felt that prosecution of those who had attempted it could only make more difficult any attempt to help them retrieve a true sense of their worth and dignity. It remains that suicidal intentions rest on what the law *must* regard as a false valuation of one's own life (as of any other human life). And that is why aiding and abetting suicide rightly remains a crime. It is not perhaps surprising that an organization such as the VES should misrepresent the implications of the decriminalization of suicide, but it is surprising to find Hoffmann LJ and Lord Goff claim (in *Bland* [1993] 2 WLR at 351–2, 367) that decriminalization of suicide 'was a recognition that the principle of self-determination should in that case [suicide] prevail over the sanctity of life'. The parliamentary debates on the Suicide Bill (see e.g. *House of Commons Debates*, 19 July 1961, col. 1425–6) make it clear that the Act's decriminalizing of the act of the suicide himself had nothing to do with a 'principle of self-determination' which is in any case incompatible with the Act's prohibition of all forms of assistance in suicide.

137

a suicidal proposal as evidence that the person in question is incompetent and to force upon him the treatment or care which is in his best interests. But it is unreasonable to treat suicidal proposals as though they were always evidence of incompetence; that would be to act as if people could never be guilty of suicide.

Consideration will be given in Section 4 (Advance Directives) to what a doctor's moral responsibilities are towards an incompetent patient who while competent had left suicidally motivated instructions for his medical treatment in specified circumstances.

2.2.3 General Grounds for Limiting Treatment

There are two quite general grounds for limiting treatment: (i) one is that a particular treatment is failing to achieve its therapeutic or palliative goal (i.e. it is inefficacious treatment); (ii) the other is that it involves burdensome consequences which it is not reasonable to expect a patient to bear. When the patient is competent his own judgement of what is a tolerable burden must be decisive.

(i) Inefficacious treatment

Since prolongation of life is not an independent goal of medicine, the possibility of continuing to prolong life does not independently create an obligation to continue to provide life prolonging treatment. If a patient is in the terminal phase of dying it will normally be the case that it is clearly inappropriate to persist with life-prolonging treatment unless that treatment has distinct palliative benefits.

More broadly, therapeutic treatment is to be judged inefficacious if the condition of the patient is such that it would be impossible to secure even an approximation to health in that patient, i.e. some desirable degree of well-functioning of the organism as a whole. It is on precisely this ground that it would be reasonable to withdraw specifically therapeutic treatment from a patient who has been securely diagnosed as irreversibly in a persistent vegetative state (PVS). For the organic condition of the patient has been rendered so seriously defective that it is impossible to achieve a desirable approximation to health (viz. the well-functioning of the organism as a whole).

To say that it may be reasonable to withdraw *therapeutic treatment* (including, for example, antibiotics for recurrent infection) from PVS patients is not to say that it is reasonable to withdraw ordinary care from them. (For a discussion of what is required in this respect see 2.3.1 below.)

Doctors do not have a duty to provide inefficacious treatment, and patients (and families of patients) cannot reasonably require such treatment of doctors. But it is very important that in answering a question about the worthwhileness of a given treatment a doctor should focus very firmly on whether the treatment can deliver medical benefits (cure, mitigation of disability, palliation of symptoms) and should not allow the basis of his answer to shift to a judgement on the worthwhileness of the patient's life, so that the question he comes to answer is whether the patient is worth benefitting. For a negative answer to that question would seem to justify not merely withholding a particular medical treatment but withholding all medical treatment and all basic care in order to end what is judged a worthless life.

(ii) Excessively burdensome treatment

Doctors do not have a duty to provide treatment which a competent patient would reasonably reject on the ground that it was in some respect excessively burdensome in its consequences. Typically treatment will hold out some prospects of benefit (specifically for prolonging a life) but will also involve burdensome consequences. There is no single right answer to the question of when those burdens become sufficiently burdensome to justify discontinuing a treatment. Providing a patient has discharged serious duties which he may have, such as duties to family, and providing he is not motivated by suicidal intentions, it may be reasonable for him to reject life-prolonging treatment because the burdens consequent upon it are more than he is disposed to put up with. Burdens may take the following forms:

(a) treatment may be excessively *costly*: the cost in question may be to an individual, to a family, or to a health service. A patient considering the financial consequences of treatment for different payers/providers may reasonably decide to forgo treatment even before a point is reached at which it would be obvious that acceptance of treatment would be unfair to others.

(b) Treatment may be excessively damaging to possibilities one cherishes. It may be reasonable to refuse chemotherapy for cancer because of its very likely effect on other bodily functions; e.g. that it renders one sterile and one is recently married and wanting a child.

(c) Treatment may be excessively painful: there will be limits to each individual's courage.

(d) Treatment may be excessively taxing psychologically: a broad species of burden, of particular relevance when considering treatment for the very elderly. When there is progressive failure of a number of systems of the body aggressive therapy can prove very oppressive.

(e) Treatment can be excessively restrictive on physical liberty: thus, doctors may promise an elderly patient a further year of life providing she remains under their constant care in hospital. She may reasonably want to spend the time remaining to her in visiting her children and grandchildren who are willing to give her ordinary nursing care.

(f) Finally, treatment may be excessively disruptive of one's inner life: thus thought, conversation, prayer may be most important to a patient, who therefore reasonably refuses the analgesia which dulls his mind.

These six categories of burden [a–f] are burdens consequent upon treatment.

139

They provide a fairly clear way of analysing the elements that can make for an acceptable or unacceptable *quality of life* when that phrase is used in a justifiable fashion to refer to the predictable consequences of treatment.[7]

A competent patient who rejects *treatment* because of its excessively burdensome consequences rejects it because of a judgement on the treatment not because of a judgement on the fundamental worth of his own continued existence. Such rejections may at times be faulted because they display a lack of prudence or courage, but they should not be faulted as euthanasiast.

2.2.4 Duties of Treatment to the Incompetent

Clearly doctors should not give inefficacious medical treatment to the incompetent. In this context a standard synonym for 'inefficacious' is 'futile'. Some judge treatment futile when they are inclined to think the life of the patient 'futile' (meaning 'no longer worthwhile'), and they think this judgement particularly well-founded if there is evidence for thinking that, in anticipation of his present condition, an incompetent patient took such a view of it while still competent. But any such judgement (and especially one invoked to justify the withholding of treatment with a view to ending the patient's life) is, for reasons already explained (see 1.3), an unacceptable basis for treatment decisions.

A doctor would be justified in withholding or withdrawing medical treatment the consequences of which a proxy decision-maker reasonably judged to be excessively burdensome. A proxy's decision would generally be reasonable if it was clear that a competent patient in similar circumstances would have good reason for refusing treatment. However, in assessing burdens a proxy needs to take account of the difference that incompetence itself may make to the burdensome character of treatment. Sometimes, sheer inability to understand what doctors are attempting and the painful, even though temporary, effects of treatment, may create considerable fear and repugnance, so that treatment which would not be excessively burdensome for the competent may become so for the incompetent. Incomprehension can also limit the ability to cooperate with certain forms of treatment.

Both a proxy decision-maker for an incompetent patient and the doctor responsible for the care of that patient owe it to the patient to secure justice in his treatment. This means in summary that –

(i) it is absolutely excluded that management of the patient should be directed to ending his life;

(ii) where there is scope for securing through a course of treatment significant medical benefits, without excessive burdens in consequence, that course of treatment should be provided;

(iii) if any suggested course of treatment which promises some medical benefits also carries with it some likelihood of unacceptably burdensome consequences then those responsible for treatment should be

---

[7] The phrase is frequently used with unacceptably euthanasiast implications to refer to the very worthwhileness of a life.

140

scrupulous in assessing the burdens of treatment. They should wish to ascertain that prospective burdens truly would be considerable before deciding that potentially beneficial treatment should be withheld.

2.3 Doctors' duties of ordinary care towards hospitalised patients

When a patient is admitted to hospital for treatment, responsibility is assumed not merely for providing him with beneficial medical treatment but also for providing him with what is ordinarily needed if the patient is to continue living: nourishment, shelter, warmth, hygiene. Dependence on a doctor in respect of such needs cannot be repudiated simply because distinctively medical goals are not achievable. No one would ordinarily doubt this. It is against this background that we should consider the question of tube-feeding of those diagnosed as irreversibly in a 'persistent vegetative state'.

2.3.1 Feeding the PVS patient

In considering what a doctor's duties of ordinary care are towards a PVS patient certain propositions should not be in doubt:

 (i) PVS patients are living human beings, albeit gravely impaired. (See 1.1. 5 above.) As living human beings they possess the ineliminable worth and dignity of our common humanity.
 (ii) Since they are living human beings it is incompatible with recognition of their dignity to judge their very existence to be without worth or value. If a PVS patient's life is judged to be without worth it will indeed seem reasonable to conclude that he would be better off dead, and, accordingly, reasonable to make his death the *object* of clinical management.
 (iii) If one aims to kill a patient by deliberate omission of treatment or care, (i.e. omission decided upon precisely to bring about death), one is intentionally killing. Such intentional killing of the innocent by planned omission is as gravely wrong as intentional killing by positive act.[8]
 (iv) Death can occur as a foreseen consequence of omitting to do something one had good reason not to do. In such a case one cannot be held to be guilty of the death.
 (v) PVS patients are entitled to the ordinary care to which any impaired and vulnerable person is normally entitled.

Given the exposition of the *limited* goals of *medical* treatment presented in this submission, one might argue that enteral feeding of a PVS patient (i.e.

---

[8] A majority of the Law Lords in *Bland* accepted the proposition that those who have the care of patients in a condition such as the judges described in the case of Tony Bland may rightly adopt a pattern of care *with the intention, purpose or aim* of terminating the lives or bringing about the deaths of those patients. See: 'the proposed conduct has the aim . . . of terminating the life of Anthony Bland; . . . the conduct will be, as it is intended to be, the cause of death' (Lord Mustill, [1993] 2 WLR at 388, 397); 'the whole purpose of stopping artificial feeding is to bring about the death of Anthony Bland' (Lord Browne-Wilkinson at 383); 'the intention to bring about the patient's death is there' (Lord Lowry at 379).

feeding by nasogastric tube or gastrostomy) is *medical* treatment, and since the limited goals of medical treatment are not achievable in a PVS patient (see 2.2.3 above) there can be no continuing obligation to supply enteral feeding once the irreversibility of the persistent vegetative state has been confirmed. Hence if one were to discontinue enteral feeding one might do so simply because there is no obligation to continue, and without entertaining any intention to cause the patient's death, even though foreseeing that discontinuance of feeding will cause his death.

The objection to this view is the weakness of the case for saying that enteral feeding is *medical treatment* rather than ordinary care. The definition of medical treatment should include *some* reference to the distinctive goals of medicine (the restoration and maintenance of health, or of some approximation to health, and the palliation of symptoms), so that medical treatment will have some identifiable therepeutic or palliative function. Enteral feeding serves neither such function but the ordinary function of nourishing the patient.

It can hardly be that just *anything* done by a doctor in the course of caring for patients is to count as medical treatment; if it were, then the distinction between medical treatment and ordinary care would collapse. Nor will it do to say that the *intrusive* or 'invasive' character of what is done to the patient makes it medical treatment.[9] Any adult finding a choking child might reach to the back of the child's mouth to pull his tongue forward. Nor is it very convincing to suggest[10] that what makes enteral feeding medical treatment in the case of PVS patients is the fact that it substitutes for an ordinary bodily function. Many PVS patients retain some degree of swallowing reflex, and they standardly possess a capacity to digest food in the normal way. Enteral feeding is an expeditious way of delivering to the PVS patient the food any human being needs, and it serves the same purpose that eating and drinking do.

It is true that it normally requires a doctor's decision to first establish enteral feeding, though it will often not require specifically medical skills to maintain feeding by nasogastric tube. It is also true that the doctor's purpose in making such a decision will normally be to sustain the patient while diagnostic investigations are carried out and an attempt is made to establish an appropriate therapeutic regimen. But the tube feeding itself is not therapy and is not reasonably discontinued on the grounds that *therapeutic* efforts have proved futile.[11]

---

[9] No member of the House of Lords in *Bland* questioned Lord Justice Butler-Sloss's remark that it is 'uncomfortable' to 'attempt to draw a line between different forms of feeding such as spoon-feeding a helpless patient or inserting a tube ...' ([1993] 2 WLR at 343).

[10] As Professor Jennett did as an expert witness before the Court in *Bland* (see [1993] 2 WLR at 325). Dr. Keith Andrews, who has very extensive experience in the management of PVS patients, maintained before the Court that enteral feeding is a part of ordinary care. His reason for doing so related to the function of enteral feeding.

[11] If it is morally acceptable to withdraw artificial ventilation from an irreversibly comatose patient why should it not be morally acceptable to withdraw artificial feeding? Artificial ventilation appears no more a therapeutic activity than artificial feeding. There is, however, a significant difference between the two activities relevant to determining whether they are properly classified as ordinary care.

Feeding people (in a variety of ways, from setting dishes before them to spoonfeeding them) is part of

In *Bland* what the Law Lords approved was discontinuing tubefeeding on the basis of a medical judgement that tubefeeding had become futile because continued existence in Tony Bland's condition was not a benefit; in other words, Tony Bland's existence was without worth or value. In consequence, as Lord Browne-Wilkinson observed:

'What is proposed in the present case is to adopt a course with the intention of bringing about Anthony Bland's death. As to the element of intention or mens rea, in my judgement there can be no real doubt that it is present in this case: the whole purpose of stopping artificial feeding is to bring about the death of Anthony Bland.'[12]

There can certainly be a sound case for stopping tubefeeding if a patient is in the final phase of dying or if tubefeeding involves gross burdens for a patient (though the latter reason hardly applies to PVS patients who are supposed to be insensate). And in certain situations of extreme scarcity or disorder (which do not obtain in our society) doctors and nurses might reasonably neglect the permanently unconscious and other severely damaged patients because of overriding duties to others.

our *ordinary care* of them. At various times in our lives, either because of underdevelopment or decline or accident, we can be helpless in regard to obtaining or ingesting food. If a mother fails to set dishes before her young children she will starve them. If she had failed to spoonfeed them when they were still younger she would have starved them. Tubefeeding (once one has embarked upon it) is most naturally understood as the *extension* of an ordinary pattern of care, and as owed to someone in the way of such care.

By contrast, 'making people breathe' is not a part of our ordinary care of people; 'oxygenating' others is not a standard part of what we do for each other. And the reason is obvious: at any normal stage of extra-uterine life we can spontaneously breathe and the air is there to be inhaled. Consequently, supplying for the inability to breathe is *not* an extension of an activity of ordinary care. It is an intervention which is more reasonably interpreted as having its justification in the achievability of properly medical goals (the restoration of health, or of some approximation to health, or the palliation of symptoms). But if those goals are not achievable there can be no obligation to continue ventilation.

[12] [1993] 2 WLR at 383.

3. Withdrawing Treatment and Intentional Killing

This section simply draws together the relevant distinctions which have already been sufficiently explained in earlier sections.

3.1 It is certainly morally unacceptable to aim or intend to bring about someone's death for a reason or reasons incompatible with recognising the basic worth and dignity of that person as a human being, and incompatible, therefore, with justice. One's intent to bring about someone's death will be equally unacceptable whether it is achieved by

    (a) a positive act, such as a lethal injection;
    (b) the omission of treatment decided upon precisely to hasten death;
    (c) the omission of care decided upon precisely to hasten death.

3.2 It can be morally acceptable to withhold or withdraw treatment precisely because it is reasonably judged inefficacious (futile) or excessively burdensome (2.2.3), even if one foresees that in consequence death will occur earlier than it might otherwise have done. One's *reason* for withholding treatment is not a judgement about the desirability of putting an end to the patient's life but a judgement about the desirability of putting an end to *treatment*, either because it is inefficacious or because it is imposing excessive burdens on the patient.

3.3 There are few circumstances (they are noted at the end of 2.3.1) in which it is reasonable to withdraw ordinary care, especially feeding, of a patient.

4. The Role of Advance Directives and Proxy Decision-makers

Here, as in previous sections, we consider the moral case for certain broad conceptions of what is desirable rather than the details of legislative proposals.[1]

4.1 Advance Directives

4.1.1 The unilateral emphasis on autonomy

(a) Many proposals for advance directive legislation are vitiated by a unilateral emphasis on autonomy in their justification, with little or no recognition that the individual in his or her self-determination may rightly be expected to acknowledge a number of moral norms. Without recognition of norms about the wrongness of suicide and euthanasia (accomplished either by act or omission), apologias for advance directives articulated in terms of the claims of autonomy must seem to justify the inclusion of euthanasia and assistance in suicide within the effective scope of advance directives.[2]

(b) A strictly unilateral emphasis on autonomy leads to the view that the *sole* determinant of how one should be treated when incompetent is the anticipatory decision one made when competent. But the consequences of such a position are fairly obviously unacceptable. All advance directive legislation provides that, while competent, makers of declarations may readily revoke them. That provision acknowledges that for a variety of reasons one may come to recognise original directives as mistaken. But why should one's family or friends be prevented by *one's present incompetence* from making decisions on one's behalf on the basis of one's *best interests*?

(c) Some defend treating as immutable and effective an unrevoked anticipatory decision about treatment made by a person when competent.[3] They often base their defence on the claim that those acting on the now incompetent person's behalf are properly confined to the role of exercising *his* right to self-determination.

The claim is based on a muddle. There are indeed rights protecting

---

[1] Some parts of this section draw verbatim on John Finnis, 'Living Will Legislation', other parts draw on Luke Gormally, 'The Living Will: the ethical framework of a recent Report' (for references see footnote 1, p.115).

[2] It cannot be true to say in general, as Lord Goff does say in *Airedale NHS Trust v Bland* [1993] 2 WLR at 367–8, that in the implementation of anticipatory refusals of life-prolonging treatment 'there is no question of the patient having committed suicide, nor therefore of the doctor having aided or abetted him in doing so'.

[3] For example, Dworkin, *Life's Dominion*, pp. 226–229. Dworkin believes a doctor would violate the autonomy of a manifestly happy patient with Alzheimer's disease if he refused to act on an advance directive made by the patient requiring that he be killed if he were to suffer Alzheimer's. Dworkin acknowledges, p.228, the shocking character of the conclusion towards which his argument drives him, but persists in his fictitious construct, so-called 'precedent autonomy', which (in tandem with the unbalanced primacy he here attributes to autonomy) impels him towards these conclusions.

145

one's fundamental interests and well-being (life, privacy, reputation, bodily integrity, etc.) which can be vindicated and, in that sense, exercised on one's behalf while one is incompetent. But a right which is a right to form one's own intentions and make and execute one's own choices, simply cannot be exercised by the choices of another. Just as the refusal (which may but need not be unjustified) to carry out a dead man's last will and testament frustrates the intentions, purposes and will which he once had but does not and cannot violate his autonomy, so the refusal to carry out a now-incompetent person's unrevoked advance directive that he be killed if permanently incompetent frustrates his earlier intention but does not and cannot violate his autonomy; he no longer has any autonomy to be exercised, though he retains his ineliminable human dignity, and the rights and interests which should be respected in virtue of that dignity.[4]

(d) The radical incoherence of the notion that the incompetent have *autonomy rights* (as distinct from dignity and welfare rights) becomes more evident when those incompetent persons who have never made any advance healthcare directive are declared to have an autonomy right exercisable on their behalf, even by an agent or 'guardian' or other 'representative' whose decision is to refuse treatment on the ground that these patients, were they competent and reasonable, would choose to refuse treatment and accept death, perhaps not for their own supposed benefit but at any rate for the benefit of others liable to the costs and burdens of caring for them.

The unbalanced primacy of autonomy is thus tightly connected with the notion of *substituted judgement*. In turn, the widespread appeal to the 'standard' of substituted judgement, in preference to the alternative standard of the patient's best interests, sets all concerned on a royal road towards decisions to bring about the death of incompetent persons on the plea that if they were reasonable they would choose to seek death, if not by 'active' then by 'passive euthanasia'.

What is characteristically missing in much modern discussion of autonomy and self-determination is any strong sense that the most fundamental expression of respect for the dignity of human beings is not respect for autonomy but respect for the good of human beings. When persons have *exercisable capacities* for self-determination then respect for their self-determination is integral to respect for their good as persons: for it is in and through choice that they have the possibility of shaping their characters for good (or ill). But when persons do not yet, or no longer, possess presently exercisable capacities for self-determination, self-determination cannot be an essential ingredient, so to speak, in what one respects in respecting their

---

[4] Writers who place a one-sided emphasis on autonomy in defending the claim that *all* advance directives should be respected will standardly admit, as does Dworkin, that even the (real) autonomy of the competent is often rightly overridden (see *Life's Dominion* pp. 192–3, 229–30). Dworkin, however, makes little or no effort to articulate a coherent account of when 'paternalism' is justified and when unjustified.

146

good. Any exercise of self-determination which seeks to determine what should (or should not) happen to one, if and when one comes to be incompetent, should be respected only to the extent that doing so in consistent with respecting the good of the now incompetent patient.

4.1.2 Advance declarations and the burdensomeness of treatment

It is certainly consistent with respecting the good of an incompetent patient to take account of the likely burdensome consequences of a course of treatment when considering it. [See 2.2.3(ii)] Now, whether certain consequences will amount to an undue burden of, say, pain or psychological stress for a patient will often depend upon the individual dispositions and circumstances of that patient. So there certainly is a role for advance *declarations* (rather than *directives*) in which a person, while competent, offers written advice on the sorts of consequence of treatment which he anticipates he would find oppressively hard to bear. That advice should then be taken carefully into account when doctors and others are deciding whether or not to proceed with a particular course of treatment which is likely to have significantly burdensome consequences.

However, the evidence supplied by the kind of advance declaration envisaged here could never be the sole determinant of the treatment decisions made. For in deciding treatment for the incompetent one would always have to make a judgement about whether it would be in the interests of the patient to bear with certain significant burdens in order to secure the benefits which treatment offered – benefits one could envisage the patient appreciating.

4.1.3 Advance directives and the refusal of ordinary care

Some patients who make advance directives, stipulating withdrawal of tubefeeding in certain conditions, do so for suicidal reasons, believing that life in the anticipated conditions would not be worthwhile and choosing (prospectively) the withdrawal of tubefeeding precisely as a means of terminating their life. When it is plain to a doctor that the intentions of a patient who has made such a directive are of this sort, the doctor should certainly not put the directive into effect, for to do so would be to aid in the carrying out of a suicidal intention.

However, it should also be recognised that an advance directive stipulating that in certain circumstances one would not want the continued provision of significantly expensive care, including tubefeeding, need not be suicidal. Persons making such directives may have in mind that even tubefeeding and nursing care, while not burdensome to them, could prove financially very burdensome to others. They might truly wish that the resources be used to meet other needs. This reason for rejecting such care is, then, not a false valuation of what their life might be at some future time. Rather it is a desire not to take up resources which they think disproportionate, to the detriment of others. That desire shows a sensitivity to the needs of

147

others, and one would not be acting in a way contrary to a person's dignity if one honoured a directive which was prompted by what is generally agreed to be an admirable desire and involved an acceptance of death rather than the choice of death as a means or an end.[5]

Many patients (perhaps a majority) who stipulate that in certain circumstances they should not receive tubefeeding will do so in terms which leave it unclear whether their intentions are suicidal or not. It seems to us that someone who has made an advance directive seeking to limit not care (or expensive care) in general but quite specifically the provision of nourishment probably has in mind that doctors should aim to bring about his death by means of this omission. And sometimes doctors will have reliable evidence from other sources that a patient's intentions were suicidal. In either kind of case, doctors should not withdraw or withhold tubefeeding. If the law as declared by the House of Lords in *Bland* is inconsistent with this, and imposes a legal duty to withhold tubefeeding in every case where consent has been withdrawn, the law should be amended by Parliament so as to restore its coherence with the principles of the Suicide Act 1961 concerning complicity in suicide (see further 6.2.2 below).

Sometimes a patient's intention in stipulating discontinuance of care, including tubefeeding, is left unclear not only by the advance directive but also by other available evidence. When that is the case, it seems to us not unreasonable for a doctor to assume that what motivated the stipulation was a desire that others should cease to undertake the burdens and costs of burdensome and costly care, accepting death as an effect of such discontinuance but not choosing it as a means to relieving them of costs and burdens. Making that assumption, the doctor can reasonably respect the patient's declared wishes, treating the patient like the patient whose motives are known to be those of self-sacrifice and whose choice is known not to have been suicidal in intent.[6]

4.1.4 Advance directives and the doctor-patient relationship

There is so much scope for doubt and conflict about whether the wording of an anticipatory decision is 'applicable in the circumstances' that it would be

---

[5] It should be noted that withholding tubefeeding in the circumstances envisaged in this paragraph is consistent not only with respect for human dignity but also with human solidarity with the deprived and the vulnerable. That is so because the reason for withholding tubefeeding is *the patient's own choice that this be an expression of solidarity* – of respect for the needs of others. But withholding tubefeeding can have this character only when the choice of the person who *suffers* deprivation of tubefeeding gives it this character; what is involved is essentially an act of *self*-sacrifice. And that is the reason why withholding tubefeeding from those who have never made such a choice cannot be turned into an expression of human solidarity by the device of substituted judgement; we cannot make acts of *self*-sacrifice on behalf of others, and the pretension that we are doing so merely masks the reality that we are engaged in sacrificing them. In the absence of a prior choice of self-sacrifice on the part of a patient while competent, withdrawal of tubefeeding from that patient when incompetent must *normally* be accounted an offence against the requirements of human solidarity.

[6] Some may think a benign interpretation of a patient's intentions when those intentions are opaque is not warranted. But the fact that there is a widespread tendency in our society to view the lives of many incompetent patients as without value should not be allowed to obscure the fact that many people have *independent* reasons for desiring to relieve others of burdens.

148

extremely imprudent to make advance directives enforceable by legislation. The proposal that doubt and conflict, where they arise, may be resolved by referring cases to a judicial forum[7] promises to introduce a degree of complexity to the decision-making process which will frequently be at odds with securing the interests of patients.

It would better accord with those interests and with sound doctor-patient relations if doctors were educated in a clear sense of those choices which are inconsistent with recognition of the dignity of patients, together with a clear sense of their obligations to try to secure medical benefits for their patients while remaining sensitive to the burdensome costs which sometimes make a treatment option undesirable.

4.2 The Proxy Decision Maker

The spurious conception of the role of the proxy decision-maker as consisting in the exercise of the incompetent patient's right to self-determination was noted in section 4.1.1.

In considering the burdensome consequences of treatment, the proxy decision-maker does have a duty to consider available knowledge about the distinctive sensibility and circumstances of the patient whose interests he represents (2.2.3/ii; 4.1.2). What is involved in doing so is something of an exercise in trying to see through the patient's own eyes. But this limited exercise of imaginative identification with the patient is justified by the unavoidably subjective element in what is to count as unduly burdensome for a given patient. An exclusive invocation of the 'claims of autonomy', however, affords no general justification for giving or withholding treatment on the basis of substituted judgement (4.1.1/d).

A substitute decision-maker who represents the interests of a patient will be concerned to act as a friend intent at least on securing justice for the patient. Friends desire the good of the person whose friends they are. What is just to a patient and what is good for a patient can in fundamental respects be determined objectively. The traditional framework for making that determination is the framework outlined and defended in this Submission.

---

[7] The Law Commission, Consultation Paper No.129: *Mentally Incapacitated Adults and Decision-Making. Medical Treatment and Research* London: HMSO, 1993, pp.41–42 (3.27–3.29).

PART TWO

5. The Courts and 'Responsible Medical Opinion'

The responsibility for ensuring that every person within the jurisdiction is treated with fundamental justice belongs in a unique way (though not exclusively) to the courts. It is the courts that, on their own initiative, developed and upheld *habeas corpus* to prevent the injustice of false imprisonment. It is the courts that have defined and enforced the law against homicide, which underwrites justice's primary demand that one person must never impose on another innocent person the radical injustice of extinction. Even today the activities of the legislature have in no way superseded the role of the courts in identifying and upholding the demands of right.

The decision of the House of Lords in *Bland* involves an abdication of the courts' responsibility. This abdication is illustrated most vividly, but not unrepresentatively, in the following passage from the judgment of the senior Law Lord, Lord Keith of Kinkel:

'... a medical practitioner is under no duty to continue to treat such a patient where a large body of informed and responsible medical opinion is to the effect that no benefit at all would be conferred by continuance. Existence in a vegetative state with no prospect of recovery is *by that opinion regarded as not a benefit*, and that, *if not unarguably correct, at least forms a proper basis* for the decision to discontinue treatment and care: *Bolam v Friern Hospital Management Committee* [1957] 1 WLR 582.

'Given that existence in the persistent vegetative state *is not a benefit* to the patient, it remains to consider whether the principle of sanctity of life, which it is the concern of the state, and the judiciary as one of the arms of the state, to maintain, requires this House to hold that the judgment of the Court of Appeal was incorrect.'

[1993] 2 WLR at 362 (emphasis added)

The significance of this judicial surrender of a vital premise (about the value of human existence) to the opinion of part of the medical profession is masked, in *Bland* itself, by the fact that the judges there seem likely to have reached the same decision even if they had not embraced the '*Bolam* principle' of deference to 'a body of responsible medical opinion'. But that principle of deference is unsound, as is stated plainly by Hoffmann L. J.[1] and noncommittally by Lord Mustill.[2]

---

[1] [1993] 2 WLR 316 at 358–9: '... the medical profession can tell the court about the patient's condition and prognosis and about the probable consequences of giving or not giving certain kinds of treatment or care, including the provision of artificial feeding. But whether in those circumstances it

Even in the area of medical negligence, there is reason to doubt the soundness of a legal rule that a doctor is not negligent if he acts in accordance with a practice accepted at the time as proper by a responsible body of medical opinion (even though other doctors adopt a different practice). That rule was disapproved by Lord Scarman, dissenting in *Sidaway v Governors of Bethlem Hospital* [1985] A. C. 871 at 876, where the issue was not one of competence in diagnostic or therapeutic procedures but involved the patient's right to be informed. In a case involving similar facts, the High Court of Australia has now unanimously disapproved the entire *Bolam* principle of determining the standard of medical care by deference to the standards of 'a responsible body of medical opinion': *Rogers v. Whitaker* (1992) 67 A. L. J. R. 47 at 50–51, a decision reached, ironically, on the same day as the President of the Family Division gave judgment in *Bland*.

Where a medical decision involves a right even more fundamental than the patient's right to be informed, the right not to be intentionally killed, it cannot be appropriate for the courts to proceed on the basis that a death-dealing course of conduct (deliberate omissions) is lawful simply because a responsible and informed body of medical opinion judges that life is no benefit to this patient, and/or that death and/or a course of conduct intended to terminate life is in this patient's best interests, and/or that tube-feeding is a medical treatment or form of 'medical care' and *therefore* may be terminated like any other medical treatment (as if it were not also an ordinary form of non-medical care). Each of these judgments is one which, though relating to the art of medicine, goes clearly beyond the expertise intrinsic and proper to that art. Each assumes a stance on the nature and meaning of human existence, the demands of justice, and/or the proper forms and limits of relationships between dependent people and those upon whom they depend.

would be lawful to provide or withhold the treatment or care is a matter for the law, and must be decided with regard to the general moral considerations of which I have spoken. As to these matters, the medical profession will no doubt have views which are entitled to great respect, but I would expect medical ethics to be formed by the law rather than the reverse. ... the plaintiff hospital trust ... has invited the court to decide whether, on medical facts which are not in dispute, the termination of life-support would be justified as being in the best interests of the patient. This is a purely legal (or moral) decision which does not require any medical expertise and is therefore appropriately made by the court.' This is a sound statement of principle.

Hoffmann L. J. also, however, made an unexplained and highly questionable concession that 'the fact that the doctor has acted in accordance with responsible medical opinion would usually be determinative' if the question related to 'some *past* act on the part of the doctor' and 'whether such an act *had* given rise to civil or criminal liability' (emphases added). As Lord Mustill implicitly indicates at p.391H, there was no basis in the context of *Bland* for this distinction between a declaration of law in relation to prospective conduct and an application of the very same law to the same facts when they lie not in the future but in the past.

2 [1993] 2 WLR 316 at 399.

151

6. Proposals to Change the Law

6.1 Proposals which should not be adopted

6.1.1 Medical Treatment (Advance Directives) Bill [H.L. Bill 73, 1993]

The wording of this Bill confirms what one would expect from a bill promoted by the Voluntary Euthanasia Society.

First, it must be observed that the form of advance directive scheduled to the Bill is purely optional (clause 1(3)) and cannot restrict the import of the Bill's own provisions for giving effect to advance directives of many kinds.

Secondly, it is clear from clause 9 of the Bill that it seeks to authorise conduct on the part of doctors intended to bring about the death of patients, the permissible conduct being limited to what is termed 'permitting the process of dying to take its course'.

Thirdly, vagueness about the definition of 'terminal condition' (clause 10) and, therefore, about 'the process of dying', means that the advanced directives which the Bill would authorise and make binding on doctors would be effective in regard to a far wider range of patients than those in the terminal phase of dying. Indeed they would be effective in regard to patients who are not, in the normal sense of the term, dying. For 'terminal condition' is defined as 'an incurable or irreversible condition which, without the use of life-sustaining treatment, will ... soon result in death.' Diabetes, for example, seems to fall within the scope of this definition of a terminal condition: it is an incurable condition, for which insulin treatment is life-sustaining and without the insulin certain patients with diabetes will soon die.

Fourthly, 'life sustaining treatment' is defined (clause 10) to mean 'any medical procedure or intervention which, when administered to a qualified patient, has the effect only of prolonging the process of dying'. Because of the definition of 'terminal condition', the notion of prolonging the process of dying is made indistinguishable from the notion of 'delaying the moment of death'. (The word 'only' in the phrase 'effect only of prolonging' is so vague and elusive that it cannot provide any effective control on the meaning of the clause.) Since treatment for any life-threatening condition delays the moment of death (perhaps for decades!), a substitute (or proxy) decision-maker may, under clause 4(1) withhold *any* life-sustaining treatment, whatever its prospective benefits, providing only that the patient who appointed him is 'comatose, incompetent or otherwise mentally or physically incapable of communication'. This is a charter for the extensive practice of non-voluntary euthanasia.

Fifthly, the provision in clause 5(2) is designed to exempt doctors from prosecution for aiding and abetting suicide in circumstances in which the natural interpretation of their behaviour would be that they were doing precisely that. For it is certain that sometimes a patient aims to bring about his own death at some time in the future by a course of planned omissions to be carried out by others on his authority, and makes it clear that that is his intention; the implementation of such a course of planned omissions on the basis of that prior authorisation and in the knowledge of that intention is, morally speaking, aiding and abetting suicide.

Sixthly, clause 4(2), read in conjunction with direction 2 in the Schedule to the Bill, makes it clear both that provision of food and fluids may be classified as 'life-sustaining treatment' in relation to a broad range of conditions, and that withdrawing food and fluid is sanctioned *whatever* the intention of the patient may have been, or the intention of a substitute decision-maker is, in authorising such withdrawal.

We respectfully urge the Select Committee to recommend that the *Medical Treatment (Advance Directives) Bill* be rejected since it would very clearly legalise (and is no doubt intended to legalise) assisted suicide and non-voluntary euthanasia.

6.1.2 Termination of Medical Treatment Bill [H.L. Bill 70, 1993]

The Bill is simply a charter for non-voluntary euthanasia (clause 2) of the incompetent (clause 1a) and assisted suicide (clause 3) of the competent (clause 1b) by the withdrawal of medical treatment or food and fluids. Its brevity has the merit of making its purpose eminently transparent. There is no need for legislation to cover the withdrawal of treatment on the grounds that it is medically otiose or unduly burdensome in its consequences.

We respectfully urge the Select Committee to recommend that any such Bill be rejected.

6.1.3 Legalizing Euthanasia: General Observations

There are a number of general objections to all proposals for legalizing euthanasia:

(1) Precisely in so far as euthanasia is considered *beneficent* to patients it involves killing on the basis of judgements about the value of their lives which are inconsistent with recognition of the dignity of the patients (1.2.2). Since recognition of the dignity of every human being is fundamental to justice, *and, therefore, to the law regulating our conduct towards each other* (1.1.4), it would be incompatible with what is basic to the law to allow euthanasiast killing.

(2) Killing the fundamental justification of which is that the patient would be better off dead (because of the disvalue of his continued existence) comprehends non-voluntary euthanasia. As clear-headed advocates of euthanasia recognise, if euthanasia is at all justified, there can be no good reason for denying the 'benefit' of killing to a patient because he is incapable of consent.[1] The evidence from the Netherlands is that doctors

---

[1] In relation to the withholding of treatment, Butler-Sloss LJ and Lord Goff both indicate that what is available as a benefit to the competent with their consent must be made available to the incompetent who cannot consent: *Bland* [1993] 2 WLR at 347G, 368D.

153

are *aiming* to bring about deaths in cases of incompetent patients much more frequently than in the case of competent patients (see Section 8 and references there).

(3) Propaganda for the legalization of euthanasia in the past heavily emphasised its desirability to deal with intractable terminal pain. But developments in pain control associated with the Hospice Movement have provided a solution, at least in principle, to the large majority of cases of intolerable pain. In consequence, the case for legalizing euthanasia has significantly shifted from drawing attention to intractable pain to emphasising 'intractable suffering'. But 'intractable suffering' is a very capacious reason for killing people, one possible effect of invoking which (see Section 7) is to encourage the cruellest pressures on those who are dependent.

(4) In so far as the legalization of euthanasia made doctors the authorised agents of euthanasiast killing, such legislation would profoundly corrupt the practice of medicine by corrupting the character of doctors.

Quite generally, intentional acts (such as deliberate killing) do not merely bring about effects external to the agent, they also shape his dispositions. If a doctor kills a patient because he judges the patient no longer has a worthwhile life then in doing so he makes himself further disposed to kill patients for that reason (unless he repents of what he did). That is why a certain kind of argument for the legalization of voluntary euthanasia is radically mistaken about what is at issue. The argument goes roughly as follows: a society should seek to prohibit only those practices which do harm to those who do not consent to the practices. But in voluntary euthanasia no party who has not consented to the practice is harmed. It is a purely private transaction between consenting doctor and consenting patient, the effects of which are contained within the confines of that relationship.

One reason that picture is false is that a doctor's character is very significantly shaped by killing patients on the grounds that their lives are now without value. A doctor disposed to think that some of his patients may lack inherent worth, and that he may therefore be justified in killing them, has seriously undermined in himself a disposition indispensable to the practice of medicine: the willingness to give what is owing to patients just in virtue of their possession of basic human dignity. The absence of that willingness is likely to be fateful for other patients, including patients who never consented to be killed or to be denied what they are owed in virtue of their basic human dignity.

For the sake of all its citizens, who all at one time or another are likely to become patients, civil society has a basic interest in maintaining a legal framework for the practice of medicine which is conducive to respect on the part of doctors for the basic dignity of all their patients.

(5) Once legalized, euthanasia would become a quick and facile technical 'fix' to dispose of certain difficult patients (whether or not at their own request) in response to the heavy demands they made on care. Medicine

would thereby be robbed of the incentive to find genuinely compassion-ate solutions to the difficulties presented by such patients. The kind of humane impulses which have sustained the development of hospice medicine and care would be undermined, because too many would think euthanasia a cheaper and less personally demanding solution. It is widely recognised that the country in which the practice of euthanasia has become widespread is a country in which palliative care medicine is very inadequately developed.

Those who protest that they advocate no more than the legalization of *voluntary* euthanasia are at best naive, though more often, it is to be feared, disingenuous. It is characteristic of certain advocates of legal reform to speak as if they could remain in control of the reform they propose once it is on the statute book. That is an illusion, as legalization of abortion has shown. What legalization of voluntary euthanasia would enshrine is the novel principle that one may be justified in killing people because, since they lack worthwhile lives, to do so is to benefit them. In enshrining such a principle in our laws we would have to contend with what Justice Cardozo described as 'the tendency of a principle to expand itself to the limit of its logic'.[2]

6.2 Proposals which should be adopted

6.2.1 The Bland ruling on lawful intention to terminate life should be overturned

By far the most serious of the immediate legal implications of the *Bland* case is, we think, the ruling by a majority of the House of Lords (neither followed nor challenged by Lords Keith and Goff) that, provided it is not 'positive action' and is adopted because, in accordance with a body of responsible medical opinion, it is considered to be in the best interests of the person whose life it terminates, it is *lawful* (and indeed may be legally required) to adopt a 'course of conduct' deliberately and precisely *with the intention, aim and purpose of terminating life.*

The basis on which Lords Lowry, Browne-Wilkinson and Mustill assumed such an intention in relation to Anthony Bland is legally obscure.[3] Be that as it may, there certainly are circumstances in which someone might decide to cease providing life support yet have no intention to terminate the life of the patient (though foreseeing and accepting that the death of the patient would be highly probable or even certain to follow in consequence of the cessation). For there can be circumstances in which those providing the support should or at least can give a higher priority to other responsibilities (e.g. to patients who can benefit more from the limited resources available).

But the tail must not be allowed to wag the dog. The fundamental and momentous issue whether intentional killing is to be allowed, ratified and

---

[2] Quoted in Yale Kamisar, 'Some Non-Religious Views against "Mercy-Killing" Legislation', *Minnesota Law Review* 42 (1958), 969–1042, at 1037.
[3] See J M Finnis, '*Bland*: Crossing the Rubicon?' in *Law Quarterly Review* 109 (1993), 329–37.

indeed commanded in our society must not be determined by the topsy turvey process of first deciding against continued life support in hard cases such as *Bland*, then deciding that that solution involves an intent to terminate life, and accordingly abandoning the hitherto central principle of our common morality and our law: *no* intentional killing of the innocent.

We do not dispute the finding of all the judges in *Bland* that what was involved was legally an 'omission'. Nor do we question the general stance of English law that omissions are unlawful only if they involve the violation of a duty of care. We do not question even the more stringent position of English law, that X's omission (e.g. to warn Y of imminent danger) deliberately chosen with malicious intent to harm Y (e.g. so as to enjoy Y's suffering or death) is not unlawful if, independently of the intent, X owed no duty to protect Y from such harm or death. But the ruling of the majority in the House of Lords in *Bland* goes far beyond these positions. For it treats as lawful the omissions of persons who admittedly had a duty to care for Anthony Bland, and who were ready and willing to continue an extensive medical, nursing and general care for him right up to the moment of his death. It treats as lawful (and sometimes, indeed, compulsory) the proposal that terminating someone's life, i.e. the bringing about of his death (by deliberate omissions), be a part of carrying out their duty of care.

The judges in question all admit that the distinction they draw is morally indefensible and leaves the law 'misshapen' or 'almost irrational'.[4] They were right to do so. The law will indeed be misshapen and indefensible for so long as it treats as criminal a harmful 'act' while treating as lawful (and indeed compulsory) an 'omission', with the *very same intent, by one who has a duty to care for the person whose life is thereby terminated.* There is nothing misshapen about a law treating acts and omissions alike when deliberately adopted with the same intention. And the settled legal (not moral) doctrine that harmful intent by itself does not make an omission criminal should not govern when the omission is by one who admittedly has a legal duty to protect the party harmed against that type of harm.

Neither in the judgments in *Bland* nor in any other legal source can we discover any reason for thinking that English law has ever, until 4 February 1993, accepted that someone who has a duty of care can carry it out by intending to terminate the life of the person in his care. We think that English law has in fact always rejected any such notion. We are surprised to note that the decided cases[5] in which English law manifested its rejection of this notion were not even cited to the judge of first instance in *Bland*, went completely unmentioned in the oral argument and the judgments in the Court of Appeal, and received mention in only two of the judgments in the House of Lords. We accept that those previous cases did not concern doctors and did

---

[4] Lord Mustill, at [1993] 2 WLR pp. 388–9: 'the distortions of a legal structure which is already both morally and intellectually misshapen'; 'the morally and intellectually dubious distinction between acts and omissions' (p.399); Lord Browne-Wilkinson at p.387: 'the conclusion I have reached will appear to some to be almost irrational.... I find it difficult to find a moral answer...'; Lord Lowry at p.379: '...a distinction without a difference...'

[5] *R. v. Bubb* (1850) 4 Cox C.C. and *R. v. Gibbins and Proctor* (1918) 13 Cr. App. R. 134.

not have to confront the arguments raised in favour of terminating Anthony Bland's life. But we think that the rule articulated in those cases sets out a legal position of principle which could and should have been reaffirmed and developed by the judges in response to those arguments. The fundamental argument, which in fact the judges accepted, was that the doctors *et al.* owed no duty to Bland to keep him alive. The fundamental answer to that argument, an answer which the judges seem never to have clearly envisaged, is that *whatever the scope of the duty of care of those caring for Anthony Bland*, they had a moral and legal duty *not to exercise their care* for him *with intent to* terminate his life.

In any event, it is now most urgently necessary, we suggest, to restore the integrity of the English law of homicide by rejecting the misshapen, almost irrational and wholly unnecessary rule or position adopted by the majority of the Lords in *Bland*. The necessary statute would not solve the problem of deciding whether and when life support can be withdrawn from incompetent patients. But it would restore one vital parameter or principle for any acceptable solution to that problem.

We respectfully ask the Select Committee to recommend the early enactment of a Bill along the following lines:

No person may in or in connection with providing to another person medical, nursing or other treatment, services or care do or omit anything with the intention[6] of terminating that other person's life. A person who by any such act or omission with such intention causes the other's death shall be guilty of murder.

A provision of this kind would not purport to settle the debate about whether withdrawal of life support from PVS patients causes their death. It would not purport to settle the debate about the extent of the duty to maintain such support. It would simply restore the integrity of the fundamental principle of the law of murder, gravely impaired by the decision in *Bland*. That principle of the law of murder is an indispensable element in the recognition and protection of the basic rights of all members of our community, and an integral part of the state's fundamental duty of justice.

6.2.2 *Unacceptable kinds of advance directive should be deprived of all legal effect*

A majority at least of the House of Lords in *Bland* went out of their way to give a blanket and indeed indiscriminate approval to the idea that advance directives to discontinue treatment or care are of binding legal effect: see Lord Goff (Lords Keith and Lowry agreeing), [1993] 2 WLR at 367H. Quite mystifyingly, Lord Goff stated, in this connection, that 'in cases of this kind,

---

[6] The concept of intention is central to the existing law of murder. A series of recent judicial decisions of the highest authority establish (in conformity with a sound philosophical understanding of intention) that there can be murder only if there is intention to kill (or cause grievous bodily harm); that there can be intention to kill without 'desire' to kill; and that one who foresees that his act will probably or even certainly cause death may, but need not, have the intention of killing. With these clarifications, the concept is to be left to the good sense of juries. See Lord Goff of Chieveley, 'The Mental Element in the Crime of Murder' (1988) 104 *Law Quarterly Review* 30.

there is no question of the patient having committed suicide ...' (p.367H). Unless he meant this, despite the syntax, to be a qualification on his ratification of advance directives, one must ask: Why is there 'no question' of suicide? Can it really be by sheer judicial fiat or stipulative definition? Suppose everyone knows that the patient's directive that on a certain date insulin (or food and water) be withdrawn was motivated simply by his intention of dying before the expiry of a term life insurance policy. On what legal principle is this not suicide?

What should be Parliament's response to this remarkable and evidently unsolicited judicial development of the law? We think it should be to legislate at an early date so as to provide that

where a patient is incompetent to give or withhold consent to medical treatment or care, the existence of a declaration made by that patient at some earlier time purporting to give directions for the withdrawal of treatment or care (or of any specified form of treatment or care) shall not be taken to require those responsible for his treatment or care to follow any course of conduct (including omission) otherwise than in accordance with their judgment as to the best interests of the patient, and shall not be taken to require or authorise any person to give any assistance in suicide (including suicide by omission).

PART THREE

7. The Hospice Movement and Advances in Palliative Care

For many ordinary people the pain associated with terminal conditions still appears the most pressing reason for allowing euthanasia in certain types of case (witness expressions of sympathy for Dr. Cox). Those actively engaged in hospice care have documented its role in controlling the pain which is associated with a number of fatal conditions, and certain carcinomas in particular. In this connection, the very success of the development of palliative medicine within the context of hospice care has had a paradoxical effect. It is this paradoxical effect that is worth remarking on here.

In so far as satisfactory control of pain is achievable with the vast majority of patients[1], the common case for euthanasia would seem to have lost its force. Investment in extending the benefits of palliative care would seem a far more rational response to the incidence of severe pain than legalization of euthanasia. And in so far as people come to know of the successes of contemporary palliative care they generally acknowledge this truth.

The response of proponents of the legalization of euthanasia, however, has been to shift from emphasising the problem of intractable pain to emphasising the problem of 'intractable suffering'. Intractable suffering, as we have already remarked, is a much more wide-ranging reason for killing patients, and covers experience that is not amenable to medical management in the way that pain has been.

It is worth remarking here on just how elastic the concept of 'intractable suffering' can be in rationalizing the practice of euthanasia. An instructive case in point (referred to again in the following section) is provided by recent research on the practice of euthanasia in The Netherlands. One informant, a leading practitioner of euthanasia, said he would be put in a very difficult position if a patient told him that he really felt a nuisance to his relatives because they wanted to enjoy his estate. Asked whether he would rule out euthanasia in such a case, [he] replied: 'I think in the end I wouldn't, because that kind of influence – these children wanting the money now – is the same kind of power from the past that ... shaped us all. The same thing goes for religion ... education ... the kind of family he was raised in, all kinds of

---

[1] A repeated figure for satisfactory pain control is in 97% of cases in the hospice setting and in 90% of cases in domicillary care.

influences from the past that we can't put aside.'[2] If the misery provoked by the knowledge that one's children want one's estate is to count as a reason for euthanasia, then there will be an open invitation to children to make the lives of their dependent parents such a misery that the 'burdensome' parents will be queuing up for euthanasia. If this were to happen then euthanasia by request would have become a facade covering a reality much closer to involuntary euthanasia.

In summary: one paradoxical consequence of the hospice movement's success in managing pain and making it seem a less pressing reason for euthanasia is that apologists for euthanasia's legalization have shifted to emphasising intractable suffering. And intractable suffering as a reason for euthanasia nominates a far wider range of candidates for euthanasia (voluntary and nonvoluntary) than intractable pain ever did.

8. The Dutch Experience[3]

8.1 The Law

The intentional killing of a person at his 'express and serious' request is an offence contrary to Article 293 of the Dutch Penal Code, and assisting suicide is prohibited by the following Article. However, in a line of cases over the past twenty years, Dutch courts have held that a doctor charged with either offence can successfully avail himself of the defence of necessity (contained in Article 40) if he acted in accordance with 'responsible medical opinion' measured by the 'prevailing standards of medical ethics'.[4]

When, according to 'responsible medical opinion', is it considered proper for a doctor to carry our euthanasia?

8.2 Medical Guidelines

In 1984 the Royal Dutch Medical Association published a report setting out conditions in which 'euthanasia' (a word which is used in Holland to mean 'voluntary euthanasia') accorded with medical ethics. It specified five:

1. The request must be made of the patient's free will, and not result from pressure by others.
2. The request must be 'well-considered', and not be based on a misunderstanding of diagnosis or prognosis.
3. The request must be 'durable', and not arise from impulse or temporary depression.
4. The patient must be experiencing 'unacceptable suffering'; he must feel the suffering to be 'persistent, unbearable and hopeless'.

[2] J Keown, 'Some reflections on euthanasia in The Netherlands' in Luke Gormally (ed) *The Dependent Elderly. Autonomy, Justice and Quality of Care* Cambridge: Cambridge University Press 1992, 70–100, at 79. See Chapter 4 below, p.203.
[3] This section draws on I J Keown, 'The Law and Practice of Euthanasia in The Netherlands' *Law Quarterly Review* 108 (1992), pp.51–78.
[4] *Ibid.*, 51–55.

5. The doctor must consult with a colleague before performing euthanasia, and report it to the legal authorities afterwards as a non-natural death.[5]

A number of highly misleading claims have been made by proponents of legalised euthanasia about the Dutch experience. It has, for example, been asserted (by the Director of the Dutch Health Council) that the guidelines are 'precisely defined' and 'strict'.

First, it is not even possible to be confident about what the guidelines are: the above five have been laid down by the Dutch Medical Association, not the courts. As Professor Leenen, a leading Dutch health lawyer (and supporter of euthanasia) has observed, different courts have listed different criteria, which has created 'much uncertainty'. It has been held by the Supreme Court, for example, that consultation is not essential for euthanasia to be lawful.

Secondly, even the five listed above are far from precise. What, for example, is meant by a 'free' request? Does it include a request made in response to a strong recommendation by a doctor or relatives? One of Holland's leading (and widely respected) practitioners of euthanasia was asked whether he would rule out euthanasia in the (hypothetical) case of a patient who asked for euthanasia because he felt a nuisance to his children who wanted him dead so that they could enjoy his estate. The doctor replied:

'I ... think in the end I wouldn't, because that kind of influence – these children wanting the money now – is the same kind of power from the past that ... shaped us all.'[6]

This illustrates how subjective, elastic and inherently vague are the guidelines requiring a 'free' request and 'unbearable suffering'.

Thirdly, far from being 'strict', the guidelines could hardly be more lax. They assume rather than ensure the expertise and good faith of the individual doctor and are quite unenforceable.[7]

8.3 Euthanasia in Practice

It comes as no surprise, therefore, that there is disturbing evidence not only of a high incidence of euthanasia in Holland but also of widespread breach of the guidelines.

In 1991 a Government Commission on Euthanasia, chaired by Attorney-General Remmelink, published its report[8] and the results of a survey it had commissioned into the practice of euthanasia.[9]

---

[5] *Ibid.*, 57–60.

[6] *Ibid.*, 63.

[7] See Carlos F Gomez MD, *Regulating Death: Euthanasia and the Case of The Netherlands* New York: Free Press 1991, p.122.

[8] *Medische beslissingen rond het levenseinde. Rapport van de Commissie onderzoek medische praktijk inzake euthanasie.* ('s-Gravenhage: Sdu Uitgeverij Plantijnstraat, 1991).

[9] *Medische beslissingen rond het levenseinde. Het onderzoek voor de commissie onderzoek medische praktijk inzake euthanasie.* ('s-Gravenhage: Sdu Uitgeverij Plantijnstraat, 1991). An English trans-

The Survey shows that for the calendar year 1990, there were 2,300 cases of (voluntary) euthanasia and 400 cases of assisted suicide.[10] There were, moreover, over 8,000 cases in which doctors administered morphine[11], and almost 8,000 cases in which they withheld or withdrew treatment[12] 'explicitly' or 'partly' *with intent to shorten life.*[13] Finally, the Survey revealed over 1,000 cases in which doctors stated that they had terminated life without the explicit request of the patient.[14] In short, the Survey, *in its own terms,* makes out that doctors admitted that it was their purpose to shorten their patients' lives in almost 20,000 cases.

Bearing in mind that there were only 49,000 deaths in 1990 in which a doctor's decision influenced the time of a patient's death[15], the finding that in over 40% the doctor purposely sought to shorten the patient's life suggests that intentional killing has become a regular feature of Dutch medical practice.

Moreover, in almost three-quarters of these cases the doctor is reported as having sought to hasten death without the explicit request of the patient.[16] The 1,000 cases in which doctors administered a lethal drug without explicit request provide particularly stark evidence of the widespread breach of the first three guidelines.

The fourth guideline, requiring that euthanasia be performed only when it is necessary, as a last resort, to end 'unbearable suffering', is also, as the remarkably high incidence itself indicates, widely ignored. Even 40% of the doctors surveyed agreed with the proposition that 'Adequate alleviation of pain and/or symptoms and personal care of the dying patient make euthanasia unnecessary'.[17] The inference from all the evidence that euthanasia is being used as an alternative to good palliative care is compelling.

Finally, the Survey also showed that of the 2,700 cases classified by the Survey as 'euthanasia' and assisted suicide, doctors certified death by natu-

---

lation has been published as P J van der Maas *et al., Euthanasia and other Medical Decisions at the End of Life* (Elsevier 1992); also published in *Health Policy* 22/1–2 (1992). (Hereafter, 'Survey')

[10] Survey, 178–179.

[11] *Ibid.,* 183. See generally chapter 7.

[12] *Ibid.,* 184. See generally chapter 8.

[13] It should be noted that these cases are explicitly distinguished in the Report from cases in which morphine is administered or treatment withheld for reasons other than that of bringing about death while *foreseeing* that death may result from the decision. The latter kind of case does fall within the bounds of acceptable medical practice. But it is misleading of VES representatives to suggest that the 16,000 cases in which, in the terms of the Survey (see footnote 9 above), there was some 'intention' to shorten life (by administering opiates or withdrawing treatment) also fall within the bounds of acceptable medical practice. It is true that about 11,000 of these cases are described by the Survey as falling within the class of choices carried out *'partly* with the intention to shorten life'. It seems not unlikely that that is an accurate description of a majority of those cases, though it should be recognised that the researchers made use of that description to cover certain cases for which it is inapplicable; namely, cases in which the only ground (mistakenly invoked) for attributing intention is that the hastening of death (resulting from the clinician's course of conduct) is regarded as 'not unwelcome' by the clinician.

[14] *Ibid.,* 182. See generally chapter 6.

[15] *Ibid.,* 187.

[16] John Keown, 'On Regulating Death', *Hastings Centre Report* 22/2 (1992), pp.39,42.

[17] Survey, p.102, *Table* 9.7.

ral causes in over 7 out of 10, thereby breaching the fifth guideline and committing the criminal offence of falsifying a death certificate.[18]

In addition to the Survey, two independent academic studies of Dutch euthanasia have also served to establish the comprehensive failure of the guidelines. The first by Dr. Carlos Gomez, an American physician[19], concludes that the Dutch attempt to control euthanasia and to provide for public accountability has failed and that attempts to protect vulnerable patients have proved 'halfhearted and ineffective at best'. The second by Dr. John Keown, lecturer in law in the University of Cambridge, concludes not only that the guidelines have been widely ignored, but that killing even without request now enjoys official approval. The evidence for this is to be found in recent publications of the Dutch Medical Association which approve in certain circumstances the killing of handicapped neonates and patients in coma, and, most recently[20], those with severe dementia. Moreover, not only did the Remmelink survey find that over half of the doctors interviewed had either performed euthanasia without an explicit request or would be prepared to do so[21] but the Remmelink Commission condoned the vast majority of the 1,000 killings without explicit request.[22]

Two main conclusions can be drawn from the Dutch experience. First, it vividly demonstrates how, when euthanasia is tolerated, it becomes practically impossible to keep it within defined limits. There is now overwhelming evidence, which has nowhere been seriously controverted, that the guidelines have proved wholly incapable of ensuring that euthanasia is confined to those who make a 'free, well-considered and durable request' and who are experiencing 'unbearable suffering'. Indeed, even Professor Leenen has observed that there is an 'almost total lack of control on the administration of euthanasia' in his country.[23]

Some twenty years ago, the then Lord Bishop of Durham, The Right Reverend J S Habgood, cautioned that the consequences of legislation to permit euthanasia would, in the long run, be 'incalculable', not least because of the likely failure of any safeguards to prevent abuse.[24] The Dutch experience confirms the prescience of this warning and reveals the baleful effects, even in the short term, of tolerating euthanasia.

Secondly, the Dutch experience lends support to the argument developed in 1.2.2 and 1.3.2 above that the case for euthanasia rests fundamentally not on respect for autonomy but on a judgement that certain lives are not worth living and that it is right to terminate them. The Dutch, who only a few years ago were seeking to justify euthanasiast killing in terms of the claims of autonomy, now accept that the absence of the ability to choose provides no reason against killing. The 1,000 cases of killing without explicit request; the

---

[18] *Ibid.*, 49, *Table* 5. 14.
[19] *Op.cit.*, p.161, n.7 above.
[20] See 'Dutch doctors support life termination in dementia', *British Medical Journal* 306 (1993), p.1364.
[21] Survey p.58, *Table* 6.1.
[22] *Op.cit.*, p.161, n.8 above: p.15.
[23] Quoted in I J Keown, *op.cit.*, p.160, n.3 above: p.78.
[24] J S Habgood, 'Euthanasia – A Christian View', *Journal of the Royal Society of Health* 3 (1974) 124,126.

approval of these killings by the Remmelink Commission, and the growing categories of incompetent patients whose lives the Dutch Medical Association now regards it as permissible to terminate, lend empirical support to the proposition that the case for euthanasia rests not on respect for autonomy but on the acceptance of the concept of 'lives not worth living'. The potential of that concept both for rationalizing grave injustice to patients and for corrupting the practice of medicine was sufficiently demonstrated in mid-century in Western Europe. Only the deepest complacency, hard to distinguish from a measure of sheer decadence, could willingly tolerate again medicalized killing, rationalized in terms fundamentally incompatible with justice, or contemplate accepting the grave damage that would be done to medicine by its involvement in such killing.[25]

---

[25] It is frequently said by contemporary proponents of euthanasia that what they seek to have legalized bears no comparison with medical involvement in euthanasia under the Nazis. The reasons advanced for the contention are weak. Some say that what they want legalized is killing justified in terms of the claims of autonomy. But no such simple justification is available (see 1.3.2). Others say that what they want justified would have a different 'motive' from medical euthanasia under the Nazis. But it is a commonplace observation, in law as in morals, that ostensibly worthy motives cannot independently render acceptable chosen behaviour which in its *intentional* character is objectionable.

Concluding Observations

In conclusion, we respectfully submit that the recommendations of the Select Committee should be governed by two broad considerations.

First, the legalization of medicalized killing, which some want the Select Committee to recommend, would necessarily find its justification in terms which are radically incompatible with recognising the equality-in-dignity of all human beings. Such killing could not be accommodated within a legal framework which recognised the basic requirements of justice. There is an urgent need, indeed, in consequence of certain judicial decisions, to introduce legislation which will restore the integrity of the law in regard to homicide (see 6.2.1 and 6.2.2).

Secondly, the traditional ethic of medicine, correctly understood, leaves very great scope for patients to refuse treatment which is likely to be found unduly burdensome, and scope for doctors to withdraw treatment on those grounds. Moreover, doctors have no moral duty to persist with *medical* treatment which is inefficacious in achieving the distinctive goals of medicine. On the other hand, a failure to achieve the therapeutic or palliative goals of medicine does not absolve doctors from the duties of ordinary care of patients.

What is to count as sound medical practice in regard to withholding and withdrawing treatment could never be exhaustively settled by legislation. But the citizens of our society, all of whom are potentially patients, do need to know that in making such decisions doctors are constrained by a framework of law which makes *absolutely* impermissible both intentional killing (by action or omission) and deliberate assistance in suicide (by action or omission). Within such a framework doctors can continue to seek to act in patients' best interests while being responsive to the reasonable desires of patients to avoid unduly burdensome treatment and respectful of the primacy of the competent patient's own responsibility for his or her health. To seek to make enforceable some wider conception of the claims of patient autonomy would be both unreasonable in itself and ultimately destructive of good doctor-patient relationships.

2

'Living Will' Legislation

JOHN FINNIS

This chapter is concerned with *advance directives*, by which individuals express their wishes as to their future health care, and/or as to future decisions by others about that health care. The directives here in question are those which request the termination, withdrawal or non-provision of health care: in most cases, they are intended to take effect in the event of the maker's becoming incompetent (i.e. unable to make rational decisions). The focus of this appendix is on legal rather than purely moral considerations, but this is an area of law in which it is rightly agreed, on all sides, that the law's concepts, distinctions and norms should tightly correspond to morality's.

Advance directives can be either (i) by *living will*, a document requesting and directing that certain measures should or, more particularly, should not be taken if one becomes incompetent, or incompetent and ill in some way specified in the document (e.g. 'terminally' or 'irreversibly' ill); or (ii) by *enduring power of attorney*, a document appointing an agent to take decisions of specified types in specified contingencies in the event of one's incompetence; or (iii) a document containing both a living will and an enduring power of attorney.

Since 1976, most states of the United States have legislated to give legal effect to living wills, and all states have provided for enduring powers of attorney. These laws almost all approximate to a common paradigm. In Australia the state of Victoria enacted in 1988/9 a Medical Treatment Act sharing many but not all the features common among the American statutes. In England the Voluntary Euthanasia Society in 1991 launched a 'Medical Treatment (Advance Directives) Bill' with the stated intent 'to enable persons to give directions to their physicians regarding the withholding or withdrawal of life-sustaining treatment in a terminal condition...'

A characteristic moral argument for giving compulsory moral and legal effect to advance directives is offered in *The Living Will: Consent to Treatment at the End of Life*,[1] the report of a working party of three lawyers and three medical practitioners (plus the Director of Age Concern), established by Age Concern England and The Centre of Medical Law and Ethics of King's College London, and chaired by Professor Ian Kennedy.

---

[1] Edward Arnold, London & New York, 1988

I

Self-determination's limits in 'here and now' directives

Before considering what directives might lawfully and effectively be given (or might authorise an agent to give) *in advance* of incompetence, it is helpful to consider the directives which individuals may lawfully and effectively give in relation to their health care here and now.

One may not say to one's doctor 'Put me to sleep for ever; give me a lethal injection'. That is an invitation to commit murder. One may not say 'Leave a lethal syringe by my bedside.' That is an invitation to commit the crime of aiding and abetting suicide contrary to section 2 of the Suicide Act 1961. One may not say 'My life insurance policy expires in a fortnight; so I henceforth refuse my insulin injections and forbid you to give me any when I lapse into unconsciousness.' That solicits the doctor to commit murder by omission,[2] or at least unlawful homicide (manslaughter) by omission.[3] The Kennedy report, in its central chapter on 'The Ethical and Legal Framework', says:

> In principle, we believe that a patient is entitled to refuse ... any ... form of treatment, even if death is the inevitable outcome. .... We take the view that even if the patient is not suffering from terminal illness from which he would otherwise die, starvation is not suicide. The patient must *positively* do something to himself before his conduct would be so regarded. Furthermore, even if the law were to regard the patient as committing suicide, the doctor's *omission* to continue artificial feeding or hydration would not be regarded as 'assistance'. This follows either because he must *act* to commit the offence and not merely omit to do something, or because the patient's refusal absolves him of any duty in law to continue treatment.[4]

Each and every one of the statements just quoted is contrary to sound moral analysis, and even after the judgments in *Airedale N.H.S. Trust* v. *Bland* in 1993 they all remain questionable in law. The pervasive error of principle is the Kennedy report's refusal to consider the significance of *intention*. The primary question is not whether death is an 'inevitable outcome', but whether death is intended, i.e. whether the patient intends to die *as a means* of escaping suffering and/or of securing some advantage. If he does, his plan to refuse medical treatment or nourishment is suicidal, and the doctor's decisions accordingly to withhold treatment or nourishment are decisions to aid and abet. The law firmly and rightly holds that those who have undertaken to provide treatment or nourishment are not absolved from their duty by the patient's adamant refusal if that refusal is either incompetent or unlawful. A refusal which is motivated by suicidal intent is unlawful, even though suicide itself is not a criminal offence; that is why assistance, and agreements to assist, in suicide are serious criminal offences.

---

[2] Cf. *R* v *Gibbins & Proctor* (1918) 13 Criminal Appeal Reports 134 (starving with intent to cause death). There are incautious remarks about self-determination, in some of the judgments of the House of Lords in *Airedale N.H.S. Trust* v *Bland* [1993] 2 Weekly Law Reports 316, [1993] 1 All England Reports 821, which might be taken to cast doubt on this proposition, but nothing sufficient to show that, if the point were raised for decision (as it was not in *Bland*), the proposition would be rejected.

[3] See *R* v. *Wilkinson*, *The Times*, 19 April 1978 (Court of Appeal); Glanville Williams, *Textbook of Criminal Law* (1983) 268. The deceased, aged 72, violently resisted offers of medical help, but her husband and 42-year old daughter were convicted of manslaughter for failing to secure assistance.

[4] *The Living Will* 29.

The judgments in the *Bland* case certainly obscure the clarity of the position as set out in the last paragraph. Many of them overlook, and some of them deny, the decisive relevance of intention; all of them in one way or another treat as decisive a distinction between omission and 'positive action'.[5] But relevance of intention was never squarely argued in the case (which concerned the withdrawal of tube-feeding from a patient after three years in 'persistent vegetative state'). And even if the common law, under siege from consequentialist ethics and euthanasiast sentiment, were to surrender its principle, the moral significance of intention will remain unimpaired. Every analysis which bypasses intention, replacing it with questions about causation and/or foreseeability and/or inevitability and/or 'positive' action, shows itself to have abandoned the fundamentals of ethics. The same must be said of every legal or moral analysis which is content to proclaim rights specified without reference to intention, e.g. 'to refuse treatment', 'to decline life-sustaining measures', and so forth.

And it is within a framework which legally and morally excludes both suicide and homicide (defined in terms of intention to bring about death as an end or a means) that the common law, like sound morality, has acknowledged the right of *self-determination*. True, the common law principle that medical treatment is unlawful unless done with the patient's consent is a principle subject to restrictions or exceptions when the patient is unable to communicate and the treatment is reasonable and in the patient's best interests. But those restrictions or exceptions do not extend to authorising treatment when a competent patient's definite refusal, here and now, to accept it is a foolish or 'irrational' refusal – not even if the refusal's foreseeable result, *as distinct from the purpose (intent)*, is the death of the patient. Such a refusal may well be morally irresponsible, a culpable failure in virtues such as prudence and fortitude and even justice. But provided it both is a genuine choice (and thus, like all free choices, an act of self-determination), and involves no unlawful e.g. suicidal *intent* (and no immediately catastrophic impact on another person, e.g. a child about to be born), the common law requires others to respect it.

II

The key concept often overlooked: Intention

The American and Australian advance declaration statutes all blur and obscure the difference between suicidal intent and other intentions. And insofar as they authorise agents or representatives to make decisions in place of the patient, they blur and obscure the difference between homicidal intent and other intentions.

True, none of these statutes has authorised any act which of its own nature

---

[5] See the critical legal commentaries by John Keown, 'Doctors and Patients: Hard Case, Bad Law, "New" Ethics' [1993] 52 *Cambridge Law Journal* 209–212; John Finnis, '*Bland*: Crossing the Rubicon?' 109 *Law Quarterly Review* [1993] 329–37.

brings about harm or death to the patient (killing by 'act' rather than 'omission'). They are all concerned with authorising the cessation or withholding or non-provision of treatment. But none of them takes care to draw to the attention of their constituency the distinction between refusing burdensome or futile treatment to avoid its burdensomeness or futility, and refusing treatment in order to secure relief from distress or despair by hastening death. After an intense campaign by some Catholics, the Victorian Medical Treatment Act 1988 was amended in 1989 so as to provide, inter alia, that inciting, aiding or abetting suicide, and homicide, would continue to be offences notwithstanding the Act's authorisation of refusals of treatment and requirement that such refusals be (on pain of criminal sanction) respected. But even then the Victorian legislature made no serious attempt to secure that those making or giving effect to certificates of refusal of treatment should clearly understand or carefully attend to the difference.

Some influential Catholics in Victoria gave enthusiastic support to the Medical Treatment Acts of 1988 and 1989, on the score that the legislation was 'consistent with Catholic principles'. In so doing, they confused legislation with a treatise on Catholic morality. Propositions which, in the context of a Catholic treatise, would have an acceptable meaning, reference and force take on a quite different sense when divorced from that context, as legislation in a pluralist community is, of course, divorced. Consider some examples of this confusion. The 1989 Act says that –

5B. (2) An agent or guardian may only refuse medical treatment on behalf of a patient if –

(a) the medical treatment would cause unreasonable distress to the patient; or
(b) there are reasonable grounds for believing that the patient, if competent, and after giving serious consideration to his or her health and well-being, would consider that the medical treatment is unwarranted.

In a Catholic context, (a) and (b) would naturally be read as reproducing the distinction between the unacceptably burdensome and the futile. Removed from that context, they extend to cover not only the burdensome and the futile but also treatment which some patient rejects precisely because he regards or (supposedly) would if conscious regard his *life* as not worth living, his further existence as yielding no net benefit. In the case where the patient is conscious, he rejects the treatment as unwarranted because he regards non-treatment as a *means* of securing death. He thus *intends* precisely to bring about his death. On a Catholic view, as on the view underlying common morality, his decision is suicidal. So too an agent's substituted decision would be complicity in suicide and homicidal. On a sound interpretation of the common law and the Victorian (and English) legislation on suicide, it would be complicity in suicide and perhaps also unlawful homicide. But on an interpretation of the law such as is proposed in the Kennedy report, and by Glanville Williams[6] and some other lawyers, it would be neither suicide nor homicide. In the Victorian statute of 1988/9 (as in the judgments in England in 1992/3 in *Bland*'s case) no care is taken to guard against the Kennedy-Williams interpretation.

6 Glanville Williams, *Textbook of Criminal Law* (Stevens, London, 1983) 268.

So casual is the Victorian Act that the statutory form of refusal-of-treatment certificate to be completed by an agent or representative contains no reminder that the only lawful grounds for refusal are (a) and (b) quoted above, and no reminder that aiding and abetting suicide, and homicide, remain offences whose reach is unaffected by the Medical Treatments Acts. The statutory forms whereby the Victorian Parliament seeks to protect consumers from high-pressure hire purchase transactions are much more careful and protective. Moreover, while the Act makes it a criminal offence for a doctor to give treatment in face of a refusal-of-treatment certificate, it fails to make it an offence for an agent or representative to refuse treatment for reasons other than those set out in (a) and (b); this failure makes successful prosecution for manslaughter, in such a case, probably impossible.

In these and many other ways, the advance directive legislation seems likely to have the 'educative' effect of undermining public consciousness of the significance of intention in the context of suicide, homicide and, on the other hand, of upright and reasonable refusal of burdensome or futile treatment.

In England, the Voluntary Euthanasia Society's draft Medical Treatment (Advance Directives) Bill (1992) makes its own contribution to this confusion by declaring that –

11. . . . nothing in this Act shall be construed to authorise or permit any act or omission to end the life of any person other than to permit the process of dying as provided in this Act.

When the tortuous logic of cl.11 is parsed out, it becomes clear that the Bill would authorise decisions to permit death *in order to* ('to') end the life of a person, i.e. with the precise intent of bringing about death.

III

Unilateral emphasis on self-determination

There is another corrosive feature of the Victorian legislation, the Kennedy report, and various *obiter dicta* in the judgments in *Bland* (this last being a case not truly involving autonomy or self-determination at all). It is the *unilateral* insistence on self-determination, autonomy, 'the patient's right to refuse *unwanted* medical treatment'. (This last phrase is the first rationale to be presented in the preamble to the Victorian Act of 1988; the essential counterbalancing rationale, 'to provide that inciting, aiding or abetting suicide, or homicide, continue to be offences', was forced into the preamble to the Act at the last minute, but will not appear in reprints of the consolidated 1988/89 legislation.)

Unrestrained by consideration of any other goods or norms, concern for 'autonomy' – more accurately, liberty to do what one pleases – is obviously an open invitation to suicide, complicity in suicide, and voluntary euthanasia of the most straightforwardly homicidal kind. But the implications and/or inevitable consequences of such a unilateral concern for autonomy go much wider.

1. Most advance directive legislation is concerned with what is to be done after the makers of such directives have become incompetent, i.e. incapable of understanding the nature and quality of their options and actions, or of acting rationally on the basis of such understanding as they may have. Such a directive, then, typically comes into effect after its maker has become incapable of performing legally significant acts such as the act of revoking the advance directive itself. Now all existing advance directive legislation provides that, *while competent*, makers of such declaration can freely revoke them, even by nod or wink. These provisions witness to the commonsense of the matter: people's assessments of their own interests and/or concerns often vary with circumstances. 'What seemed a good idea to me then no longer seems so.' But the inner logic of advance directives is this: Once one becomes incompetent, it is one's *past* assessments and directives that prevail over one's own present desires, however urgently felt and expressed, and over any assessments of one's best interests that may be made by one's friends, family, and attending doctors and nurses.[7]

2. The notion that the incompetent have *autonomy* rights (as distinct from dignity and welfare rights) becomes radically incoherent when those incompetent persons who have never made any advance healthcare directive are declared to have an autonomy right exercisable on their behalf, even by an agent or 'guardian' or other 'representative' whose decision is to refuse treatment on the ground that these patients, were they competent and reasonable, *would* choose to refuse treatment and accept death, perhaps not for their own supposed benefit but at any rate for the benefit of others liable to the costs and burdens of caring for them.

   The unbalanced primacy of autonomy thus is often given effect to *via* a notion of *substituted judgment*. In turn, the widespread appeal to the 'standard' of substituted judgment, in preference to the alternative standard of the *patient's best interests*, sets all concerned on a royal road towards decisions to bring about the death of incompetent persons on the plea that if they were reasonable they would choose to seek death, if not

---

[7] Ronald Dworkin, *Life's Dominion* (Harper Collins, London, 1993) 228–9, argues: 'A competent person's right to autonomy requires that his past decisions about how he is to be treated if he becomes demented be respected even if they contradict the desires he has at that later point.' As he says, this conclusion 'has great practical importance' and 'very troubling consequences'. 'We might [sic] consider it morally unforgivable not to try to save the life of someone who plainly enjoys her life, no matter how demented she is, and we might think it beyond imagining that we should actually kill her. . . . We might have other good reasons for treating [her] as she now wishes, rather than as . . . she once asked. *But still, that violates rather than respects her autonomy.*' (emphasis added). On p.232, Dworkin adds that if we refuse to carry out the advance directive which the person now happily demented gave while competent, 'we cannot claim to be acting for her sake.' The practical conclusion of Dworkin's argument (though he carefully abstains from ever clearly expressing or repudiating it) is that those who when competent have willed that they should die if they become incompetent have a right to be put to death when incompetent even though, at that time, they enjoy life and firmly wish to stay alive.

172

by 'active' then by 'passive euthanasia'.[8] Section 5B(2)(b) of the Victorian statute, quoted above, is a mild example of the appeal to substituted judgment.

IV

Is a 'terminally ill' patient really dying?

The Victorian statute differs from the American state statutes (and the VES Bill) in one particularly important way. At least down to 1986, every American statute provided that advance directives should take effect only if and when the patient is *terminally ill*.[9] The Victorian statute contains no such provision. (On the other hand, an advance directive in Victoria takes effect only in relation to a stated medical condition 'current' at the time of the making of the directive, and the directive certificate becomes inoperative if and when that condition ceases to be current.)

Moreover, half of the American statutes define terminal illness as one which will soon result in death *whether or not* (i.e. even if) life-sustaining treatments are employed. American euthanasiast writers are impatient with this:

If the patient will shortly die with or without life-supporting treatment, there is little reason to engage in euthanasia. Further, if the intent of living will statutes was to permit the 'natural death' of persons who would otherwise linger for years maintained by modern machinery in a vegetative but 'alive' state, then the requirement that death be imminent whether or not treatment is withdrawn nullifies the purpose of such statutes.[10]

In line with this dissatisfaction, the English VES Bill defines a terminal condition as

an incurable or irreversible condition which, *without* the use of life-sustaining treatment, will ... result in death in a relatively short time. (emphasis added)

The Bill defines 'life-sustaining treatment' as any medical procedure or intervention which, when administered to a patient in a terminal condition, 'has the effect only of prolonging the process of dying'. These definitions of 'terminal' and 'life-sustaining', being thus logically interdependent, are

---

[8] Of course, English law's preference for the 'best interests' over the 'substituted judgment' standard does not of itself offer secure protection against euthanasiast interpretations of best interests. Thus it was decided in *Bland* that it was in *his* best interests to be killed by withdrawal of food and water, even though his life was no burden *to him*. His life itself was treated as if it were of *no* value.

[9] American courts have gone well beyond this, and in 1989 the Supreme Court of Georgia concluded a judgment by suggesting that 'the legislature might well choose to legislate in this area to provide appropriate non-judicial procedures for competent adult patients who do not have "terminal conditions", but who wish to exercise their rights to refuse medical treatment by the withdrawal of life-sustaining procedures.': *State of Georgia* v *McAfee* 259 Ga. 579; 385 S. E. 2d 651 (1980).

[10] Gregory Gelfand, 'Living Will Statutes: The First Decade', [1987] *Wisconsin Law Review* 737–822 at 741–2. In Gelfand's view, all the American state statutes (rightly) provide for passive euthanasia (p.748), and he notes with apparent irritation that, because many of the statutes require that death be imminent, 'a patient like Karen Quinlan, who lingered in a coma (unaided by the life-prolonging treatments that living will acts would allow to be discontinued) during virtually the entire first decade of living will statutes, could not be terminated under any of these provisions' (p. 744 n.20). His own model statute would allow active euthanasia ('death hastened' by 'administration of medication to affirmatively induce death') for all patients whether dying or not: pp. 802, 805, 819.

173

confusingly elusive. Is a condition terminal if it is irreversible (like diabetes) and would soon result in death unless treatment were used which is life-sustaining not merely in the Bill's special sense but in the ordinary under-standing of the term? It is impossible to say.

What one can say is that American euthanasiast lawyers have expressed scepticism about the notion (used in over 30 state statutes) of treatments which 'serve only to postpone the moment of dying': as these lawyers observe, 'such a provision would be far too broad if taken literally.' For, they say, 'most medical interventions serve only to postpone the moment of death, even in an otherwise healthy patient'.[11] This objection assumes, of course, that medicine is precisely about preserving life and postponing death. In truth, however, medicine is about restoring and preserving health. At the core of the good of health is the integrated organic functioning which we call life; psychosomatic fitness to participate in other basic human goods is health's fruition or fullness.

Are those patients terminally ill who can no longer participate in any good activity or experience (e.g. because they are irreversibly unconscious), but who will survive for a long time (e.g. many years) if given food and fluids and elementary nursing care? On this key question, the VES Bill is, at best, ambiguous. Does giving such patients food and water 'only prolong the process of dying'? Doubtless the euthanasiasts who sponsor the VES Bill answer that question affirmatively, like all those American and now English judges and jurists who declare that life in such a condition is mere scare-quotation-marked 'life', and/or is tantamount to death, and/or is the death of the person, and/or is of no benefit to anyone, and is certainly not 'worthwhile' or 'worth living'.[12] Indeed, the phrase 'only prolong the process of dying', though it has an acceptable sense and application, is likely in its context and current usage to corrode the sense that human life itself remains a good even when as deeply wounded and inadequately instantiated as in the permanently comatose. The fact remains that feeding and caring for such persons does not merely prolong the process of their dying, since they are not yet dying in the common-sense meaning of 'dying'.[13] And that common-sense is the last link between the real human world and the definitions of the VES Bill and many other advance directive statutes, whose subtlety and artificiality is an open door to abuse, i.e. to deliberate killing, as a means to an end.

[11] Gelfand at 743.
[12] See e.g. Ronald Dworkin, 'The Right to Death', *New York Review of Books*, 31 January 1991, 14–17; *Cruzan* v. *Director Missouri Department of Health* 110 Supreme Court Reports 2841 (1990) per Stevens J (dissenting); *Airedale N.H.S. Trust* v. *Bland* [1993] 2 W.L.R. 316 at 330, 353, 372; cf. 367.
[13] Of course, it is not the *word* that matters. The confusion created by artificial definitions of 'terminally ill' can be replicated in the case of 'dying'. Thus Richard McCormick SJ, who thinks that medical technology ought to be used if it will bring about '(1) a return to relatively normal health; (2) ultimate independence from the technology', states that 'in some instances, the difference between a dying and a nondying patient is rooted in a *value judgment* about whether we *ought* to use the available technology or not'; patients 'are "not dying" only if we judge that we *ought* to feed them artificially'! See Richard A. McCormick, *The Critical Calling* (Georgetown U. P., Washington DC, 1989) 378–82.

V

May nutrition and hydration be refused?

A vital question, therefore, in considering any advance directive (or legislation concerning such directives) is whether the authorised refusal of 'treatment' extends to nutrition and hydration. If it does, one can be sure that – unless the directive applies only to someone *dying* in the real commonsense sense – suicide and homicide are in play. For, in an affluent society which can afford to feed, even artificially (e.g. intravenously), all its members, what reason can there be to refuse nutrition and hydration, or withdraw them, in the case of someone who could assimilate them and whose death is otherwise not imminent? The only reason can be: in order to bring about death, as a means (e.g. of alleviating suffering or saving the expenses of continued life).

The majority of American states exclude from the provisions of advance directives (i) comfort care, (ii) the alleviation of pain, and (iii) nutrition and hydration. These cannot be refused in advance, or withdrawn by an agent. The legislative trend has been to *add* the third category,[14] obviously for fear of suicide and homicide.[15] A majority of *these* states, however, permit the refusal etc. of 'mechanical' or 'artificial' treatments, which is taken to include intravenous or naso-gastric tubal provision of food and water.[16] And meanwhile the judicial trend has been towards judging that all the exclusions, and especially the third, are unconstitutional restrictions of the supposed 'constitutional right' to refuse treatment.[17]

The Victorian statute gives no right to refuse or withhold or withdraw 'palliative care', which is defined as including (a) the provision of reasonable medical procedures for the relief of pain, suffering or discomfort, or [sic] the reasonable provision of food and water. It is impossible to predict the interpretation of the key words 'reasonable' and 'or' in this somewhat opaque provision.

The VES Bill provides only that it 'shall not affect the duty of the attending physician to provide for a patient's comfort and care and the alleviation of pain'. The silence about food and water, or nutrition and

---

14 Gelfand at p. 750.

15 Gelfand, however, says: 'The reluctance of most states to permit ... a choice [to refuse food and water] is undoubtedly the result of the non-too-merciful image of a patient slowly and painfully starving to death ... In those cases where the patient can feel pain ... such a death is an extremely cruel one. So much pain is quite a price to pay for an emotional desire to avoid active euthanasia. This problem, of course, would not arise if living will statutes permitted active euthanasia' (pp. 751–2).

16 See Gelfand at p. 752. He comments that the distinction between natural and artificial feeding seems unsustainable. From an entirely different moral perspective, a similar conclusion is reached in two important papers: Germain Grisez, 'Should Nutrition and Hydration Be Provided to Permanently Comatose and Other Mentally Disabled Persons?' *Linacre Quarterly*, 57 (2) (1990), 30–43; William E. May et al., 'Feeding and Hydrating the Permanently Unconscious and Other Vulnerable Persons' *Issues in Law & Medicine* 3 (1987) 203–217. See likewise the careful Statement of the Catholic Bishops of Pennsylvania, 12 December 1991, 'Nutrition and Hydration: Moral Considerations' *Linacre Quarterly* 59 (1992) 8–30.

17 *Bouvia* v. *Superior Court*, 179 California Appeals 3d 1127, 225 Cal. Reptr. 297 (1986); *Corbett* v. *D'Alessandro*, 487 Southern 2d 368 (Florida District Court of Appeals 1986); *Zant* v. *Prevatte* 246 Georgia 832, 286 SE 2d 715 (Georgia Supreme Court, 1982)

hydration, is eloquent indeed. Moreover, the model advance directive appended as Schedule 1 to the Bill (and more widely distributed by the VES independently of their Bill) directs that 'any distressing conditions (*including any caused by lack of food or fluid*) are to be fully controlled by appropriate analgesic or other treatment ...' (emphasis added). In short, though the Bill expressly provides only for the refusal of 'medical procedures or interventions', it carries the strong implication (or implied intent) that food and fluid may be refused, certainly when they could only be administered artificially, and quite possibly also in other cases too. It is, after all, a Bill sponsored by overt euthanasiasts.

Should English law, supposing it were to give legal effect to advance directives,[18] follow the common American route of allowing refusal of *artificial* nutrition and hydration? The Bishops of Pennsylvania give a pertinent answer:

It is not ... the question of whether a type of care is artificial or natural that makes the difference in terms of its continuance or discontinuance. The fact is that every mode of taking in food and drink is, to some extent, artificial. ... If the supplying of nutrition and hydration is of benefit to the patient and causes no undue burden of pain or suffering or excessive expenditure, then it is our duty to take and to provide that nutrition and hydration.[19]

Save when the pathological condition which caused a persistent vegetative state or which is concurrent with it threatens imminent death, supplying nourishment to the permanently unconscious 'is clearly beneficial in terms of preservation of life'; it is not a matter of simply prolonging the dying process without actually preserving life.[20] In short, it is morally ordinary (obligatory) treatment, which neither the patient nor the surrogates of the patient have the moral right to withhold or withdraw. 'Neither does the physician have the right to do so simply because the patient or the surrogates demand this.'[21]

What is 'excessive expenditure'? Although human life even in irreversible unconsciousness is of intrinsic value, and may not be intentionally destroyed by act or omission, that value wholly lacks the further goods which normally accompany it (knowledge, friendship, play and skill, communication in prayer, etc). Might not someone contemplating being in so radically deprived a state reasonably decide that any use of hospital and specifically medical resources would be excessive? If so, he could judge that the duty to give and accept ordinary care requires no more than this: the giving of such food, water and nursing care as can be provided from the resources available in one's home.

[18] *Obiter dicta* of the Law Lords in *Bland* treat them as having legal effect already, by common law.
[19] Statement of December 1991, 59 *Linacre Quarterly*. at p.17.
[20] Ibid., at p. 18.
[21] Ibid., at p. 23.

3

The BMA Report on Euthanasia and the Case Against Legalization

LUKE GORMALLY

1. Introduction

The most important document on euthanasia to have appeared in the UK in the decade since *Euthanasia and Clinical Practice* was published in 1982 is the British Medical Association Working Party Report on *Euthanasia*[1]. This is a substantial document[2] which is more comprehensive in scope than *Euthanasia and Clinical Practice*, which concentrates almost exclusively on the *ethics* of clinical practice.

By contrast the BMA Report specifically discusses, among other questions, whether voluntary euthanasia should be *legalized*. Nonetheless, it is the view which the BMA Working Party took of the ethical considerations that should govern clinical practice which also determined the case they make against legalization of euthanasia. Concern with the ethics of clinical practice is central to both documents. This chapter seeks to analyse and evaluate the case which the BMA Report makes against the legalization of voluntary euthanasia.

The Working Party which produced the Report was chaired by Sir Henry Yellowlees, a former Chief Medical Officer of The Department of Health and Social Security, and comprised two specialists in community medicine, a general practitioner, a consultant paediatrician, a professor of geriatric medicine, and the medical director of a hospice. It was served by officers of the British Medical Association, and there were three 'observers': one a solicitor who was a former chief nursing officer of a district health authority, one a barrister, and the third a professional philosopher who is also a neurosurgeon[3]. The seven members of the Working Party were, then, all members of the medical profession and, apart from what came to them in the form of submissions and evidence, had access to advice on legal and philosophical questions from the 'observers'.

---

[1] *Euthanasia, Report of the Working Party to review the British Medical Association's guidance on euthanasia.* London, British Medical Association, May 1988.

[2] The main part of the document is ordered consecutively in 271 paragraphs, organized into 14 chapters. A final Chapter 15 contains 16 conclusions. References in the text of the present chapter to the BMA Report will be by paragraph number (e.g. para.16) or to a numbered conclusion (e.g. Conclusion 16).

There are frequent cross-references in the present chapter to the Linacre Centre's *Submission to the Select Committee of The House of Lords on Medical Ethics* (pp.111–165 of the present volume). Such references are indicated by the short title *Submission*, followed by the section number.

[3] Dr Grant Gillett. For some evidence suggestive of his influence on the Working Party Report see footnote 9 to this chapter.

The Working Party was established early in 1987 in response to a resolution passed at the 1986 Annual Representative Meeting of the British Medical Association urging that the Association 'reconsider its policy on euthanasia'. To this end the Working Party held 15 meetings in a period of as many months, publishing the Report in May 1988.

The Working Party undertook to review a wide range of considerations with some bearing on the question of whether euthanasia should be legalized: ethical and legal considerations, the teaching of religious bodies, practices in other countries, as well as professional views about what is appropriate in those areas of clinical practice in which the issue of euthanasia can arise.

The primary objective of the Working Party was to define a general rule of appropriate professional conduct in regard both to voluntary and non-voluntary euthanasia. The position advanced is that euthanasia, whether voluntary or non-voluntary, is *generally* undesirable, and, accordingly, the Working Party concludes that killing patients for euthanasiast reasons should remain a criminal offence.

In section 2 of this Chapter I shall outline the main ethical considerations which lead the Working Party to conclude that euthanasia should not be legalised. In section 3 I shall identify what seem to be the weak points in that case. Those weaknesses are sufficiently grave to be damaging to a coherent professional ethic. The framework of principle required for a coherent ethic has been analysed in the *Submission* (Book II, Chapter 1 of the present volume), and in some respects is explored in greater depth in *Euthanasia and Clinical Practice: trends, principles and alternatives* (Book I).

2. The Working Party's case against legalizing voluntary euthanasia

2.1 Euthanasia and the value of the individual

The Working Party claim that a constant and core feature of the ethos of medicine is 'the conviction that human life is of inestimable value and ought to be protected and cherished' (para.72). An ethos dominated by that conviction leads one to embrace the arduous task of finding value in the lives of patients suffering pain and severe disability; to end those lives would be a comparatively easy option (para.62). The view that someone would be 'better off dead' is linked to being 'discriminatory about the kind of worth that attends a life' (para.56). In being asked to kill patients doctors are being asked to abandon the conviction that human life is of inestimable value and ought to be protected and cherished (para.72). The principal reason for rejecting 'a change in the law to permit doctors to intervene to end a person's life' derives from recognition 'of the supreme value of the individual, no matter how worthless and hopeless that individual may feel' (Conclusion 16).

One strand in the thinking of the Working Party involves distinguishing between the *objective* value of individual human beings, which remains 'inestimable', and the *subjective* sense of value an individual experiences, which may wax and wane. The 'inestimable' objective value does not permit us (it is at least suggested) to discriminate between the value of individual lives in such a way as to provide justification for ending some of those lives on the grounds that the individuals concerned would be 'better off' dead. To take that view of a human life would be to abandon the conviction that human lives are of 'inestimable value'.

Here we have the sketch of a line of reasoning for opposing euthanasiast killing. It needs a more developed and systematic statement, but seems clearly to represent one strand in the thinking of the Working Party. However, there are other elements in that thinking which are at odds with the reasoning sketched here and which tend to undermine the conclusion the Working Party seek to advance. It will be necessary to discuss those elements in the next section (see 3.1 below).

2.2 The importance of an unambiguous rule against euthanasiast killing for maintaining the true character of the doctor's commitment to patient care.

The second point presupposes and develops from the first. A sense of the inestimable value of individual human lives is essential if doctors are to 'maintain a dedication to care of patients and the preservation of life' (para.238). But if they do not have this dedication, 'if patients were to perceive that doctors were ready to kill where they cannot cure' (ibid.), then patients would cease to have confidence in the commitment of doctors. The destruction of trust in the character of doctors' commitment would undermine the doctor-patient relationship. To permit euthanasia would be to create a climate in which certain patients are perceived 'as lingering nuisances whose worth and well being are no longer significant' (ibid.) In so far as euthanasiast killing rests on the view that those to be killed would be better off dead because they no longer have lives worth living, it is premised on a valuation of human life incompatible with that valuation which is essential if doctors are to maintain a positive, creative commitment to the care of patients. For the sake of supporting that commitment doctors need to be forbidden to engage in killing which rests on the assumption that the lives of some human beings are not of inestimable value. For in so far as they engaged in such killing they would have ceased to grasp the *practical import* of the belief that each human life is of inestimable value.

The reasoning of the Working Party here connects *practical* belief in the inestimable value of individual human lives with the *character* of doctors. 'If the profession is seen as sometimes curing and sometimes killing depending on a rather complex set of guidelines ... the patients may well have some apprehension *about the nature of the individuals* who are supposed to be jealously preserving their lives.' (para.77, emphasis added)

For reasons explained in the *Submission* (section 1.2.2), the Working Party is right to see a close connection between euthanasiast killing and the valuation of human life.

179

However, it is not clear that the Working Party's understanding of the kind of prohibition of euthanasiast killing they support will do the job they think required: the job of sustaining doctors in their commitment to the care of patients. For though the Working Party wish to see maintained a legal prohibition on euthanasiast killing they do not support their case by arguing for an *absolute* moral prohibition, i.e. a prohibition which does not allow of exceptions. The Working Party readily concede that a doctor may be confronted by cases in which, however rarely, he may justifiably kill a patient. It will be important to discuss the reason for allowing such exceptions and to ask whether the logic of doing so does not undermine a general prohibition (i.e. one which is meant to hold *for the most part*) and consequently the role of such a prohibition in protecting the character of doctors in their commitment to the care of patients (see 3.4 below).

2.3 The insensitivity of euthanasia

In a number of places the Working Party Report advances the following consideration against permitting euthanasiast killing: euthanasia carried out as a solution to problems of pain and suffering is very often insensitive to the underlying significance of a plea to be killed and to the potentially transient character of the outlook which prompted the patient to make the plea (para.92.2; see para.61). Evidence for the frequently transient character of the desire that one's life be brought to an end is seen in the fact that 'failed suicides rarely repeat their attempts and that most are glad that their lives were saved' (para.42).

Considerations of this kind are not insignificant in considering the effect legalization of voluntary euthanasia would have on the practice of medicine. If it were legalized there should be little doubt that ostensible pleas to be killed which are covert pleas for considerate and committed care will be treated as providing sufficient justification for killing patients. The Netherlands has now provided us with ample evidence of how doctors are likely to behave when euthanasia is not in fact treated as a criminal offence.[4]

Nonetheless, someone might doubt whether a consideration of this kind provides sufficient reason for a blanket prohibition of euthanasia. In conjunction with the two other reasons offered it is indeed a powerful consideration. But those two reasons carry the main burden of the case for a blanket prohibition and so it is important to examine how well-grounded and consistent is the Working Party's presentation of those reasons.

3. Weaknesses in the Working Party's case.

3.1 Which human beings are of 'inestimable value' and why are they?

The key assertion on which the Working Party's case against euthanasia hangs is that 'human life is of inestimable value'. At first sight this might be taken to mean that *any* human life is of inestimable value. But a reading of

---

[4] See the two chapters by John Keown in this volume.

the sections of the Report on Brain Death (paras.29–33) and the Persistent Vegetative State (paras.34–39) undermines this interpretation.

The Working Party think that acceptance of 'brain death as a criterion for the end of life' indicates 'that it is the distinct functions provided by the human brain that make human life of unique ethical importance' (para.31). This confuses two questions which are quite distinct (though they may have a single correct answer): (1) When is X dead? and (2) When does X's life cease to have special moral significance?

A particular understanding of the meaning of death and certain physiological claims about the role of the brain stem in the human organism, together provide grounds for accepting that diagnosis of 'brain stem death' (which is what the UK protocol purports to establish[5]) is an adequate basis for diagnosing death. The understanding of death referred to here is 'the cessation of the bodily life of the human individual'. By a living human individual is meant (given the falsehood of dualism[6]) a living human organism. For something to cease to be an organism is for it to cease to be an integrated whole; death is loss of the capacity for integrated functioning. Given the truth of the physiological claim about the role of the brain stem as the key organ in the integration of the human organism, it is reasonable to hold that *total* destruction of the brain stem amounts to irreversible loss of the capacity for integrated organic functioning. On this account 'brain stem death' is a decisive indicator of death because in establishing the existence of 'brain stem death' one establishes that there no longer is a living organism.

The Working Party, however, speaking more broadly of 'brain death' (rather than 'brain stem death') think of its significance as lying not in the loss of integrated organic functioning but in the loss of the capacity for distinctively human experience (para.31). On this account of why someone may be dead, death is compatible with a functioning brain stem, for it could be declared on the basis of establishing irreversible destruction of the neocortex. It is indeed the view of the Working Party that all that stands in the way of declaring someone dead on the basis of establishing 'neocortical death' is the technical difficulty of establishing 'that irreversible and complete loss of all neocortical function has occurred' (para.34).

Discussing the case of a child with hydranencephaly, Dr. Christopher Pallis has written: 'There is a spinal cord, a brain stem, and perhaps some diencephalic structures but certainly no cerebral hemispheres. The cranial cavity is full of cerebrospinal fluid and transilluminates when a light is applied to it. The child can breathe spontaneously, swallow, and grimace in response to painful stimuli. Its eyes are open. The heart can beat normally for months. No culture would declare that child dead.'[7] That last obser-

---

[5] The protocol is contained in Conference of Medical Royal Colleges and their Faculties in the UK. 'Diagnosis of Brain Death'. *British Medical Journal* 2(1976) 1187–1188. See further Conference of Medical Royal Colleges and their Faculties in the UK. 'Memorandum on the diagnosis of death'. *British Medical Journal* 1(1979) 322.

[6] See the *Submission*, section 1.1.5

[7] Christopher Pallis. *ABC of Brain Stem Death* London, British Medical Association 1983, 3. Dr Pallis, who has been the principal apologist for UK practice in the diagnosis of brain stem death, specifically repudiates neocortical death as an indicator of death; *ibid.*, 2.

vation does not appear to be one which the Working Party would dismiss as irrelevant since they state that '... it is important for doctors to be clear as to what they mean by death and to ask whether that is commensurate with what the community at large believes' (para.29).

Why did the Working Party come to think that the determination of an appropriate criterion of death should be based on an understanding of what is *valuable* in human life, as if loss of value were equivalent to death? Some indication of the source of this confusion may be found in the discussion of the Persistent Vegetative State (PVS): 'To be a human life of the type that we all regard as being of special ethical importance we require that there be a persisting capacity for sentience. Where we know that any such capacity has been irreversibly lost we conclude that there is no ethical reason to prolong the biological functions that remain ...' (para.32) Here loss of the capacity which makes for 'ethical significance' is seen as a reason for not seeking to prolong 'biological functions'. Whatever the merits of this consideration as a reason for ceasing life-prolonging treatment it is not as such a reason for saying that the remaining 'biological functions' are not the functions of a living human organism.[8] In one breath the Working Party recognises this (para.35) but in another they seek to justify the brain death criterion by reference to what functions are valuable to an individual[9]: 'Where an individual can no longer have the experiences of a human being and never will again we think that the functions that remain are of no further value to that individual. *That is why controversy over whether the brain stem is completely and in every part dead and whether the whole brain can be said not to be functioning just on the basis of the accepted battery of tests, are beside the point.*' (para.31; emphasis added)

In fact our sense of the 'unique ethical importance' of human beings is not based on their possession of 'sentience'. *All* forms of animal life possess sentience. It is the exercise of the capacities to understand and know the truth and to make free choices which *exhibit* the distinctive dignity and worth of human beings. But the BMA Working Party, along with most people, would be disinclined – for the present – to declare someone dead who, through partial brain damage, had exclusively lost the material vehicles of just those capacities. So they retreat to the view that it is loss of sentience which renders someone dead. But in doing so they are not entitled to defend that claim by explaining that sentience is that distinct function provided by the human brain that makes human life of unique ethical importance.

The dangers of conflating questions about whether or not a human being's life has lost its unique value or significance with the question about whether that human being is dead ought to be obvious. It is quite clear that there is a

[8] The conflation of grounds for discontinuing treatment with grounds for declaring someone dead may be said to have occurred already in the change of position that occurred between the 1976 Report and the 1979 Memorandum of the Conference of Medical Royal Colleges and their Faculties in the UK.

[9] There is reason to think that this strand in the Working Party's thought derives from one of its 'observers', Dr Grant Gillett. See Grant Gillett, 'Why let people die?' *Journal of Medical Ethics* 12 (1986), 83–86, and 'Euthanasia, letting die and the pause' *Journal of Medical Ethics* 14 (1988), 61–68. His position is stated more fully in Grant Gillett, *Reasonable Care*, Bristol: The Bristol Press 1989, especially pp.15–19, 56–68, 93–94, 99–105, and 145.

variety of conflicting views in our society about the conditions under which human beings may be said to have lost unique value or significance. If death is to be defined as the loss of such significance, then an adverse view about the value of a human being's life can find expression in the judgement that that human being is dead. Declarations of death would then be the expression of merely qualitative discriminations between human beings, that is discriminations based on the fact that a human being lacked some significant qualitative attribute.

One effect of acting in this way would be to disguise from people the extent to which they were involved in unjust discrimination between living human beings. It is clear that the Working Party is disposed to adopt this disguise in regard to PVS patients: as already noted, they consider the only obstacle to moving from 'brain death to neocortical death' is our technical inability 'to establish that irreversible and complete loss of all neocortical function has occurred' (para.34). Hence there is said to be a 'vast clinical and philosophical distinction' between terminating the life of a PVS patient and terminating 'the life of a sentient person'. While it is recognised that with PVS 'In one sense there is a human being still alive . . . in another the situation is often best described when a relative remarks that the person they love is no longer there.' The testimony of a distressed relative is invoked to give plausibility to the distinction advanced nowadays by certain philosophers between 'personal life' and 'mere biological life'. If one can be said to enjoy only the latter, then, these philosophers would say, one does not exist as a person.[10]

Philosophical thinking along these lines was undoubtedly influential in the composition of the Report. For when considering the case for killing a patient 'in a state that can no longer be called human life' (para.98), in which 'there is no prospect of restoring the patient to sentient life', the Report observes: 'The situation is not the same as one in which a sentient person is killed.' It immediately adds, however, that 'a patient in the UK who is in a persistent vegetative state, and, consequently, who is non-sentient, is not killed.' (para.101) This has somewhat the force of a detached ethnographic observation rather than a report on practice which the Working Party has given convincing reasons for maintaining. Indeed, when they say

... some patients have permanently lost all capacity for *the conscious quality of life that constitutes being fully human* . . . We have stopped short of saying that such a state ought to be terminated by a *positive* act. (para.131.1; emphasis added)

the position stated sounds decidedly pragmatic, temporary and insecure. Two further points should be noted about this statement. First, many more patients than those in PVS have 'lost all capacity for the conscious quality of life that constitutes being fully human'. Certainly, on one interpretation of that formula (whether or not intended by the Working Party) patients with advanced senile dementia have lost the sort of 'conscious quality of life that constitutes being fully human'. Secondly, the Working Party merely stops

[10] Speaking of malformed babies held to be incapable of giving 'an appreciative response to care-giving', the Report says there is a 'threshold' below which 'there is only a biological vestige of life which it is pointless and cruel to preserve in its distorted state' (para.175).

short of recommending that these patients be killed by a *positive* act. But it does not oppose killing them by a planned course of omissions. That, however, is to raise another major point about the unsatisfactory character of the Working Party's case against legalizing euthanasia, a point to be considered more fully in the next section (3.2 below).

The *qualitative* discrimination between patients that the Working Party introduces in its discussion of patients in a PVS also plays an important role in its discussion of the treatment of 'severely malformed infants'. Some of these are clearly likened in status to PVS patients. The paediatrician's duty is said to be that of ascertaining 'whether there is any hope that the child will have a life that could reasonably be called the life of a person'. In regard to children with severe brain damage this is treated as equivalent to asking whether the child has 'the capacity to love and be loved. If this is not present and is never going to be then it is clear that the child lacks that crucial engagement with persons that constitutes a basis for ethically significant life. Where a child is responsive to human care and contact in some sentient way then the child must be treated as a person, however poorly developed.' (para. 132) Some children, however, are said to lack 'the capacity for meaningful human life' (para 133)

Which human beings are, then, of inestimable value? Those with the distinctive brain-related capacities which confer 'unique ethical importance' on human beings. It is wholly implausible to suggest that sentience is the relevant capacity. Whatever developed level of ability is required for a 'meaningful human life' is also required if one is to be a human being of inestimable value.

Which abilities, and what degree of development of those abilities, are requisite will inevitably be contentious. In consequence the exercise of distinguishing between those who may not be intentionally killed (because they are of inestimable value) and those who may (because they lack that value) will unavoidably be arbitrary and therefore unjust.[11]

3.2 What counts as intentional killing?

The Working Party are commendably clear in recognising

The law's deep seated adherence to intent rather than consequences alone [as] an important reference point in the moral assessment of any action. A decision to withdraw treatment which has become a burden and is no longer of continuing benefit to a patient has a different intent to one which involves ending the life of a person. We accept drug treatment which may involve a risk to the patient's life if the sole intention is to relieve illness, pain, distress or suffering. [Conclusion 14]

Accepting the central importance of intention to the characterization and, therefore, the evaluation of chosen actions, the Working Party reject the view that it is only outcomes or consequences which should count in the moral evaluation of actions. [see paras. 94–97] On this latter, characteristically utilitarian view there is no significant moral distinction between

---

[11] See further the *Submission*, section 1.1.4

hastening death as a foreseeable consequence of the administration of drugs aimed at controlling pain, and bringing about death as a result of administering a lethal dose of drugs aimed precisely at bringing about death.

While the Working Party's insistence on the basic importance of intention is clear, their treatment of the important topic of intentional omissions is unsatisfactory. They tend to discuss decisions to terminate life as if they could be implemented only by positive acts. Thus at para.92 we read:

There is a distinction between a decision to terminate someone's life and a decision not to prolong a person's life. The former involves an act or intervention which causes death and the latter involves the cessation of life-prolonging treatment.

But a 'decision to terminate someone's life' may be carried out by a planned course of omissions as well as by a positive act. This fact is never sufficiently clearly recognised by the Working Party.[12] Indeed one of their conclusions explicitly contrasts nontreatment decisions with 'active interventions by a doctor to terminate life' as if the former were in all cases no more than decisions 'not to prolong life' [Conclusion 3].

Having recognised the centrality of intention to the law's characterization and assessment of action, the Working Party should have also taken account of the law's recognition of homicidal omissions.[13]

3.3 Limits of the duty to treat

Some decisions to omit life-prolonging treatment are morally acceptable and some are morally unacceptable for reasons other than that they are aimed at hastening a patient's death. While a comprehensive discussion of the limits of a doctor's duty to treat would be inappropriate here, it is necessary to give some consideration to the views of the Working Party about when omission of treatment is acceptable and to enquire whether those views are compatible with a principled opposition to euthanasia.

Under the general title 'Quality of life' the Working Party outline the kinds of situation in which differing quality of life considerations provide reasons for withholding treatment. They are:

(1) When '... patients have permanently lost all capacity for the conscious quality of life that constitutes being fully human' (para. 131.1). The

[12] Paras. 261 and 262 do not provide clear evidence of such a recognition.

[13] Perhaps the clearest direction, of obvious relevance to certain medical practices, is the one approved by the Court of Criminal Appeal in *R v Gibbins and Proctor* (1918) 13 Criminal Appeal Reports 134 at 137–8:

'... if you think that one or other of the prisoners wilfully and intentionally withheld food from that child so as to cause her to weaken and to cause her grievous bodily injury, as the result of which she died, it is not necessary for you to find that she intended or he intended to kill the child then and there. It is enough if you find that he or she intended to set up such a set of facts by withholding food or anything as would in the ordinary course of nature lead gradually but surely to her death. '

This direction was of the clearest relevance in *Regina v Arthur*, but the issue was regrettably obfuscated by the trial judge in his summing up in that case.

The court in *Gibbins and Proctor* was aware of many earlier directions to like effect, and specifically approved that given in *R v Bubb and Hook* (1850) 10 Cox C.C. 455 att 459. The concept of murder by omission is fully confirmed by the Infanticide Act 1938, s.1(1), and the Homicide Act 1957, s.2(1).

quality of life judgement made here to characterise the condition of the patient is one which determines in effect whether the kind of life someone has is worth preserving. The Working Party are disposed to ask whether a patient has 'the capacity for meaningful human life' (para. 133). If the answer is no, they clearly believe that life-prolonging measures should be withheld, though they stop 'short of saying that such a state ought to be terminated by a positive act' (para. 131. 1)

(2) When the burdens consequent upon treatment greatly exceed the benefit secured by treatment, so that in effect the treatment is inflicting 'prolonged suffering then it is correct and wise to take the kinder course and ... settle for comfort and care rather than further intervention.' (para. 131. 2)

(3) When 'life as a whole' has become 'an intolerable burden' to a patient, it is not the treatment as such which is a burden but the medical prolongation of life; then 'the right thing to do is to agree not to take any measures which merely prolong life and cannot relieve the patient's condition'. (para. 131. 3)

Of these three kinds of reason for limiting treatment, (1) is clearly euthanasiast; for the reason offered purports to be a comprehensive judgement on the very value of a human being's existence such that, if the judgement is adverse, death may be presented as 'a good to be pursued by the doctor'.[14]

By contrast (2) offers a clearly non-euthanasiast reason for limiting treatment: treatment is limited precisely to avoid imposing unwarranted burdens consequent upon treatment and not with a view to hastening death.

The formulation of (3) as it stands is unsatisfactory, for two reasons: (a) because it does not distinguish between judgements made by a competent patient which give a doctor reason to limit treatment, and any parallel grounds there may be for limiting treatment of the incompetent; and (b) because it does not sufficiently distinguish between a construal of the suggested reason for limiting treatment which, in the mouth of a competent patient, would be clearly suicidal and any possible non-suicidal construal of the reason. [A clarification of these issues is offered in the Endnote to this chapter.]

The Working Party does briefly consider the question of cooperation with a patient's suicidal decisions when, in relation to high spinal injuries, they discuss what a doctor's response should be to a patient's refusal to consent to continuing respiratory support. At this point they show themselves aware of the fact that death may be intentionally hastened by deliberate omission, for they observe:

As the law stands it is impossible to maintain a hard and fast distinction between withdrawal of such support and assisted suicide. (para. 84)

Accordingly, they hold that '... in this situation, doctors should make their position clear by both acting and being seen to act according to a court decision'. (ibid.,)

[14] See Linacre Centre Working Party Report in the present volume, Book I, chapter 3, sec.5, pp.43–5.

The Working Party's endorsement of comprehensive quality of life judgements in clinical practice along with their general reluctance to recognise the reality of intentional killing by planned omission, show most clearly their joint influence in what the Report is prepared to accommodate in the field of paediatric care. It will be evident to anyone familiar with the debate about management of handicapped newborns[15] that para. 134 of the Report, in referring to 'a practical decision not to offer life-prolonging treatment', includes omission of adequate nutrition. It is made evident from what is specified as the appropriate treatment of children judged to be incapable of 'meaningful human lives': 'Hydration should be provided and the patient should not be deprived of the normal cuddling that expresses a fundamental human concern' (para. 134); in other words, it is hydration and cuddling which alone should be given. Of course the condition of some irreversibly dying infants may be such that attempts at feeding may be an unwarranted burden. But 'the practice of sedation and demand feeding' (para. 172) is applied to infants with malformations not because the provision of adequate nutrition would be burdensome but precisely as a method of bringing about the death by starvation.

The Working Party (at para. 135) seek to resist the logic of the position they have adopted in countenancing comprehensive quality of life judgements:

'The profession's moral stance ought to be that human life is generally worth saving and any slide toward the view that quality of life can be used to exercise "quality control" so that parents or society can opt to keep only "top quality" infants should be strongly resisted. If the medical profession was ever to allow such an attitude to influence our treatment of children then this would clearly undermine our commitment to preserve and enhance human life. The soundness of medical judgement is intimately dependent on a reverence for human life, and any erosion of our intuitive feelings for the young, the weak and the helpless carries great potential for making a fundamental difference to the ethos of medical practice.' (para. 136)

Much of this is well said, but unfortunately the Working Party have disabled their own case against these undesirable developments both by countenancing comprehensive quality of life judgements and by their intellectual evasiveness about the moral character of policies of sedation and starvation.

3.4 General Rules and Exceptions

It will be obvious enough from the points surveyed in 3.1–3.3 that the Working Party have not provided a case for an absolute *moral* prohibition on the practice of euthanasia. But this observation may be thought to be beside the point since the Working Party did not think of themselves as constructing such a case but rather of arriving at a clear general rule of conduct which would serve to sustain the character of the doctor's commitment to the well-being of patients and thereby retain the trust of patients in doctors (see section 2.2 above). As the Report observes: 'If the profession is seen as sometimes curing and sometimes killing depending on a rather

---

[15] For some summary documentation of the debate as it had taken shape over a decade ago see the Linacre Centre Working Party Report, chapter 2, pp.15–22 in this volume.

complex set of guidelines ... the patients may well have some apprehension about the nature of the individuals who are supposed to be jealously preserving their lives.' (para. 77) So what is at issue is the character of doctors as the necessary guarantor of the character of clinical practice.

The Working Party clearly does not think that an exceptionless (or absolute) moral rule is necessary to foster the kind of character they think desirable in doctors. Following the advice of Professor Hare, they seem to think that what is required is a fairly simple and clear general rule. Hare is quoted as saying:

Doctors would do well, having adopted some fairly simple set of principles which copes adequately with the cases they are likely to meet, to dismiss from their minds (at least when they are doctoring) the possibility of their being *further* exceptions to their principles. For doctors, like all of us, are human, and if once they start thinking, when engaged on a case, that this case might be one of the limitless and indeterminate set of exceptions to their principles, they will find such exceptions everywhere ... The temptation to special pleading is too great. A doctor once said to me in connection with the proposal to allow euthanasia: 'We shall start by putting patients away because they are in intolerable pain and haven't long to live anyway; and we shall end up putting them away because it's Friday night and we want to get away for the weekend'. [Quoted in para. 12; emphasis added.]

So Hare's advice is that one formulate a clear moral rule which has built into it clear and unambiguous exceptions of a kind that do not require much on-the-job reflection about whether the case confronting one is covered by those exceptions. Clearly it is also required that the rule should draw the line about what is impermissible in a fashion sufficiently credible not to excite on-the-job doubts about its reasonableness.

The Working Party addresses the topic of exceptions to a general rule against euthanasia at two points. At para. 76 it is allowed that there may be 'highly unusual and circumscribed situations' in which 'it may well not be appropriate to regard a doctor's actions as totally and solely answerable to the general rule'; which seems to mean that it may be reasonable for a doctor to act on the basis of the judgement that the case he is dealing with is a justifiable exception to the rule. But the Working Party then go on to say that in such situations the doctor should 'seek a second opinion and explore one of the many other recourses we have suggested ... We believe that if the unusual problem is shared with a colleague the doctor will almost always find a way to deal with it which does not involve killing the patient'.

At paras. 115–120 the Working Party consider what they believe to be a circumscribed kind of situation in which 'mercy killing' is justifiable, and the practical implications such an exception may be thought to have for the practice of medicine. The situation they have in mind is one in which

a person, usually not medically qualified, kills a companion in order to avoid inevitable suffering before an equally inevitable death. Such a situation could occur in wartime where one of two companions is wounded and certain to be found by the enemy who will perpetrate acts of cruelty before death is inflicted. It is only the certain knowledge that a person will fall in the way of terrible and malicious suffering that can justify a 'mercy killing'. The Working Party did not feel that such an action could be justified when there was any chance of the suffering being averted in some other way or of some unpredictable 'good' befalling the victim. Such a mercy killing can be condoned only where the strongest humanitarian motives act in accord with *an uncontestable factual prediction*. (para. 115)

The Working Party believe that the situation which may arise in warfare provides no precedent for what a doctor should do in the face of situations in which euthanasia is demanded, both because there can be no certainty about what might eventuate before natural death and because terminally ill patients can normally expect to be well cared for. Others, however, may well think that the terms in which the Report expressed its justification of mercy killing in warfare also provide justification for killing in situations which may arise in clinical practice.[16] According to the Report: 'It is only the certain knowledge that a person will fall in the way of terrible and malicious suffering that can justify a "mercy killing".' That a person's suffering is inflicted from malice may indeed make it more terrible, but it is the certain knowledge that suffering will be *terrible* which provides the purported justification of 'mercy killing'. Many people think one can be as certain in clinical situations that terrible suffering will overtake people as one can be in military situations. So the Working Party is likely to seem unreasonable in resisting the logic of the justification of 'mercy killing' which it concedes at para. 115.

However, it should be clear from 3.1–3.3 that the Working Party has conceded much wider grounds for mercy killing than just the certain knowledge of terrible suffering. For they take no principled stand against killing by planned omission, and they allow that comprehensive and adverse quality of life judgements may provide grounds for making a patient's death the proper object of clinical management. Such judgements are inevitably arbitrary (see 3.1 above).

All this means that, despite their protestations to the contrary, the Working Party have conceded grounds on the basis of which doctors might well feel they are justified in carrying out euthanasia on an extensive scale. That being so, it is difficult to sustain the Working Party's opposition to the legalization of euthanasia, an opposition which assumes that the situations in which euthanasia may be called for are so circumscribed, marginal and infrequent that there is no case for legalizing it.

If the present reading of the Report is correct, then the intellectual concessions made by the Working Party would accommodate extensive

[16] The members of the BMA Working Party very clearly felt (as would a majority of people in our society) that it is intolerable to maintain an absolute prohibition on euthanasia in face of harrowing situations of the kind which are recorded as having arisen in the Burma campaign in the Second World War (para. 117 and reference). But we need to reflect on the terms in which the Working Party express their reason for making exceptions: it is the certain knowledge that suffering will be *terrible* that provides the purported justification of 'mercy killing'. Even if this were the only ground for mercy killing conceded by the Working Party (and it is not) many would think it a ground that in principle allowed extremely wide scope for euthanasia in clinical practice. For the logic of conceding the exception is to allow that there are circumstances in which it is reasonable to treat the human dignity of the person to be killed as a value which can be nullified by the entirely predictable evils which are about to overtake a life (see *Submission*, section 1.2.2). But it is the standard case for euthanasia that incontestably predictable evils of suffering and loss of faculties rob so many lives of dignity and value that the ending of such a life is a benefit.

Absolute norms do confront us with hard cases where pressures of sympathy and compassion can make the norm seem intolerable. But the choice of euthanasia as the solution to intolerable suffering has implications that go far wider than the relief of hard cases and extends to the introduction, willy nilly, of very great evils. Among these evils is certainly to be included the corruption of the character of doctors in respects fundamentally subversive of the commitment to patient care that we require of them.

euthanasiast practice, particularly of non-voluntary euthanasia. It is difficult, therefore, to see that they have provided a solid moral case for a legal prohibition of euthanasia. Moreover, in so far as the argument of the Working Party implies that a doctor may choose to kill patients on the grounds that they lack lives of value or that they lack 'the capacity for meaningful human life', they allow behaviour of a kind calculated to undermine precisely that disposition which we need doctors to have: the disposition to respect human beings simply because they are human. Lacking this fundamental requirement of justice, doctors will not 'stand by the commitment that leads us to preserve life and meet suffering creatively' (para. 75).

The reasoning of the Report fails, then, convincingly to articulate and defend the moral norms or rules which would support the cultivation of those dispositions which the Working Party recognise to be indispensable to the practice of good medicine. And that failure makes the Working Party's insistence on a blanket legal prohibition seem ill-supported.

The dispositions we require in doctors cannot be cultivated without conformity to a different normative framework for clinical practice from that envisaged by the Report. The elements of the necessary framework are discussed and analysed in other parts of this volume.

Endnote: Euthanasia and the limits of the duty to treat

The case outlined in the *Submission* is both a case for an exceptionless (i.e. absolute) moral prohibition on the practice of euthanasia as well as a case for a blanket legal prohibition: the justification of euthanasia is too radically subversive of the foundations of just law to be legally accommodated in any form.

The absolute moral prohibition is implicit in what is called a sanctity of life ethic. Critics of a sanctity of life ethic are apt to caricature it by claiming that it requires a commitment to prolonging human lives whatever the circumstances.[17] No such commitment is a requirement of traditional morality. Some of the limits, consistent with a sanctity of life ethic, to a doctor's duty to treat are discussed in chapters 5 and 6 of the Linacre Centre Working Party Report (Book I in this volume, pp.61–71). Here it will be useful to recall some of the clarifications established in those chapters which have a bearing on elements of the BMA Working Party's thinking which were surveyed earlier (at 3.3 above).

At that point it was noted that, whereas the first reason given for limiting treatment was euthanasiast (the judgement that someone lacks 'the capacity for meaningful human life'), and the second reason (that the burdens

---

[17] The caricature makes its most recent appearance in *Medical Ethics Today. Its Practice and Philosophy* London: British Medical Association, 1993. The volume, produced by the Medical Ethics Committee of the BMA, offers 'practical advice . . . in order to guide doctors in any aspects of their practice where ethical considerations arise'. (p. xxvi). At p.165 we read: 'The BMA does not espouse a strict vitalist "sanctity of life" approach although it recognises some of its members do.' This approach has been introduced in the text as requiring that 'life is . . . to be indefinitely sustained in all circumstances, for example, where its prolongation by artificial means would be regarded as inhumane and the treatment itself burdensome'.

consequent on treatment greatly exceed the benefit secured by it) was consistent with opposition to euthanasia, the character of the third reason was in this respect not entirely clear.

The third reason envisaged by the BMA Working Party for limiting treatment is that 'life as a whole' may become 'an intolerable burden' to a patient, so that it is not treatment as such which is burdensome but rather the medical prolongation of life. In those circumstances the Working Party took the view that 'the right thing to do is to agree not to take any measures which merely prolong life and cannot relieve the patient's condition'. (para. 131.3)

A number of quite distinct lines of reasoning might be covered by what the Working Party has in mind at this point. In distinguishing them it would be useful, first of all, to separate the reasoning a *competent* patient might offer to a doctor as grounds for limiting treatment, from comparable reasoning about limiting treatment for an incompetent patient.

If patients are not in the ordinary sense of the term dying, the fact that they may be 'in pain, distressed, incontinent, upset at their insight into the fact that they are severely deformed or disabled, or becoming demented' (para. 131. 1) would not provide grounds for discontinuing a treatment for some other condition (such as insulin for diabetes) when the treatment does nothing to alleviate precisely what is burdensome in the patient's condition. For what could motivate discontinuing it other than the thought: My life is miserable and I can put an end to it by refusing insulin treatment? To proceed on that basis is to choose suicide by omission.

Similarly, when a patient who is dying and wretched decides to refuse treatment for some supervening condition which may hasten death precisely so that death will come sooner, it is clear that his attitude is suicidal.

But *Euthanasia and Clinical Practice* envisages the following scenario in which a patient who is dying is overcome by a supervening condition (e.g. pneumonia) which may hasten death. He reflects, after taking stock of the unalleviated wretchedness of his condition, on whether he has a duty to continue to strive to prolong his life and decides that he has not and *for that reason* declines treatment for the supervening condition. This line of reasoning is to be distinguished from the suicidally motivated reasoning of the previous patient.[18]

At one point *Euthanasia and Clinical Practice* seems firmly to rule out the possibility of a parallel judgement being made (by a doctor or others) in respect of an incompetent patient.[19] But this impression is belied a few pages later by what is implicit in the management of the patient with Parkinson's disease.[20] For what the doctor does implies that he has come to the decision that he does not *have* to keep on treating the repeated supervening bronchitis in a patient who is manifestly dying. Why? Not (as some have assumed[21]) because he judges the patient no longer has a worthwhile life. Rather, what

[18] See the careful analysis in sections 6 and 7 of chapter 5. [pp.64–66 in this volume]

[19] See section 3 of chapter 6. [pp.69–70 in this volume]

[20] Chapter 7 [pp.77–78 in this volume]

[21] Such as Helga Kuhse, who thinks that implicit in the Linacre Centre Working Party's description of this case is a comprehensive quality-of-life judgement on the life of the patient: treatment is discon-

he judges is that curative treatment is no longer effectively securing some approximation to health in his patient. The recurrence of bronchitis is evidence in this case of the inexorable decline we call dying. It is not the purpose of medicine to seek to prolong life irrespective of whether it is possible to restore the patient to some approximation to health. (See *Submission* 2.1) And if that is so, one may judge, in respect of an incompetent patient, that one no longer has a duty to treat a life-threatening supervening condition (just because it is life-threatening[22]) when the patient is already irreversibly dying.

These brief analyses of differing lines of reasoning which may determine clinical treatment are significant not because they always lead to obviously different overt behaviour but precisely because of the different character of the reasoning: some is compatible with recognition of human dignity, some is not. And the differences matter not only because of the large consequences they can have for the treatment of patients but also because of their significance for the moral integrity of doctors, which is undermined by choices to act for reasons incompatible with the recognition of human dignity.

tinued allegedly because he is judged no longer to have a worthwhile life. See Helga Kuhse, *The Sanctity-of-Life Doctrine in Medicine. A Critique* Oxford: Clarendon Press 1987, pp.193–194.

[22] Consideration of what is required for proper palliative care may of course suggest that one ought to treat the supervening life-threatening condition.

4

Some Reflections on Euthanasia in The Netherlands*

JOHN KEOWN

Introduction

Drawing on empirical research which I have been carrying out in The Netherlands since 1989,[1] this chapter examines critically the Dutch euthanasia experience.

Part I deals with the offence of taking a person's life at his request contained in article 293 of the Penal Code and the extent to which the courts have allowed doctors a defence to this charge. Part II considers the guidelines for voluntary euthanasia which have been set out by the Royal Dutch Medical Association (KNMG). Part III examines the extent to which the Dutch experiment confirms or confutes a major ethical argument against the legalisation of voluntary euthanasia, namely, the 'slippery slope' argument.

Part I: The offence of killing a person at his request and the defence of necessity

1 The offence of killing a person at his request

Killing a person at his 'express and serious request' is punished by article 293

* Reprinted with permission, and with some modifications, from Luke Gormally (ed) *The Dependent Elderly. Autonomy, Justice and Quality of Care* Cambridge: Cambridge University Press, 1992, pp. 70–100.

[1] This research was generously funded by the British Academy whose support I gratefully acknowledge. I also appreciate supplementary sums provided by the Dutch Ministry of Education and by my Department. Thanks are also due to the following for their invaluable assistance: Dr Maurice de Wachter, Hub Zwart and Ingrid Ravenschlag of the Instituut voor Gezondheidsethiek, Maastricht; Therese te Braake, Nicole de Bijl (of the Department of Health Law) and Jurgen Worestshofer, Job Cohen and Louise Rayar (of the Department of Law) at the State University of Limburg; Henk Jochemsen of the Lindeboom Instituut, Ede; Dr Martens, of the Royal Dutch Medical Association (KNMG); Drs Admiraal, Cohen, van der Meer and Gunning; Mrs Tromp-Meesters and Professor Dupuis of the Dutch Voluntary Euthanasia Society (DVES); Eugene Sutorius, Counsel to the Society; Mrs Borst-Eilers, Vice-President of the Dutch Health Council; H J J Leenen, Emeritus Professor of Social Medicine and Health Law at the University of Amsterdam; two public prosecutors, one in Rotterdam, the other in Alkmaar; Attorney-General Remmelink and his Secretary Mr den Hartog Jager; Mr Stryards and Mr Kors, legal advisers at the Ministry of Justice; and Professor J M Finnis of University College, Oxford, who commented on an earlier draft of this paper.

Unless the contrary is apparent, all translations are by Hub Zwart, to whom I owe a special debt of thanks. All references to 'interviews' refer to interviews I conducted between July 1989 and December 1991. Unless attributed to another, the views expressed in this paper are mine and I remain solely responsible for the accuracy of the paper.

of the Penal Code.[2] It is one of the 'Serious offences against human life'[3] in Title XIX of the code. Article 287 provides that a person who intentionally takes another's life without premeditation commits 'homicide'[4], but a person who intentionally and with premeditation takes the life of another is guilty of murder: article 289.[5]

Article 294 punishes assisting suicide.[6] Suicide itself is not criminal; nor is aiding attempted suicide, evidently because the legislature feared that the imposition of criminal liability might encourage a further attempt.[7] In short, voluntary euthanasia, or the intentional acceleration of a patient's death at his request as part of his medical care, is prohibited by article 293. The intentional killing of an incompetent person (non-voluntary euthanasia) or of a person against his wishes (involuntary euthanasia) would constitute either murder (contrary to article 289) or 'homicide' (contrary to article 287).

2 The defence of necessity

(i) The Supreme Court decision of 1984

Notwithstanding the apparently clear terms of article 293, the criminal courts have come to interpret the Code as providing a defence to a charge of voluntary euthanasia under that article and equally to a charge of assisting suicide under article 294. The line of relevant cases stretch from the decision of a District Court in 1973 to decisions of the Supreme Court in 1984 and 1986.[8]

The Supreme Court decision of 27 November 1984, the *Alkmaar* case, involved the killing of an elderly woman, a 'Mrs. B', at her request by her GP. The doctor was acquitted by the Alkmaar District Court but, on an appeal by the prosecution, was convicted by the Court of Appeal at Amsterdam. He then appealed successfully to the Supreme Court[9] which held

---

[2] Quotations from the Penal Code are taken from an unpublished translation of the Code by Louise Rayar.

[3] *Ibid.*

[4] B Sluyters, 'Euthanasia in The Netherlands' (1989) 57(1) *Medico-Legal Journal* 34, 35.

[5] *Ibid.*

[6] Rayar, *op. cit* n2, *Supra.*

[7] Jurgen Woretshofer, 'Current Court Decisions and Legislation on Euthanasia in The Netherlands' (pages 25–51 of an unpublished manuscript on euthanasia) 26. (Page references correspond to those in the manuscript.) Articles 293 and 294 were added to the Penal Code in 1891. H J J Leenen. 'Euthanasia in the Netherlands' in Peter Byrne (ed) *Medicine, Medical Ethics and the Value of Life* (1990) 10.

[8] See generally H J J Leenen, 'Euthanasia, assistance to suicide and the law: developments in the Netherlands' (1987) 8 *Health Policy* 197, 200–2; *op. cit.* n7. *supra*, 4–6.

The pyramidal structure of the criminal court system rises from the sixty-two Cantonal Courts, which deal with minor offences, through the nineteen District Courts, each covering three or four cantons, to the five Courts of Appeal, each of which covers three or four districts. At the apex is the Supreme Court, which is concerned solely with questions of law. See Peter Zisser, 'Euthanasia and the Right to Die: Holland and the United States face the Dilemma' (1988) 9 *New York Law School Journal of International and Comparative Law* 361, 365 n.53.

[9] *Nederlandse Jurisprudentie* (hereafter *NJ*) (1985) No 106.

that the Court of Appeal had wrongly rejected the doctor's defence that he had acted out of necessity. The Supreme Court held that the Court of Appeal had not given sufficient reasons for its decision and that, in particular, it should have investigated whether 'according to responsible medical opinion' measured by the 'prevailing standards of medical ethics' a situation of necessity existed.[10]

The defence of necessity is contained in article 40 of the Penal Code, which provides that a person who commits an offence as a result of 'irresistible compulsion or necessity [*overmacht*] is not criminally liable.'[11] The defence takes two forms: first, 'psychological compulsion' and secondly 'emergency' (*noodtoestand*) or choosing to break the law in order to promote a higher good.[12] Commenting on the latter form of the defence as applied by the Supreme Court to euthanasia. Professor Mulder, an expert on criminal law, explains that it refers to the situation where a doctor, faced with the dire distress of his patient, is faced with a 'conflict of interests' which results in the doctor breaking the law to promote a higher good.[13]

The Supreme Court observed in the *Alkmaar* case that whether a situation of necessity existed would depend on the circumstances of the case and that the Appeal Court could have taken into account, for example, the following matters:

whether and to what extent according to professional medical judgement an increasing disfigurement of the patient's personality and/or further deterioration of her already unbearable suffering were to be expected;

whether it could be expected that soon she would no longer be able to die with dignity under circumstances worthy of a human being;

[10] J K M Gevers, 'Legal Developments concerning active Euthanasia on Request in The Netherlands' (1987) 1 *Bioethics* 156, 159. The case report reads as follows:

'At the trial ... counsel for the accused appealed to necessity [*overmacht*] in the sense that the accused found himself confronted by a "conflict of duties, in which he came to a right choice in a well-considered manner". This appeal to a conflict of duties, which should be distinguished from the accused's appeal to necessity in the sense of constraint of conscience [*gewetensdrang*], can hardly be interpreted otherwise than as an appeal to emergency [*noodtoestand*], which amounts to the accused carefully weighing the duties and interests which faced each other in this case, especially in accordance with the norms of medical ethics and with the expertise which he, as a physician, can be expected to possess; and making a decision which – considered objectively and in view of the special circumstances in this case – was justified.' (*NJ* (1985) No 106, 451 at 452)

The report continues (at 452–3) that the Court of Appeal had properly rejected the defence of 'constraint of conscience' but that its rejection of the defence of 'emergency' was unsound as it failed to take into account the condition of Mrs B. and the fact that the accused in his 'competent judgement as a physician' felt that she experienced each day of life as 'a heavy burden under which she suffered unbearably'. In view of this, the Supreme Court continued (at 453):

further clarification is needed as to why the Court of Appeal ... still comes to the judgement that it "has not become sufficiently plausible" that the suffering of B. at the very moment the accused terminated her life ... should be considered so unbearable that the accused in fairness had no other choice than to spare her this suffering by means of euthanasia ... Rather it should have gone without saying that the Appeal Court, after having determined the facts and circumstances ... [relating to B's condition], would have further investigated whether, according to well-considered medical judgement and in accordance with medico-ethical norms [*nader zou hebben onderzocht of naar verantwoord medisch inzicht, getoetst aan de medische ethick geldende normen*], it was a matter of emergency as claimed by the accused.

[11] Rayar, *op.cit.* n2, *supra*.

[12] Woretshofer, *op. cit.* n7, *supra*, 38.

[13] 'The High Court of the Hague', Case No. 79065, October 21, 1986'; (edited and translated by Barry A Bostrom and Walter Lagerwey) (1988) 3 *Issues in Law & Medicine* 445, 448. Bostrom and Lagerwey attribute this and other passages from the 'Note', appended to the report of the case, to

whether there were still opportunities to alleviate her suffering.[14]

The case was referred to the Hague Court of Appeal with a direction that it investigate whether, on the facts, the performance of euthanasia by the doctor 'would, *from an objective medical perspective*, be regarded as an action justified in a situation of necessity'.[15] On 11 September 1986, the Court of Appeal acquitted the accused on the basis that the defence of necessity applied.[16] Having noted that the accused maintained that he had done nothing contrary to medical ethics, the Courts added that he had, on the basis of his expertise as a physician and his experience as Mrs. B's doctor, and after careful consideration of conflicting duties in the light of medical ethics, made a choice which had to be regarded as justified according to 'reasonable' medical opinion.[17] Advocate-General Feber has noted the substitution of 'reasonable' for 'objective' medical opinion[18] and that the Court raised for discussion the question of the degree to which euthanasia could be justified by a normal psychological reaction to physical deterioration.[19]

(ii) The Supreme Court decision of 1986

On 21 October 1986, one month after the decision of the Hague Court of Appeal, the Supreme Court delivered a second judgment on euthanasia.[20] This case[21] concerned the prosecution of a doctor, who, after repeated requests, euthanatised a 73 year-old friend suffering from advanced multiple sclerosis. The doctor was convicted by the Groningen District Court and her conviction was upheld by the Court of Appeal at Leeuwarden. The Supreme Court, however, allowed her appeal, holding that the Court of Appeal had wrongly failed to consider two defences raised at trial. The first was that the accused acted because of her patient's 'dire distress'; the second that she acted out of 'psychological necessity' because she 'was confronted with the suffering of her patient and found *herself* under duress and could not arrive at any other decision than to grant the assistance requested'.[22] The Supreme

A.-G. Remmelink. As the initials 'G.E.M.' at the end of the Note indicate, however, it is in fact by Mulder.

14 *NJ* (1985) No 106451 at 453 (translated by Gevers, *op. cit.* n10, *supra*, 159–60).

15 Abstract (prepared from a translation and summary by Dr Walter Lagerwey) of H R G Feber, 'De wederwaardigheden van artikel 293 van het Wetboek van Strafrecht vanaf 1981 tot heden' ('The Vicissitudes of article 293 of the Penal Code from 1981 to the Present') in GA van der Wal, ed, *Euthanasie: Knelpunten in Een Discussie* ('*Euthanasia: Bottlenecks in a Discussion*') (1987) 54–81 in (1988) 3 *Issues in Law & Medicine* 455, 458. (Emphasis in original.)

16 *NJ* (1987) No 608.

17 Feber, *op. cit.* n15, *supra*, 462.

18 *ibid.*

19 *ibid*, 463–4.

20 *NJ* (1987) No 607.

21 See *op. cit.* n13, *supra*. 445.

22 *ibid*, 445–6. (Emphasis in translation.) The Court held: 'The Court of Appeal should have considered whether the accused, as she arrived at her decision and proceeded to execute it, acted in emergency [*noodtoestand*] or psychological compulsion [*psychische overmacht*]'. *NJ* (1987) No 607 at 2124. In his 'Note' appended to the report of the case, Mulder observes that two differences strike him between the Supreme Court decisions of 1984 and 1986. One is that in the 1984 case the accused was the patient's physician whereas in the 1986 case she was not. The other is that in the latter decision, the Court

Court remitted the case to the Court of Appeal at Arnhem for further investigation[23]; the doctor was convicted.[24]

(iii) The criteria for lawful euthanasia: a summary

The criteria laid down by the courts to determine whether the defence of necessity applies in a given case of euthanasia have been summarised by Mrs. Borst-Eilers, Vice-President of the Health Council (a body which provides scientific advice to the Government on health issues), as follows:

1 The request for euthanasia must come only from the patient and must be entirely free and voluntary.
2 The patient's request must be well considered, durable and persistent.
3 The patient must be experiencing intolerable (not necessarily physical) suffering, with no prospect of improvement.
4 Euthanasia must be a last resort. Other alternatives to alleviate the patient's situation must have been considered and found wanting.
5 Euthanasia must be performed by a physician.
6 The physician must consult with an independent physician colleague who has experience in this field.[25]

Whether consultation must be with an 'independent' physician is, however, doubtful: in the *Alkmaar* case the defendant GP had merely consulted his assistant. Further, it has been pointed out by Eugene Sutorius, counsel to the Dutch Voluntary Euthanasia Society (DVES), that the Supreme Court has stated that consultation is not always essential. He has explained that, although the Court did not elaborate on this point, in his view, as the purpose of consultation is to obtain a second opinion about the medical aspects of the case, consultation is not necessary when there is no doubt about these aspects and when witnesses are available to verify that the non-medical criteria have been satisfied.[26]

(iv) Liability for falsifying the death certificate

Necessity is not, however, a defence to a charge of falsely certifying the cause

'provides an appeal to psychological compulsion [*psychische overmacht*] a chance of success'. *NJ* (1987) No 607 at 2129.
23 *Op. cit.* n13, *supra.* 446.
24 Because, says, Leenen, she did not consult another doctor, *op. cit.* n8, *supra.* 202. A further appeal to the Supreme Court was dismissed *NJ* (1989) No 391. Attorney-General Remmelink informed me that in the light of this case, psychological compulsion is only a 'theoretical' defence especially for doctors, whom the courts expect to act in a professional manner (Interview, 26 November, 1991).
25 E Borst-Eilers, 'The Status of Physician-Administered Active Euthanasia in The Netherlands' (Unpublished paper delivered at the Second International Conference on Health Law and Ethics, London, July 1989) 3. See also Leenen, *op. cit.* n8, *supra*, 200; Sluyters, *op. cit.*, n4, *supra*, 41; Gevers, *op. cit.* n10, *supra*, 158.
26 Interview, 10 July 1989. In the *Alkmaar* case the Appeal Court ruled that although the accused had consulted his assistant and Mrs B.'s son, their opinions were insufficiently independent. The Supreme Court held that this did not prevent the euthanatising of Mrs B. from being an act in 'emergency' according to 'objective medical judgement'. *NJ* (1985) No 106 451 at 453. Again, A N A Josephus Jitta, a public prosecutor, has written that the requirement of a second opinion was 'abandoned once by the Dutch Supreme Court in 1987' when it dismissed the case against a doctor who had been prosecuted solely because he had not consulted. 'The Right to Euthanasia in the Terminal Period' in *The Right to*

of death. In a case decided by the Court of the Hague (Penal Chamber) in 1987, the defendant doctor admitted that, having performed euthanasia, he had certified that death was due to natural causes[27]. The Court of Appeal upheld the trial court's decision that death by euthanasia was not death by natural causes and that the doctor could not rely on necessity as a defence to falsifying the death certificate. The Appeal Court declared that it was a matter of great public concern that non-natural deaths should be investigated by officials such as the coroner and prosecutor and that this was especially so in cases of euthanasia in view of the proven danger of abuse.[28]

Part II: Medical Guidelines

The judgment of the Hague Court of Appeal in the *Alkmaar* case gave striking weight to the views of a 'considerable number of medical doctors' against whom, it said, a judge could not 'make a choice in this matter'.[29] In fact, the medical profession, or at least its main representative body, the Royal Dutch Medical Association (KNMG), to which some 60% of the 30 000 Dutch doctors belong, has played a significant role in the relaxation of the law and practice of euthanasia.

1 The KNMG Criteria

In 1973 the KNMG issued a provisional statement which said that euthanasia should remain a crime but that if a doctor shortened the life of a patient who was incurably ill and in the process of dying, a court would have to judge whether there was not a conflict of duties which justified the doctor's action.[30] In August 1984, three months before the decision of the Supreme Court in the *Alkmaar* case, the central committee of the KNMG produced a Report setting out the criteria which the KNMG felt should be satisfied in cases of euthanasia.[31] As Borst-Eilers has pointed out, there is a close correspondence between these criteria and those laid down by the courts.[32]

Self-Determination: Proceedings of the 8th World Conference of the International Federation of Right to Die Societies (1990) 47, 48.

[27] 'Court of the Hague (Penal Chamber) April 2, 1987', (edited and translated by Barry A. Bostrom and Walter Lagerwey) (1988) 3 *Issues in Law & Medicine* 451.

[28] *Ibid*, 452. Affirmed, *NJ* (1988) No 811.

[29] Feber, *op. cit.* n15, *supra*. 462. The Prosecutor had sought the advice of the KNMG about the defence of necessity and, when the Association replied that euthanasia was permissible if the patient was suffering unbearably and had made a free and well-considered request, had moved for the prosecution to be dismissed. *Ibid*, 461.

[30] Gevers, *op. cit.* n10, *supra*, 158.

[31] 'Standpunt inzake euthanasie' (Position on euthanasia) (1984) 39 *Medisch Contact* 990. Quotations from the Report are taken from an unpublished translation by the KNMG entitled 'Vision on Euthanasia' (hereafter 'Vision'). The translated version states that it has updated the Report on a few points to take account of developments in law, politics and within the KNMG until the end of 1986.

[32] *Op. cit.* n25, *supra*, 3.

Subsequently, the KNMG formulated[33] certain 'Guidelines for Euthanasia'.[34]

The Report lists five criteria: 'voluntariness'; 'a well-considered request'; 'a durable death-wish'; 'unacceptable suffering'; and 'consultation between colleagues'[35]. These are reproduced in the Guidelines.[36]

(i) Voluntariness

The Report stresses that the request must be made of the patient's free will and must not be the result of pressure by others.[37] Conceding that it will not always be possible to be completely sure that the request is not influenced by others, the Report says that the doctor should talk privately with the patient and that, after a 'number of conversations', he must be able to get a 'fairly reliable impression' of the voluntariness of the request.[38] The Guidelines, by contrast, state that there need only be 'a' conversation with the patient to verify voluntariness.[39]

(ii) A well-considered request

To ensure that the request is well-considered the Report urges that the doctor should give the patient a 'clear picture of his medical situation and the appropriate prognosis' and, because a request for euthanasia is 'not uncommonly found to be an expression of fear – such as fear of pain, deterioration, loneliness', the doctor should also examine the extent to which these fears influence the request, and should dispel them as far as possible.[40]

Similarly, the Guidelines state that a doctor must guard against granting a request which arises essentially from 'other problems than the will to terminate life' such as the feeling of being superfluous or a nuisance to the family. A request made on such grounds should first of all be an occasion for a consultation with the patient about alternative solutions; in no case should euthanasia be granted because of problems which could be resolved in another way.[41]

(iii) A durable death wish

The Report declares that requests arising out of 'impulse or a temporary depression' should not be granted but adds that it is not possible to indicate what time span should have elapsed before a request becomes 'durable'.[42]

---

[33] In collaboration with the National Association of Nurses.
[34] 'Guidelines for Euthanasia' (translated by Lagerwey) (1988) 3 *Issues in Law & Medicine* 429. Hereafter 'Guidelines'.
[35] Vision, 8–11.
[36] Guidelines, 431–3.
[37] Vision, 8.
[38] *Ibid.* 9.
[39] Guidelines, 431.
[40] Vision, 9.
[41] Guidelines, 432.
[42] Vision, 9.

The physician is advised to 'steer mostly by his own compass' but that 'durable', in the opinion of the committee, does not simply mean more than once.[43]

(iv) Unacceptable suffering

The Guidelines state that the patient must experience his suffering as 'persistent, unbearable, and hopeless' and they add that the relevant case-law indicates that an important consideration is whether the patient will be able to die 'in a dignified manner'.[44]

The Report, however, states that the committee, while aware that the courts indicated that the suffering must be persistent, unbearable and hopeless, declined to support this definition of the criterion because it felt that these concepts overlapped and were unverifiable.[45] It continues that although the degree of suffering is an important criterion, there are only limited possibilities for verification since the unbearable and hopeless character of a person's situation is so dependent on individual standards and values that an objective assessment is difficult.[46]

Suffering, says the Report, can have any of three causes: first, pain; secondly, a physical condition or physical disintegration without pain; and thirdly, suffering without any physical complaint which could be caused either by 'social factors and the like' in a healthy person or by a 'medical-psychiatric syndrome'.[47] Pain, the Report continues, can be controlled to such an extent that, in general, it is not a primary cause of unbearable suffering. And as to suffering caused by social factors, a doctor usually cannot assess the unbearability of the patient's situation or the prospects of its alleviation.[48]

The Report adds that, although the KNMG's 1973 statement had raised the question whether euthanasia was justifiable if the patient were incurably ill and in the process of dying,[49] the committee felt that, quite apart from the fact that the 'dying phase' could not be clearly defined, it was not reasonable to deny a patient who was suffering unbearably the 'right to euthanasia' solely because he was not dying. Consequently, it could no longer support the 'dying phase' as a criterion.[50]

(v) Consultation and reporting

The committee considered consultation with a colleague with experience in this field to be 'indispensable' to promote well-balanced decision-making[51]

---

43 *Ibid*. 10.
44 Guidelines, 432.
45 Vision, 10.
46 *Ibid*.
47 *Ibid*. 11.
48 *Ibid*.
49 See text at n30.
50 Vision, 12.
51 *Ibid*.

and the Report recommends that the doctor consult first a colleague with whom he is professionally involved and later an independent doctor.[52]

Finally, having noted that it was 'not unusual' for cases of euthanasia to be reported as a natural death in order to protect the relatives and/or the doctor from police investigation, the Report urges that this 'improper' practice be discontinued and stresses the Committee's advocacy of due openness in the reporting of death.[53]

2 Current Medical and Legal Procedures

Procedures followed by doctors who have performed euthanasia vary throughout the country. At one of the leading centres for euthanasia, the Reinier de Graaf Hospital in Delft, the procedure is that the doctor does not certify a natural death but informs the police.[54] The municipal medical examiner comes to inspect the body and a policeman to interview the doctor. Both the officials then file reports with the prosecutor who, if satisfied that the legal criteria have been met, gives permission for the corpse to be handed over to the relatives.[55] As Borst-Eilers comments: 'This whole procedure after death need only take a few hours. Only if the public prosecutor suspects that all the criteria have not been met with, he orders further interviews with nurses, members of the family etc.'[56] If the prosecutor's suspicions are not allayed, he may then ask an examining magistrate to investigate. In November 1990, however, the Minister of Justice and KNMG agreed that the doctor need only report to the medical examiner, and the Minister of Justice directed prosecutors that on receiving the examiner's report they should ask the police to investigate euthanasia cases only when there are grounds for suspecting that the appropriate criteria have not been met.[57]

The final decision whether to prosecute is taken at a meeting of the country's five Chief Prosecutors (*Procureurs-Generaal*) according to the criteria laid down by the courts. The Chief Prosecutors, each of whom is attached to one of the five regional Courts of Appeal, meet every three weeks, together with a representative from the Ministry of Justice, to discuss prosecution policy in relation to crimes in general and to decide, according to the criteria laid down by the courts,[58] whether to prosecute in each notified case of euthanasia. In practice, they simply approve the decision of the local prosecutor.[59]

Part III: Sliding Down a Slippery Slope?

Having set out in Part I the legal and in Part II the medical criteria for

---

[52] *Ibid*, 12–13.
[53] *Ibid*, 14.
[54] Borst-Eilers, *op. cit.* n25, *supra*, 5.
[55] *Ibid*.
[56] *Ibid*.
[57] Interview with public prosecutor, Alkmaar, 7 December 1990.
[58] Leenen, *op. cit.* n8, *supra*, 200.
[59] Interview with public prosecutor, Rotterdam, 31 July 1989.

voluntary euthanasia, I can now examine the extent to which the experience of euthanasia in The Netherlands confirms or confutes the 'slippery slope' argument, an argument which has been deployed in major reports opposing the legalisation of voluntary euthanasia, such as those of the Working Party of the Church of England's Board for Social Responsibility (1975),[60] the Canadian Law Reform Commission (1983),[61] and the Working Party of the British Medical Association (1988).[62] On this argument, even if euthanasia in certain circumstances (in particular that of a free and well-considered request by the patient) is not intrinsically wrong, its legalisation will result in a slide down a 'slippery slope' to non-voluntary and possibly even involuntary euthanasia. It will do so, the argument runs, either because any safeguards which might prevent such a slide could not in practice be made effective or, more fundamentally, because the ethical (and/or legal) reasoning underlying the case for voluntary euthanasia also supports euthanasia without request.

1 The 'Practical Slope'

Are the criteria for voluntary euthanasia laid down by the Dutch courts and endorsed by the KNMG adequate to prevent instances of euthanasia which do not satisfy the criteria, especially the requirement of a free and well-considered request? It has been stressed by defenders of the Dutch criteria, such as Henk Rigter, Executive Director of the Health Council, that the guidelines for lawful euthanasia are both 'precisely defined' and 'strict'.[63] Are they?

(i) Identifying the criteria

Before deciding whether the criteria are precise and strict it is necessary accurately to identify them. The Supreme Court decided that necessity could operate as a defence to a charge under article 293 but omitted to state with any exactitude the criteria to be satisfied for the defence to apply. Even taking into account the decisions of lower courts, the criteria are not easy to determine. For example, Professor Leenen has written that each court decision has its own set of criteria, which creates 'much uncertainty'.[64]

(ii) 'Strict' and 'precise'?

Even if, say, Borst-Eilers's list of criteria were definitive there would still remain the question of the precision and strictness of those criteria. As for

---

[60] Working Party of the Church of England's Board for Social Responsibility, *On Dying Well: An Anglican Contribution to the Debate on Euthanasia* (1975), 62.

[61] Law Reform Commission of Canada, *Euthanasia, Aiding Suicide and Cessation of Treatment* (Report 20: 1983) 18.

[62] *Euthanasia: Report of the Working Party to review the British Medical Associations' guidance on euthanasia* (1988) 4; 6; 31; 59.

[63] Henk Rigter, 'Euthanasia in The Netherlands: Distinguishing Facts from Fiction' (1989) 19(1) *Hastings Center Report* 31.

[64] H J J Leenen, 'Dying with Dignity: Developments in the Field of Euthanasia in the Netherlands' (1989) 8 *Medicine and Law* 517, 523. See also M A M de Wachter, 'Active Euthanasia in the Netherlands' (1989) 262 *Journal of the American Medical Association* 3316, 3317.

their supposed precision, Dutch jurists, such as Leenen, have remarked upon their vagueness. He defines euthanasia as a 'deliberate life-shortening act – including an omission to act – by a person other than the person concerned, at the request of the latter'.[65] He observes that other elements such as 'unbearable pain' are sometimes included but objects that they cannot form part of the definition – first, because they introduce judgements on which people disagree, and secondly because 'these elements cannot be delineated precisely'.[66] He continues that to include 'unbearable pain', whether physical or psychological, is to render the definition of euthanasia 'vague and useless' by stretching it to cover a broad range of human suffering.[67] Moreover, far from clarifying these inherent ambiguities the Supreme Court in the *Alkmaar* case appears to have compounded the problem by introducing such opaque concepts as 'death with dignity'.[68]

As for Rigter's claim that the criteria are 'strict', this too is difficult to sustain, not only because of their imprecision but also because of the absence of any satisfactory procedure, such as an effective independent check on the doctor's decision-making, to ensure that they are met.

Take, for example, the first criterion, that the request must come only from the patient and be 'entirely free and voluntary'.[69] What this means is not explained, and although the KNMG Guidelines state that the request must not be the result of pressure by others, they do not prevent either the doctor or nurse from mentioning euthanasia to the patient as an option or even strongly recommending it. Further, although the Guidelines provide that a request for euthanasia on the ground of being a nuisance to family should be an occasion to discuss alternative solutions, and that euthanasia is not to be administered because of problems which can be resolved in another way, they by no means rule out euthanasia in such a case.[70] Herbert Cohen, a GP who is one of Holland's leading practitioners of euthanasia, has said that he would be put in a very difficult position if a patient told him that he really felt a nuisance to his relatives because they wanted to enjoy his estate. Asked whether he would rule out euthanasia in such a case, Dr. Cohen replied: 'I . . . think in the end I wouldn't, because that kind of influence – these children wanting the money now – is the same kind of power from the past that . . . shaped us all. The same thing goes for religion . . . education . . . the kind of family he was raised in, all kinds of influences from the past that we can't put aside'.[71]

Even if the meaning of 'entirely free and voluntary' were clear, do doctors possess the expertise to determine whether a request fulfills this requirement?

---

[65] H J J Leenen. 'The Definition of Euthanasia' (1984) 3 *Medicine and Law* 333, 334.
[66] *Ibid.*
[67] *Ibid.*
[68] See text at n14.
[69] See text at n25.
[70] Guidelines, 432.
[71] Interview, 26 July 1989. 'Not wanting to be a (continued) burden on family/surroundings' was mentioned by 22% of patients in van der Wal's survey as a reason for requesting euthanasia. *Op. cit.* n78, *infra.*, 214 Table 5.

If they do, can the recommended procedure for ascertaining whether a request is free – the Guidelines merely recommend 'a' conversation[72], of unspecified length and content – ensure that any such expertise is effectively deployed? Leenen, observing that a doctor can never know that a request is free and not the result of pressure from relatives, has commented: 'He does not know about emotional influence from the family ... He never knows about the annoyance which patients can be to the nursing staff sometimes. All these factors can ... be true'.[73]

Turning to the second criterion, that the request be 'well-considered, durable and persistent', the question again arises how all this is to be determined. How is the doctor to decide whether the request is the result of rational reflection or the influence of pain or drugs? As Kamisar has observed:

Undoubtedly, some euthanasia candidates will have their lucid moments. How they are to be distinguished from fellow-sufferers who do not, or how these instances are to be distinguished from others when the patient is exercising an irrational judgment is not an easy matter,

particularly when no psychiatrically-trained personnel assist in the assessment of the request.[74] He continues by asking whether, even if the mind of the 'pain-racked' patient is clear, it is not likely to be 'uncertain and variable'?[75]

The Guidelines merely state that one request is insufficient;[76] presumably two requests, even if made during the same consultation, would suffice. It is difficult to maintain that this is sufficient to meet Kamisar's point. Moreover, in assessing the practitioner's ability to ensure that a request is free, well-considered and durable, it is relevant to note that, on average, each GP in The Netherlands sees thirty patients per day in consultations lasting only seven to ten minutes.[77]

Doubts about whether the Guidelines can ensure that a request is well-considered and enduring have not been dispelled by a recent survey of GPs about euthanasia. The survey was carried out in 1990 by medical examiner van der Wal et al. It concluded that the interval between the first request for euthanasia and its performance was no more than a day in 13% of cases, no more than a week in another 35%, and no more than a fortnight in a further 17%, and that the interval between the last request for euthanasia and its performance was, in three out of five cases, no more than a day. The survey also found that in 22% of cases there was (contrary to the guidelines) only a single request and that in a further 30% of cases the interval between the first

[72] See text at n39.
[73] Interview, 24 July 1989.
[74] Yale Kamisar, 'Some Non-Religious Views against Proposed "Mercy-Killing" Legislation' (1958) 42 *Minnesota Law Review* 969, in Dennis J. Horan and David Mall (eds). *Death, Dying and Euthanasia* (1980) 406, 425.
[75] *Ibid.*
[76] Guidelines, 432.
[77] Interview, Dr Martens, 24 July 1989.

and last requests was between an hour and a week. Finally, in almost two-thirds of cases the request was purely oral.[78]

Further, Kamisar asks whether, even if the patient's request could be said to be clear and incontrovertible, other difficulties do not remain: 'Is this the kind of choice, assuming that it can be made in a fixed and rational manner, that we want to offer a gravely ill person? Will we not sweep up, in the process, some who are not really tired of life, but think others are tired of them . . . ?'[79]

Moving to the third criterion, 'intolerable suffering', the KNMG's Report declared that the concept is imprecise, not susceptible to objective verification, and can be caused by non-medical factors.[80] Moreover, van der Wal's survey found that although in 56% of official notifications 'intolerable suffering' was certified by doctors as the most important reason for euthanasia, only 42% of the patients had mentioned it as a reason and only 18% as their most important reason, 29% of patients gave 'senseless' suffering as their most important reason, and 24% 'fear/anticipation of mental deterioration'.[81]

One argument against entrusting the euthanasia decision to the patient's doctor is that the doctor is fallible and that he may make errors in diagnosis or prognosis which could lead him to conclude, mistakenly, either that the patient's suffering is unbearable or that there is no means of palliation.[82] Here one may mention a report of the Health Council, published in 1987, on palliative care in The Netherlands. It concluded that 54% of cancer patients who were in pain suffered unnecessarily because doctors and nurses had insufficient understanding of the nature of the pain and the possibilities for its alleviation.[83] There is, moreover, the related argument that the doctor's objectivity can be swayed by emotional pressures; as Kamisar has commented: 'no man is immune to the fear, anxieties and frustrations engendered by the apparently helpless, hopeless patient'.[84]

Is the danger of fallibility, whether due to medical ignorance or emotional stresses, countered by the sixth criterion: consultation? It is questionable whether this criterion provides an effective safeguard against mis-interpretation and mis-application of the other criteria.

First, *if* consultation is a legal requirement at all, it may well only be required when there is doubt about the *medical* aspects of the case.[85] Now in

---

[78] G van der Wall *et al.*, 'Euthanasie en hulp bij zelfdoding' (Euthanasia and Assisted Suicide) (1991) 56(7) *Medisch Contact* 211, 212–14 Tables 2, 3, 4, & 7. This paper is the third of four published in the KNMG journal in February 1991 which contain the methodology and results of van der Wal's survey. The papers have been translated by the Hemlock Society. Quotations are taken from this unpublished translation; page references are to the journal.

[79] *Op. cit.* n74, *supra*, 427.

[80] Vision, 10–11.

[81] Van der Wal, *op. cit.* n78, *supra*, 214 Table 5.

[82] See generally Kamisar, *op. cit.* 74, *supra*, 430–5.

[83] Interview, Gunning, 2 August 1989. Dr P. Sluis, a founder in 1987 of the Dutch Hospice Movement, has observed that palliative care is not very good in The Netherlands: 'The Dutch Hospice Movement', in *op. cit.* n26, *supra*, 97, 103.

[84] *Op. cit.* n74, *supra*, 429.

[85] See text at n26.

a large proportion, if not the vast majority, of cases the doctor may well believe that there is no such doubt. Moreover, if consultation is not required when the diagnosis is clear, this suggests that when consultation is required, the requirement is satisfied if the second opinion is sought solely on the medical aspects of the case. The requirement of consultation is, then, hardly apt to allay concern about the difficulty of ensuring that the non-medical criteria are satisfied. Secondly, the consultation procedure recommended by the KNMG committee in 1984 has not been implemented. Nor has any court set out the form which consultation should take.[86] Thirdly, there is no requirement that the second doctor concur with the first doctor's interpretation of the criteria on which the second doctor is consulted or with their application to the patient in question. Further, the second doctor could adopt an interpretation of the criteria at least as relaxed as the first.

Even were consultation a universal practice it would, therefore, seem, of limited value as a check on the judgment or integrity of the first doctor. It is, moreover, far from universal. Van der Wal reports: 'One quarter of the general practitioners said they had not had *consultation* prior to euthanasia/assisted suicide . . . More serious is the finding that 12% . . . manifestly had no form of *discussion* with any other care givers either'.[87] When consultation did occur the second opinion was in most cases a colleague rather than an independent doctor. Further, the second doctor already knew the patient in about 60% of cases and only put his opinion in writing in about a quarter of cases. Finally, fewer than half of the GPs consulted the patient's district nurse about his request for euthanasia.[88]

(iii) Empirical evidence

Another of Rigter's claims is that if a doctor were to press euthanasia on a patient 'this would surely be discovered, and the doctor would have to face charges of murder or manslaughter'.[89] Empirical evidence does not substantiate this claim.

Estimates of the number of cases of medical euthanasia in The Netherlands, which has a population of some 15 million and some 130 000 deaths per year, put the figure at at least 2000.[90] The survey by van der Wal estimates the annual number of cases of euthanasia and assisted suicide by general practitioners at 2000. However, the survey excludes cases in hospital, mainly on 'the assumption that the incidence of euthanasia and assisted

---

86 This was stated by Sutorius in an interview on 10 July 1989. There is, indeed, no legal requirement that the second doctor should even see the patient and a public prosecutor told me that it has by no means been a universal practice for the second doctor to see the patient. Interview, Rotterdam, 31 July 1989.

87 G van der Wal *et al.*, 'Toetsing in geval van euthanasie of hulp bij zelfdoding' (Verification in Euthanasia or Assisted Suicide) (1991) 46(8) *Medisch Contact* 237, 239. (Emphasis in original.)

88 *Ibid*, 240.

89 Henk Rigter *et al.*, 'Euthanasia across the North Sea' (1988) 297 *British Medical Journal* 1593, 1594.

90 See de Wachter, *op. cit.* n64, *supra*. 3316. Jitta has written that according to the estimate of the Central Medical Inspection of National Health, euthanasia is performed at least 6000 times per year in general practice and that if hospitals and nursing homes are added, the total is 10 000–12 000 cases: quoted in C I Dessaur and C J C Rutenfrans, 'The Present Day Practice of Euthanasia' (1988) 3 *Issues in Law & Medicine* 399, 400.

suicide is greatest in the home situation'; it also excludes cases of the 'discontinuation of or failure to institute a treatment' at the patient's request.[91] Finally, in September 1991, a government committee, chaired by Attorney-General Remmelink, reported that its own survey of doctors revealed that in 1990 there were 2300 cases of voluntary euthanasia; 400 cases of assisted suicide; 1000 cases of life termination without an explicit request, and 16850 cases in which it was the doctor's 'explicit' or 'partial' purpose to shorten life, either by administering pain-killing drugs (8100 cases) or by withholding or withdrawing treatment (8750 cases). In short, in the terms of the Survey, doctors had it as their 'explicit' or 'partial' purpose to shorten life in over 20 000 cases.[92]

It is difficult to determine how many cases of euthanasia satisfy the legal criteria, not least because it appears that the overwhelming majority of cases are falsely certified as death by natural causes and are never reported and investigated. Reported cases for the years 1987–90 totalled 122; 181; 336 and 454 respectively.[93] Even if the lowest estimate of 2000 euthanasia cases per year were accurate, this would still mean under-reporting by over 90% in 1988; over 80% in 1989, and over 70% in 1990. This fact places a large question mark against Rigter's claim that if the situation in The Netherlands is at all unique, 'it is perhaps in the wish of physicians to subject their actions to public scrutiny'.[94]

Borst-Eilers has stated that in unnotified cases there is no guarantee of propriety and that it is impossible to evaluate what the doctors have done.[95] Similarly, Mrs. Tromp-Meesters, a spokesman for the DVES, has observed that under the present law 'there is no control', that the purpose of notification is merely statistical and that it is not an adequate safeguard against abuse.[96]

In short, notwithstanding the permissive character of the Dutch criteria for permissible euthanasia, there would appear to be no hard evidence that these criteria are being widely observed; on the contrary, the fact that, as just

[91] G van der Wal et al. 'Euthanasie en hulp bij zelfdoding door huisartsen' (Euthanasia and Assisted Suicide by GPs) (1991) 46(6) Medisch Contact 171. See also ibid, 174–6. The study's assumption, even if true, seems an odd reason for ignoring euthanasia in hospitals.

[92] Richard Fenigsen, 'The Netherlands: First Reactions to the Report of the Committee on Euthanasia' (1991) (Unpublished summary of Medische beslissingen rond het levenseinde: Rapport van de Commissie onderzoek medische praktijk inzake euthanasie (Sdu Uitgeverij Plantijnstraat, s-Gravenhage, 1991) 1–2. See also Paul J van der Maas et al., 'Euthanasia and other medical decisions concerning the end of life' (1991) 338 Lancet 669; K F Gunning, ibid., 1010. See also Richard Fenigsen, 'The Report of the Dutch Governmental Committee on Euthanasia' (1991) Issues in Law & Medicine 339. On the question of what is meant by 'explicit' and 'secondary' see pp.225–7 of the following chapter.

[93] Personal communication from Stryards, 6 September 1991, citing Javerslaag Openbaar Ministerie 1990 (1991) 59.

[94] Op. cit. n63, supra, 32. Remmelink reported that three-quarters of GPs and almost two thirds of specialists who carried out euthanasia or assisted suicide in 1990 had falsely certified death by natural causes. Fenigsen, op. cit. n92, supra, 343. Almost half of the GPs in van der Wal's study had made no record of their last euthanasia case and, of those who had, fewer than half had done so in the form of a separate record, op. cit. n87, supra, 240. His general conclusion is that 'a substantial proportion of general practitioners is not (yet) operating in accordance with current procedural precautionary requirements'. ibid. 241.

[95] Interview, 1 August 1989.

[96] Interview, 11 July 1989.

noted, the vast majority of deaths from euthanasia are illegally and incorrectly reported as natural deaths itself casts doubt on the lawfulness of much of the euthanasia which is being carried out. Moreover, it does not follow that the doctor who notifies the authorities has complied with the criteria; a doctor who has acted in breach of the law is no more likely to admit having done so in his report than a tax evader is likely to reveal his dishonesty on his tax return.

The limited prospects that may have existed for detecting abuse in reported cases have been further reduced by the Minister of Justice's directive to prosecutors that they should order a police investigation only if the medical examiner's report reveals suspicious circumstances. One prosecutor regarded the directive (which, he revealed, had been introduced against the advice of the Chief Prosecutors) with dismay. He explained that the medical examiner does not have the necessary investigative expertise and conducts an inquiry which is 'just a chat between doctors and no inquiry at all'. The prosecutor added that the examiner's perfunctory certificate stating the cause of death was hardly of assistance in deciding whether the police should be asked to investigate. Under the previous system, he said, the prosecutor insisted on 'some hard facts' before deciding not to order an investigation. He continued that the directive had been welcomed by the medical profession because they saw it as an indication of the Minister's agreement with them that decisions about euthanasia should be made by doctors rather than by lawyers. 'So it can be', I asked, 'a little chat between the medical examiner and the doctor and that's how they would like it?' 'Yes, yes', he replied, adding that in the countryside there were some towns with only two or three doctors: 'What's the use', he said, 'of asking one of those two or three to judge the handling of a euthanasia case by the other one? How objective can that be? I don't see it'. He concluded that the new directive required prosecutors to lower their professional standards to what he regarded as below even the 'absolute minimum'.[97]

It is evident that the statistical evidence does nothing to refute allegations of non-voluntary and involuntary euthanasia which have been made by several Dutch experts. For example, Dr. Fenigsen, a cardiologist at the Willem-Alexander Hospital, 's-Hertogenbosch, maintains that there is widespread public and professional support for euthanasia without request, as well as ample evidence of the practice.[98] Drawing on his own observations he declares: 'Doctors whose actions I observed, repeatedly tried to justify euthanasia by making reference to false data – citing a non-existent lung cancer, or a presumed, but never made, family request ... '.[99] He refers also to the work of experts such as Drs. Hilhorst and van der Sluis. Dr. Hilhorst, a sociologist who conducted empirical research in Dutch hospitals, reported that doctors and nurses told him that requests for euthanasia came more frequently from the family than the patient and he concluded that both the

[97] Interview, public prosecutor, Alkmaar, 7 December 1990.
[98] 'A Case against Dutch Euthanasia' (1989) 19(1) *Hastings Centre Report* 22, 25.
[99] *Ibid.* 30. See also Richard Fenigsen 'Euthanasia in the Netherlands' (1990) 6 *Issues in Law & Medicine* 229, 235–242.

family and the doctors and nurses often pressured the patient to request euthanasia.[100] Dr. van der Sluis, a dermatologist involved with the treatment of AIDS patients, states that non-voluntary and involuntary euthanasia are common and openly defended in medical journals.[101]

Moreover, in a survey by medical lawyer Professor van Wijmen, 123 doctors, or 41% of the respondents, admitted that they had performed euthanasia without the patient's request, 88 had done so in 1–4 cases: 24 in 5–10 cases: 4 in 11–15 cases: and 7 in more than 15 cases.[102]

Further, the Remmelink Committee reported that in 1000 cases in 1990, life was terminated without an explicit request from the patient and that in 14,258 cases the doctor's 'explicit' or 'secondary' intention was to shorten life without request, either by withholding or withdrawing treatment (8750 cases) or by administering pain-killing drugs (5508 cases). In short, doctors intended to shorten life without request in some 15,000 cases.[103]

Other evidence of euthanasia without request is provided by a number of criminal prosecutions. Professor Sluyters, a medical lawyer, mentions one case in 1985 involving a doctor who was convicted of killing several patients in a nursing home in The Hague and who was sentenced to one year's imprisonment; his conviction was quashed because the police had improperly seized incriminating documents and he was awarded 300000 guilders (approximately £85,000) compensation for the six months he had already spent in prison. Sluyters also refers to cases in which nurses were convicted of killing handicapped children. Although expressing his support for 'the Dutch solution of restrained liberalisation' of the law relating to euthanasia, he concedes: 'In the Netherlands we have seen some cases in the courts in recent years which could perhaps be illustrating the adverse consequences of the liberalisation of euthanasia'.[104] Again, Borst-Eilers has commented that, although she did not believe that voluntary euthanasia led logically to involuntary euthanasia, 'if I am honest I must admit that I cannot judge whether the fact that euthanasia is openly talked about does not bring about a kind of feeling that it's something that you are allowed to do' and that this might have influenced the doctor and nurses in the above cases to perform euthanasia without request.[105]

In sum, the legal and medical criteria for euthanasia would not appear to constitute an effective safeguard against the practice of non-voluntary and

---

[100] Quoted in Barry A Bostrom, 'Euthanasia in the Netherlands: A Model for the United States?' (1989) 4 *Issues in Law & Medicine* 467, 477.

[101] I van der Sluis, 'The Practice of Euthanasia in the Netherlands' (1989) 4 *Issues in Law & Medicine* 455, 463.

[102] F C B van Wijmen, *Artsen en het Zelfgekozen Levenseinde* (*Doctors and the Self-Chosen Termination of Life*) (1989) 24, Table 18. Van Wijmen observes that as cases of 'pseudo-euthanasia' (such as the withdrawal of futile treatment) were expressly excluded in the question, the answers are 'amazing'. *Ibid*. Again, in their book on euthanasia published in 1986, Professor Dessaur and Dr Rutenfrans, of the Criminology Department at the University of Nijmegen, maintain that genuinely voluntary euthanasia amounts to no more than 10% of the 6000–12000 cases per year. *Op. cit.* n90, *supra*, 401–2.

[103] See the Table on p.224 of this volume.

[104] Sluyters, *op. cit.* n4, *supra*, 42. See also Ph. Schepens, 'Euthanasia: Our Own Future?' (1988) 3 *Issues in Law & Medicine* 371, 376–7; Fenigsen, *op. cit.* n98, *supra*, 25.

[105] Interview, 1 August 1989.

involuntary euthanasia. Moreover, the evidence of critics of the Dutch euthanasia experience, such as Fenigsen and van der Sluis, suggests that what the criteria are sufficiently loose to permit is indeed taking place. There is, moreover, a dearth of evidence to support contrary claims that the criteria are being generally observed; as the KNMG indicated in its report, the failure of doctors to notify would mean the legality and propriety of what was happening in practice would be 'absolutely unverifiable'.[106]

2 The 'logical slope'

Even if doubts about the meaning and enforceability of the criteria for lawful euthanasia were dispelled, there would remain the question whether these criteria state necessary as opposed to merely sufficient conditions for lawful euthanasia. Is the legal reasoning of the Supreme Court and the ethical reasoning of the Dutch proponents of euthanasia based upon a principle which entails that some or even all of the existing criteria are not strictly necessary conditions for the legality of euthanasia and which would, if accepted, justify euthanasia without request?

(i) The legal slope

In fact, in the *Alkmaar* case, the Supreme Court did not lay down a list of necessary criteria for lawful euthanasia; its judgment was framed in more general terms. It held that necessity was available as a defence to euthanasia and that in determining the availability of the defence in a given case, a crucial question was whether there was a situation of necessity according to 'responsible medical opinion', tested by 'prevailing standards of medical ethics'.[107]

This suggests that the existence of necessity in a given case is to be determined primarily by criteria fashioned by the medical profession rather than by the courts. Commenting on the case Sutorious observes that according to the Supreme Court 'the primary judgment should remain with the medical discipline, the second judgment is a legal one and should rest with society' and he adds that in his opinion the court 'wishes to have euthanasia problems solved where they arise, notably in the medical discipline'.[108]

However, it is doubtful whether there is a consensus within the profession about the conditions justifying euthanasia and in the absence of an agreed set of criteria there will only be disparate bodies of medical opinion. Medical opinion is often divided over purely technical matters such as diagnosis and treatment, a fact recognised by the common law's test for medical negligence which refuses to hold a doctor negligent merely because he acted in accordance with one responsible body of medical opinion rather than another.[109]

---

[106] Vision, 14.
[107] See text at n10.
[108] Eugene Ph R Sutorius. 'A Mild Death for Paragraph 293 of the Netherlands Criminal Code?' (Unpublished paper, 1986), 7.
[109] *Bolam v. Friern Hospital Management Committee* [1957] I WLR 582.

Medical opinion is likely to be at least as split over an ethical issue such as euthanasia. Presumably, a doctor performing euthanasia will not incur criminal liability if he acts in accordance with a body of medical opinion. But, does this not render the current criteria essentially provisional? Moreover, how is a court in determining what amounts to a 'responsible medical opinion' to select expert witnesses and how is it to proceed if they disagree?

The centrality attached by the Supreme Court to medical opinion has attracted the criticism of a number of Dutch jurists. Feber concludes that the court's decision to cede so much influence to medical opinion leaves insufficient room for the judge to arrive at an independent decision.[110] Leenen has observed: 'By referring to medical ethics the Supreme Court left the problem of the criteria for the acceptability of euthanasia on request in essence unsolved. Moreover, the reference is useless because of the ... disagreement within the medical profession upon ethics'.[111]

However, even if doctors were unanimous about the appropriate criteria, there would still be several weighty objections to the Supreme Court's reasoning. First, if the Court is effectively entrusting the determination of the lawfulness of euthanasia to the medical profession, does this not amount to an abdication of judicial responsibility? Mulder argues that the legal boundaries of euthanasia should be made by the judiciary as representatives of society and not by the medical profession.[112]

Secondly, are doctors, whose training is in medicine, not ethics or law, competent to determine when, if ever, euthanasia is justifiable?

Thirdly, are the existing criteria, which are presumably in line with 'reasonable' medical opinion, consistent with the principles informing Dutch criminal law, particularly that instantiated in article 293, which requires the protection of human life? Mulder points out that whereas an act intended to alleviate the suffering of a dying patient which has the foreseen consequence of accelerating the death of the patient has been permitted by Dutch law, to allow the intentional killing of a patient to alleviate suffering is a new departure.[113]

Fourthly, the decisions of the Court contain no adequate analysis of the doctor's duty to the patient nor reason why the alleviation of suffering

[110] Op. cit. n15, supra, 458.
[111] Op. cit. n8, supra, 201.
[112] Op. cit. n13, supra, 449.
[113] Ibid. 446. Dr Admiraal has stated that he sees no moral difference between intentionally killing a patient and accelerating his death by administering analgesic drugs, even though the hastening of death is merely foreseen. He regards drawing any moral distinction as hypocritical and as a 'ridiculous way out of responsibility'. (Interview, 25 July 1989) He thus elides a distinction which can be crucial for both legal and moral purposes. For example, in English law, the doctor who intentionally kills his patient to alleviate pain commits the offence of murder; by contrast, if the doctor intends solely to alleviate pain and the acceleration of death is an undesired side-effect, even though it is foreseen as certain, he does not. See Robert Goff, 'The Mental Element in the Crime of Murder' (1988) 104 Law Quarterly Review 30, 446. For a discussion of the ethical distinction which can exist see The Principle of Respect for Human Life (Linacre Centre Paper 1) London: The Linacre Centre, 1978 and Is there a morally significant difference between killing and letting die? (Linacre Center Paper 2) London: The Linacre Centre, 1978. See generally John Finnis, 'Intention and side-effects' in R G Frey and Christopher W Morris (eds), Liability and Responsibility: Essays in Law and Morals. Cambridge: Cambridge University Press 1991, 32.

should override the clear terms of article 293. The decisions are all the more remarkable when it is recalled that the very terms of the article emphasise that the victim's earnest request, let alone consent, is no defence to a charge of homicide. Sluyters has written that article 293 was enacted primarily 'to leave no doubt that the killing of a person is unlawful even if that person desires death'.[114] Moreover, the Explanatory Memorandum to article 293 explains that, although one who takes the life of another at his request should be punished 'considerably less severely than those guilty of plain murder', the victim's consent 'cannot abolish the criminality of taking someone's life'. It continues: 'the law so to speak no longer punishes the assault on the life of a particular person, but rather the violation of the respect due to human life in general irrespective of the offender's motive. The criminal offence against life remains, the assault against the person expires'.[115] Again, Mulder, having noted that life has value to the community as well as to the individual, observes that it is 'certain that the Lawgiver considered life worth protecting, even when it no longer has any value to the individual'.[116]

Neither the letter nor the spirit of the Code, then, appears to give any support to the Supreme Court's decision that a defence to a charge under article 293 is implicit in article 40. Indeed, had the legislature intended to provide a defence to article 293 it could have done so expressly. There seems no evidence or reason to doubt that the legislature decided that the protection of life took priority over the autonomy of the individual or the alleviation of suffering. By holding that a doctor may choose to kill in order to relieve suffering, the Court inverted (without any show of juridically sufficient reason) the legislature's ordering of values.

But perhaps the legislature did not foresee the acute suffering which can be imposed on patients by, or as a side effect of, modern medical technology? Perhaps the prohibition in article 293 is outdated and could not have been intended to apply in contemporary Holland? But, in 1891 as today, the legislature must have been well aware that people typically seek euthanasia precisely to avoid suffering. There is no reason to think that the legislature was willing to allow the alleviation of even 'unbearable' suffering to take priority over the protection of life, or that the suffering experienced today is greater than when article 293 was enacted. As Driesse observes:

Despite the fact that people were deeply persuaded that life could bring much and serious suffering, and despite the fact that in those days there were also people who requested death, the lawgiver in Article 293 ... did not abrogate punishment.[117]

Moreover, it would be reasonable to conclude that, with modern palliative care, the suffering which leads people to request euthanasia is substantially less today than it was when article 293 was enacted. Driesse concludes:

---

[114] Op. cit. n4, supra, 35.
[115] NJ (1985) No 106, 451 at 452.
[116] Op. cit. n13, supra, 449.
[117] Marian H N Driesse et al., 'Euthanasia and the Law in the Netherlands' (1988) 3 Issues in Law & Medicine 385, 386–7.

To change this article ... by declaring killing on request, or alternatively rendering assistance in self-killing, to be non-punishable in certain instances, is not the adaptation of an obsolete regulation which is required by changed circumstances. It is the concretization of a fundamental change of attitude in regard to the inviolability of the human individual and of respect for human life.[118]

To all this one must add that the legal position thus reached in 1984 would be rendered all the more far-reaching if the Supreme Court were clearly to hold that the defence of duress in euthanasia cases could extend to 'mental duress' *suffered by the defendant healthcare professional.* Mulder has commented that the courts should not be too eager to allow this type of defence as it paves the way to 'euthanasia-like' acts by other experts, especially nursing personnel.[119] But one must go further: to allow this defence of mental duress is already, in principle, to have accepted *in*voluntary euthanasia, since the request or the consent of the person killed is quite irrelevant within the framework of such a defence.

(ii) The ethical slope

The main argument advanced in The Netherlands for legalising voluntary euthanasia has been that it respects the individual's right to self-determination. Leenen, for example, argues that interference with that right can only be justified if it is to protect essential social values, which is not the case where patients suffering unbearably at the end of their lives request euthanasia when no alternatives exist. He adds: 'Not allowing people euthanasia would come down to forcing them to suffer against their will, which would be cruel and a negation of their human rights and dignity'.[120] Echoing other proponents of legalisation,[121] he observes that modern medicine has contributed to the prolongation of suffering and the 'disfigurement of dying'[122] and he advances arguments in favour of the *statutory* legalisation of euthanasia such as the need to protect self-determination by ensuring that euthanasia is only carried out at the free, explicit and serious request of the patient, and the need to guarantee that doctors, who may be influenced by emotion, exercise great care in making the decision. He points to the legislative proposals of the State Commission on Euthanasia which reported in 1985 and which recommended that article 293 be amended to provide that it would not be unlawful to terminate the life of another at his express and serious request when he was in an 'untenable situation without any prospects' and when the termination was carried out by a doctor 'within the framework of careful medical practice'.[123]

[118] *Ibid*, 387.
[119] *NJ* (1987) No 607 at 2131. In his annotation of the *Alkmaar* case, Professor van Veen comments: "there might be situations in which also the non-physician might appeal successfully to necessity. In his case, an appeal to psychological constraint [*psychische dwang*] would much rather apply than an appeal to emergency in the sense of 'conflict of duties'." *NJ* (1985) No 106, 451 at 467.
[120] *Op. cit*. n7, *supra*, 10.
[121] See e.g. Henriette D C Roscam Abbing, 'Dying with Dignity, and Euthanasia: A View from the Netherlands' (1988) 4 *Journal of Palliative Care* 70.
[122] *Op. cit*. n7, *supra*, 1.
[123] *Ibid*. 7.

Dutch advocates of legalisation take pains to stress that they support *voluntary* euthanasia but oppose *in*voluntary euthanasia. Their position on *non*-voluntary euthanasia is often obscure, largely because of a tendency to confine discussion to the voluntary type. This is often effected by adopting Leenen's definition of euthanasia as *voluntary* euthanasia[124] and declining to regard as euthanasia the termination of life without the patient's request.

Notwithstanding the difficulty of ascertaining their complete ethical position, there is some evidence that many of the Dutch proponents of euthanasia in fact regard the existing criteria for legal euthanasia as sufficient but by no means morally necessary conditions. For example, in relation to the criterion of 'unbearable suffering', Tromp-Meesters has stated that the DVES would ideally like the law to allow anyone to ask their doctor for euthanasia even in the absence of such suffering: 'If you can convince your doctor that you have good reasons to want to die, the doctor should feel free to help you'.[125] *She* felt that ideally it would be like ancient Rome where (she says) once a year citizens could ask to be put to death.[126]

Again, there is widespread support for euthanasia even though the patient is incompetent. The State Commission, for example, recommended that 'the intentional termination of the life of a person unable to express his or her will should not be an offence provided this is performed by a physician in the context of careful medical procedure in respect of a patient who, according to the current state of medical knowledge, has irreversibly lost consciousness, and provided also that treatment has been suspended as pointless'.[127] Further, the KNMG Report in 1984 did not condemn euthanasia without request but simply confined itself, for the time being, to euthanasia for those who were capable of expressing their will. Indeed, it did not even address the ethics of euthanasia but merely observed that euthanasia was practised and that in a pluralistic society views on the subject would always differ.[128] This approach could, of course, also be used to approve euthanasia without request. Indeed, in 1988 a KNMG working party condoned euthanasia for malformed infants,[129] concluding that in certain situations the doctor ought to terminate life.[130] In 1991, a KNMG committee considering 'Life-Ending

---

124 See text at n65, *supra*. An example of this is to be found in a letter to the editors of the *Hastings Center Report* in reply to the article by Fenigsen. *Op. cit.* n98, *supra*. Signed by many of the leading defenders of the Dutch approach to euthanasia it cites Leenen's definition and then states that 'euthanasia' is, therefore, necessarily voluntary, and adds that the killing of incompetent patients is not a part of the euthanasia problem. 'Letter', (1989) 19(6) *Hastings Center Report* 47–9.

125 Interview, 11 July 1989.

126 *Ibid.*

127 'Final Report of the Netherlands State Commission on Euthanasia: An English Summary', (1987) 1 *Bioethics* 163, 168.

128 Vision, 3.

129 *Discussienota inzake levensbeeindigend handelen bij wilsonbekwame patienten, deel l: zwaar-defecte pasgeborenen (Discussion paper on the termination of life of severely handicapped new-born infants)* (1988), cited by Sluyters, *op. cit.* n4, *supra*, 35.

130 Interview, Gunning, 2 August 1989.

214

Treatment of Incompetent Patients' advocated the killing of patients in persistent coma.[131]

Finally, leading proponents of euthanasia have occasionally expressed support for euthanasia without request. Asked whether he saw any moral distinction between removing artificial feeding from a comatose patient and actively killing him, Dr Admiraal replied: 'No, I should kill the patient as well ... In a coma there is no ... suffering ... and there is no consciousness so there is no ... reason to stop life immediately but I should do [so] and not wait for the starving of that patient for the next weeks. Oh no, I should say if I made the decision to stop tube-feeding, I should give active euthanasia ...'. He added that it was the same situation with a neonate: 'You can't speak about voluntary euthanasia, it's only the parents asking for ... the judgement of the doctors and you are just killing that baby'. Asked whether there was anything wrong with that, he replied that he did not think so.[132]

The above considerations suggest that a substantial number of the most prominent Dutch advocates of voluntary euthanasia in fact support non-voluntary euthanasia. They may, moreover, be logically committed to this position, for the basis of their case for voluntary euthanasia, namely, respect for self-determination, may well be thought to provide little or no ground for judging wrongful the euthanatising of those who do not possess autonomy, whether because they are infants, senile adults, mentally handicapped, or comatose. The widespread condonation of euthanasia in the case of the comatose is particularly revealing, for it undermines the need for either a request or for suffering (whether unbearable or not) and suggests that the right to self-determination is, notwithstanding the emphasis commonly placed upon it, an incomplete explanation of the case for euthanasia which is advanced in The Netherlands. The case would appear fundamentally to rest on the principle that lives which fall below a certain 'quality' are not worth living. This principle has evidently been openly adopted by some of the leading Dutch exponents of euthanasia. For example, Professor van der Meer, former Head of Internal Medicine at the Free University of Amsterdam, has written that it is obvious that the 'quality of life' of a person rendered permanently comatose has fallen 'below the minimum'.[133]

Of course, if the Dutch case for voluntary euthanasia is, as it would appear

[131] Personal communication from Gunning, 27 April 1991, about the second report (entitled 'Treatment of Patients in Prolonged Coma') of the KNMG's Committee on the Acceptability of Life-ending Treatment.

[132] Interview, 27 July 1989. Similarly, H M Dupuis, Professor of Medical Ethics at the University of Leiden and ex-President of the DVES, has said that she accepts that in some cases in which the diagnosis was clear, the life of an irreversibly comatose patient ought to be terminated as when stopping treatment merely increased the patient's suffering and there was a consensus that the patient's life was senseless. (Interview, 28 July 1989. See also 'The Right to a Gentle Death' in *op. cit.* n26, *supra*, 53, 55–6). Again, Tromp-Meesters, asked whether the requirement of a request did not deprive those too young or too old to make a request of a right to be relieved of suffering replied: 'Yes, I think so, and that could never be, in my view, the decision of one doctor: that should be a team of two or three people'. She added that her Society had not ruled out non-voluntary euthanasia and was still considering the matter. (Interview, 11 July 1989).

[133] C van der Meer, 'Euthanasia: A Definition and Ethical Conditions' (1988) 4 *Journal of Palliative Care* 103, 104.

to be, based on the principle that certain lives are not worth living, then it raises the questions whether this principle is defensible and whether it does not logically permit non-voluntary and even involuntary euthanasia. One of the unfortunate consequences of the emphasis in the Dutch euthanasia debate on the right of self-determination has been that these important questions have not received the attention they deserve. They have, however, been addressed by opponents of legalisation, notably Kamisar. He concludes that there is a real danger of sliding down the 'slippery slope', first because it has already taken place this century and started with the acceptance of the attitude that there is such a thing as a life not worth living[134] and secondly because, as he demonstrates, many supporters of voluntary euthanasia have historically shared this attitude.[135] He argues, moreover, that reasons which have been advanced by proponents of voluntary euthanasia for not extending euthanasia to the senile and the defective are much more tentative and unpersuasive than the arguments they deploy for legalising euthanasia in the first place.[136]

Conclusion

The significance of the Dutch euthanasia experience for law, medicine and social policy in other countries is considerable, not least in respect of the support it lends to the 'slippery slope' argument. Some have argued that the danger of a slide into non-voluntary and involuntary euthanasia would be reduced if the criteria were statutory. It will be recalled that Leenen listed arguments in favour of legislation, such as the need to ensure that euthanasia was only performed at the patient's request.[137] He omits, however, to explain *how* legislation would provide more effective safeguards against abuse. Moreover, as medical lawyer Professor Gevers has cautioned: 'It is impossible to delineate precisely the situations in which euthanasia should be allowed; therefore, a new law cannot add very much to what has already been developed by the courts, and will only partially reduce legal uncertainty'.[138] Further, the legislative proposals contained in the report of the State Commission on Euthanasia are, as Leenen himself has observed,[139] essentially the same as those developed by the courts. Indeed, it is arguable that the central criterion proposed by the Commission, an 'untenable situation' with no prospect of improvement[140], is even looser than the existing criterion of unbearable suffering which cannot be alleviated.

It could, of course, be argued that although euthanasia without request may be practised in The Netherlands, it is also carried out in jurisdictions where euthanasia is unlawful, such as the UK, and that the legalisation of

[134] *Op. cit.* n74, *supra*, 468–9.
[135] *Ibid.* 451–67.
[136] *Ibid.* 467.
[137] See text at nn122–3.
[138] *Op. cit.* n10, *supra*, 162.
[139] *Op. cit.* n7, *supra*, 7–8.
[140] See text at n123.

voluntary euthanasia helps prevent the carrying out of euthanasia without request. As a spokesman for the KNMG put it, there is a choice between on the one hand prohibiting euthanasia and not knowing how often it is carried out and, on the other hand, legalising it and knowing how most of it is carried out. The KNMG, he explained, wanted it to be controlled, and if it were prohibited, it could not be controlled.[141] But it is clear from the evidence set out in Part III 1 (iii) above that all that is known with certainty in The Netherlands is that euthanasia is being practised on a scale vastly exceeding the 'known' (truthfully reported and recorded) cases. There is little sense in which it can be said, in any of its forms, to be under control. As Leenen has observed, there is an 'almost total lack of control on the administration of euthanasia'[142] and 'the present legal situation makes any adequate control of the practice of euthanasia virtually impossible'.[143] And there is little reason to suppose that the legalization of euthanasia, involving the translation of the current criteria into statutory form, would result in more effective control. While it is reasonable to think that legalization might encourage more doctors to report, since they would no longer be reporting a criminal act, it would neither cure the vagueness of the criteria, reduce the largely untrammelled discretion of the doctors, nor render the reporting procedure any more effective a check on the exercise of that discretion.

The lack of any effective control over the practice of euthanasia in Holland has recently been confirmed by Dr Carlos Gomez. The extent to which the Dutch control euthanasia is the central concern of his book *Regulating Death: Euthanasia and the Case of the Netherlands*[144] which documents Dr Gomez's empirical investigation of this question.

He begins by asking: 'How will we assure ourselves that the weak, the demented, the vulnerable, the stigmatized – those incapable of consent or dissent [will] not become the unwilling subjects of such a practice?'[145] He observes that it is commonly agreed that prosecutors review only a small minority of cases and he concludes that, therefore, the 'formal, juridical level' of the Dutch regulatory system is 'routinely bypassed'.[146] As for the 'informal' regulatory criteria laid down by the KNMG, Gomez concludes: 'not only are they not enforced, they are probably unenforceable'.[147] He adds that the role of regulated and regulator has fallen to doctors with the tacit consent of Dutch society and that this bespeaks not only a remarkable trust in the medical profession but also an 'almost cavalier attitude toward those – however many or few their numbers – who cannot challenge a decision to have euthanasia performed upon them'.[148] He concludes that 'on

---

[141] Interview, Martens, 11 July 1989.
[142] 'Legal Aspects of Euthanasia, Assistance to Suicide and Terminating the Medical Treatment of Incompetent Patients' (Unpublished paper delivered at a Conference on Euthanasia held at the Instituut voor Gezondheidsethiek, Maastricht, 2–4 December 1990) 6.
[143] *Ibid.* 11.
[144] Free Press, 1991. My review of this book appears in 22/2 (1992) *Hastings Center Report* 39–43.
[145] *Ibid.* xiv.
[146] *Ibid.* 121.
[147] *Ibid.* 122.
[148] *Ibid.* 124–5.

the core issues of the controversy – how to control the practice, how to keep it from being used on those who do not want it, how to provide for public accountability – the Dutch response has been, to date, inadequate'.[149]

---

[149] *Ibid.* 133.

5

Further Reflections on Euthanasia in The Netherlands in the Light of The Remmelink Report and The Van Der Maas Survey*

JOHN KEOWN

Since the original publication of my article on euthanasia in The Netherlands,[1] the euthanasia Survey carried out at the request of the Dutch Government's Commission on Euthanasia has been published in translation.[2] The Survey, carried out by a team led by P J van der Maas, Professor of Public Health and Social Medicine at the Erasmus University, opens a revealing window on euthanasia in Holland and invites further reflections, in the light of its findings, on Dutch euthanasia. Moreover, the British Government has established a House of Lords Select Committee on Medical Ethics to consider, *inter alia*, whether euthanasia may be justified and the Committee has solicited evidence about the experience of other countries, particularly in Western Europe. Further analysis of the Dutch experience is, therefore, particularly timely.

First, a word about terminology. 'Euthanasia' is commonly understood to connote the intentional killing of a patient, by act or omission, as part of his medical care. The word will be used in this sense in this paper. In The Netherlands, however, the word is used in a narrower sense to mean intentional killing, by act or omission, *at the patient's request*.[3] The use of the word in this sense will be flagged in this paper by inverted commas.

I. The Origins of the Remmelink Commission and the van der Maas Survey

The Dutch coalition government which assumed office in 1989 decided to appoint a Commission to report on the 'extent and nature of medical euthanasia practice'. A Commission under the chairmanship of the Attorney-General, Professor Remmelink, was appointed on January 17 1990 by the Minister of Justice and the State Secretary of Welfare, Health and Culture and asked to report on the practice by physicians of 'performing an

* The research resulting in this paper was funded by the Research Board of the University of Leicester, whose support I gratefully acknowledge.
1 I J Keown, 'The Law and Practice of Euthanasia in The Netherlands' (1992) 108 *Law Quarterly Review* 51. An updated version of this paper appears as 'Some reflections on euthanasia in The Netherlands' in Luke Gormally (ed.) *The Dependent Elderly* (Cambridge University Press, 1992) 70 and is reprinted as the preceding chapter in this volume.
2 P J van der Maas *et al.*, *Euthanasia and other Medical Decisions Concerning the End of Life* (Elsevier, Amsterdam: 1992). (Hereafter 'Survey'.) Also published in (1992) 22 (1) / (2) *Health Policy*. A summary of the Survey was published in (1991) 338 *Lancet* 669.
3 See n20 and nn36–39, *infra*. For standard definitions see n.46, *infra*.

act or omission ... to terminate [the] life of a patient, with or without an explicit and serious request of the patient to this end'.[4]

To assist the discharge of this responsibility, the Commission asked Professor van der Maas to carry out a survey which would produce qualitative and quantitative information on the practice of euthanasia. The Commission and van der Maas agreed that the survey should embrace all medical decisions affecting the end of life so that euthanasia could be seen within that broader context. The umbrella term 'Medical Decisions Concerning the End of Life' ('MDELs') includes 'all decisions by physicians concerning courses of action aimed at hastening the end of life of the patient or courses of action for which the physician takes into account the probability that the end of life of the patient is hastened'.[5] MDELs comprise the administration, supply or prescription of a drug; the withdrawal or withholding of a treatment (including resuscitation and tube-feeding), and the refusal of a request for euthanasia or assisted suicide.[6] The Commission's Report[7] and the Survey[8] were published in Dutch in September 1991. One year later, the Survey was published in English.[9]

My earlier article suggested that the Dutch experience lends support to the 'slippery slope' argument in both its 'logical' and 'practical' forms. Do the Report and Survey require that suggestion to be qualified? The answer, on a simple reading of the Report would be Yes. But a reading of the Report in the light of its Survey yields a contrary answer. Indeed, taken together, the Survey and Report tend to confirm the application of both forms of the slippery slope argument to euthanasia in Holland.

II. The Findings of the Survey and the Conclusions of the Commission

It is proposed, after outlining the Survey's findings about the incidence of euthanasia, to consider what light the Survey and the Report throw on the extent to which the criteria laid down by the courts and the Royal Dutch Medical Association (KNMG) are being observed in practice. Attention will, for two reasons, focus on the Survey rather than the Report. First, the Report contains the Commission's conclusions in the light of the Survey but the Survey is a comprehensive empirical study which stands independently

---

[4] Survey, 3–4.

[5] *Ibid.*, 19–20

[6] *Ibid.*, 20.

[7] *Medische beslissingen rond het levenseinde. Rapport van de Commissie onderzoek medische praktijk inzake euthanasie.* Sdu Uitgeverij Plantijnstraat, 's-Gravenhage (1991). (Hereafter 'Report').

[8] *Medische beslissingen rond het levenseinde. Het onderzoek voor de Commissie Onderzoek Medische Praktijk inzake Euthanasie.* Sdu Uitgeverij Plantijnstraat, s-Gravenhage (1991).

[9] See note 2, *supra.* Oddly, the Report has not been translated, though a brief English summary has been produced by the Ministry of Justice: *Outlines (sic) Report Commission Inquiry into Medical Practice with regard to Euthanasia* (nd) (hereafter 'outline'). Dr. Richard Fenigsen's unpublished 'First Reactions to the Report of the Committee on Euthanasia' (1991) contains a translation of key passages of the Report. I am grateful to Dr. Fenigsen for permission to rely on his translation. His paper 'The Report of the Dutch Governmental Committee on Euthanasia' is published in (1991) 7 *Issues in Law & Medicine* 3.

of the Report. Secondly, the conclusions drawn in the Report are not infrequently difficult to square with the findings of the Survey.

1. Methodology

Before turning to the Survey's findings, a summary of its methodology is appropriate. The Survey comprised three studies.

(i) the retrospective study[10]

A sample of 406 doctors was drawn from GPs, specialists (concerned with MDELs) and nursing home doctors, of whom 91% agreed to participate. The doctors were interviewed on average for two and a half hours and almost always by another doctor.[11] The respondent was asked about relevant types of decision. If he had made a decision of a given type, the last occasion on which he had done so was discussed in greater detail. At most, ten cases were discussed with each.[12]

(ii) the death certificate study[13]

This study examined a stratified sample of 8500 deaths occurring in Holland from July to November 1990 inclusive. The treating doctor was identified from each death certificate and was sent a short questionnaire which could be returned anonymously. The response rate was 73%[14]

(iii) the prospective study[15]

Each of the doctors interviewed in the retrospective study was asked at interview if he would complete a questionnaire (identical to that in the second study) about each of their patients who died in the following six months. This study had several advantages: there would be little memory distortion because the questionnaire would be completed soon after the death; it would provide additional information to strengthen the quantitative basis of the interview study, and the carefully planned selection of respondents meant that the responses were representative of 95% of all deaths. The study ran from mid-November 1990 to the end of May 1991.

---

[10] See generally Survey, Part II (chapters 4–10).

[11] *Ibid.*, 14–17;191. The authors considered whether those who refused to participate formed a select group which could lead to serious bias and concluded that, in the light of the total number of refusals (41) and the variety of reasons for refusing (mainly lack of time), this could hardly be so. The 15 who indicated that they disapproved of the Survey, did not wish to comment or opposed euthanasia could only introduce a 'very modest' bias. *ibid.*, 228. This reasoning is unpersuasive; does not the conclusion that there is no risk of bias rest on answers which are unverified? Is it not possible that some of the 41 who declined to participate frequently performed euthanasia and equally possible that some of these cases fell outside the guidelines?

[12] *Ibid.*, 33.

[13] See generally Part III (chapters 11–13)

[14] *Ibid.*, 15; 121–125; 191.

[15] See generally Part IV (chapters 14–15)

80% of those involved in the first study participated, completing over 2250 questionnaires.[16] In all, each of some 322 doctors supplied information about, on average, seven deaths.[17] The method of collection of data in all three studies was such that anonymity of participants could be guaranteed.[18]

2. Incidence of euthanasia

In 1990, the year covered by the Survey, there were almost 130,000 deaths in Holland from all causes, of which 49,000 involved a MDEL.[19] Both the Report and the Survey adopted the Dutch definition of euthanasia as the *intentional* termination of another's life at his request.[20] How many cases of 'euthanasia' so defined were there in 1990?

The three studies differed as to the incidence of euthanasia, yielding respective figures of 1.9%, 1.7% and 2.6% of all deaths. The researchers felt that the difference between the second and third estimates was 'probably due to the existence of a boundary area between euthanasia and intensifying of the alleviation of pain and/or symptoms' and to the probability of the third study counting cases of pain alleviation as cases of 'euthanasia', thereby exaggerating its incidence.[21]

It is, however, arguable that, of the three studies, it is the third which produces the most accurate estimate of 'euthanasia'. As the authors of the Survey point out, whereas the respondents in the second study had no information other than the questionnaire and an accompanying letter, those in the third had participated in the physician interviews, discussing one or more cases from their practice and the crucial concepts in the questionnaire for over two hours with a trained interviewer. The authors, noting that a 'great number' of interviewees commented that the interview had clarified their thinking about MDELs, suggest the possibility of a learning effect: familiarity with the questionnaire, in which the question about euthanasia followed those relating to other MDELs, may have led the respondents to reply negatively to the earlier questions knowing that the question about euthanasia was to come. The authors conclude that the most important fact was that the respondents in the third study 'changed their approach with respect to their intention when administering morphine due to their recent intensive confrontation with thinking about this complex of problems'.[22] If the thinking of participants in the third study had been clarified by their participation in the first study, are their responses not likely to be more reliable than those in the second study particularly as, the second study being retrospective, there was less risk of memory distortion?

[16] *Ibid.*, 15; 149–151;192.
[17] *Ibid.*, 160.
[18] *Ibid.*, 16.
[19] Report, 14.
[20] 'the intentional action to terminate a person's life, performed by somebody else than the involved person upon the latter's request'. Report, 11 (see also Outline, 2); 'the purposeful acting to terminate life by someone other than the person concerned upon request of the latter'. Survey, 5; see also *ibid.*, 23;193.
[21] Survey, 178.
[22] *Ibid.*, 162.

The authors' conclusion is, however, that in the light of all three studies, 'euthanasia' occurred in about 1.8% of all deaths, or about 2300 cases,[23] and that there were almost 400 cases of assisted suicide, some 0.3% of all deaths.[24] More than half the physicians regularly involved with terminal patients indicated that they had performed 'euthanasia' or had assisted suicide and only 12% of doctors said they would never do so.[25]

So much for euthanasia in its narrowest sense: intentional termination of life *at the patient's request*. But the authors of the Survey themselves go on, rightly, to consider euthanasia in a somewhat wider but still precise and realistic sense. They estimated that in a further 1000 cases (or 0.8% of all deaths) physicians administered a drug 'with the explicit purpose of hastening the end of life without an explicit request of the patient'.[26]

And beyond this, there lies a range of evidence yielded by the Survey, but not adequately considered by the authors in their commentary. For many other MDELs also involved an intent to hasten death. Palliative drugs were administered in 'such high doses ... that ... almost certainly would shorten the life of the patient'[27] in 22,500 cases (17.5% of all deaths).[28] In 65% (or 14,625) of these cases the doctor administered the medication merely 'Taking into account the probability that life would be shortened', but in 30% (or 6750 cases) it was administered 'Partly with the purpose of shortening life' and in a further 6% (or 1350 cases) 'With the explicit purpose of shortening life'.[29]

Moreover, doctors withdrew or withheld treatment in another 25,000 cases and, by the time of the survey, some 90%, or 22,500, had died.[30] In 65% (or 16,250 cases) the treatment was withdrawn or withheld 'Taking into account the probability that life would be shortened', but in 19% (or 4750 cases) 'Partly with the purpose to shorten life' and in a further 16% (or 4000 cases) 'With the explicit purpose to shorten life'.[31]

Further, physicians received some 5800 requests to withdraw or withhold treatment when the patient intended at least in part to hasten death.[32] In 74% of these cases the doctor withdrew or withheld treatment 'Partly with the purpose of shortening life' and in 26% 'With the explicit purpose of shortening life'.[33] By the time of the interview, some 82% (or 4756) had died.[34] The above figures are reproduced in the following *Table*.

---

[23] *Ibid.*, 178.
[24] *Ibid.*, 179.
[25] *Ibid.*, 40, *Table* 5.3
[26] *Ibid.*, 182. The third study returned a figure of 1.6%. *ibid.*, 181
[27] *Ibid.*, 71. The authors were not concerned with cases where palliative drugs were used which had no chance of shortening life. *ibid.*, 72. Life was shortened by up to one week in 70% of cases and by one to four weeks in 23%. *ibid.*, 73, *Table* 7.3.
[28] *Ibid.*, 183.
[29] *Ibid.*, 73, *Table* 7.2.
[30] *Ibid.*, 85; 90, *Table* 8.14.
[31] *Ibid.*, 90, *Table* 8.15.
[32] *Ibid.*, 81.
[33] *Ibid.*, 84, *Table* 8.7.
[34] *Ibid.*, 82, *Table* 8.6.

		Acts or omissions with intent to shorten life (cases of 'explicit' intent to shorten life in bold) (cases without explicit request in parentheses)
Total deaths (all causes)	129,000	
'Euthanasia'^		**2300**
Assisted suicide		**400**
Intentional life-terminating acts without explicit request+		**1000 (1000)**
Alleviation of pain/symptoms~	22,500 with the 'explicit purpose' of shortening life 'partly with the purpose' of shortening life	**1350 (450)** 6750 (5058)
Withdrawal/withholding of treatment without explicit request *	25,000 with the 'explicit purpose' of shortening life 'partly with the purpose' of shortening life	**4000 (4000)** 4750 (4750)
Withdrawal/withholding of treatment on explicit request**	5,800 with the 'explicit purpose' of shortening life 'partly with the purpose' of shortening life	**1508** 4292
SUB-TOTAL#		**10,558 (5450)**
TOTAL##		26,350 (15,258)

^ No shortening of life occurred in 1% of these cases. Survey, 49, *Table* 5.13.
+ No shortening of life occurred in 4% of these cases. *ibid*, 66, *Table* 6.10.
~ No shortening of life occurred in 8% of these cases. *ibid*, 73, *Table* 7.3.
* 90% of these patients (22,500) had died by the time of the interview and there had been no shortening of life in 20% of these cases. *ibid*, 90, *Table* 8.14.
** 82% of these patients (4756) had died by the time of the interview and there had been no shortening of life in 19% of these cases. *ibid*, 82, *Table* 8.6.
# This sub-total refers to cases where doctors 'explicitly' intended to shorten life by act or omission.
This total refers to cases where doctors intended ('explicitly' or 'partly') to hasten death by act or omission. Both it and the preceding sub-total therefore include (as does the Survey) cases where life may not in fact have been shortened and cases in the asterisked categories where patients had not died by the time of the survey.

Thus it becomes clear that, while the Commission stated that the figure of 2700 cases of 'euthanasia' and assisted suicide 'does not warrant the assumption that euthanasia in the Netherlands occurs on an excessive scale ...'[35] the total number of euthanasiast acts and omissions in 1990 was in reality far higher than the Commission claims. To clarify and confirm this conclusion it is necessary to look more closely at the definitions used by the authors of the Survey in classifying their data to produce the figures given above.

The definition of euthanasia adopted by the Commission was the '*intentional* action to terminate a person's life, performed by somebody else than the involved person upon the latter's request'.[36] Similarly, that adopted in the survey was 'the *purposeful* acting to terminate life by someone other than the person concerned upon request of the latter'.[37] These definitions echo that embraced by the central committee of the Royal Dutch Medical Association (KNMG) in its 1984 report on euthanasia as all actions 'aimed at' terminating a patient's life at his explicit request.[38] This report added that a majority of the committee had rejected a sub-division into 'active' and 'passive' as 'morally superfluous' and undesirable: 'All activities or non-activities with the purpose to terminate a patient's life are defined as euthanasia'.[39]

The authors of the Survey distinguished the following states of mind:

(acting with) the explicit purpose of hastening the end of life;
(acting) partly with the purpose of hastening the end of life;
(acting while) taking into account the probability that the end of life will be hastened.[40]

They explained that the first category, unlike the third, applied where the patient's death was the intended outcome of the action. The second category was used because sometimes an act was performed with a particular aim (such as pain relief) but the side-effect (such as death) was 'not unwelcome'. Strictly speaking, stated the authors, this side-effect should be categorised as intentional because in order to be considered unintentional, death 'should in fact not have been desired'.[41] However, the second category was used because sometimes doctors felt that neither the first nor third category described their intention. The second category 'relates to a situation in which death of the patient was not foremost in the physician's mind but neither was death unwelcome'. It was a 'type' of intention.[42]

As the *Table* reveals, doctors are stated by the Survey to have intended to accelerate death in far more than the 2700 cases classified by the Commission as 'euthanasia' and assisted suicide. There are the 1000 cases of intentional killing without request. There are, in addition, three additional categories where there is said to have been some intention to shorten life: firstly, the

[35] Report, 31; Outline, 2.
[36] See note 20, *supra*. (Emphasis added.)
[37] *Ibid.* (Emphasis added.)
[38] *Vision on Euthanasia* (a translation by the KNMG in 1986 of its Report 'Standpunt inzake euthanasie' published in [1984] 39 *Medisch Contact* 990) 15. Hereafter 'Vision'.
[39] *Ibid.*
[40] Survey, 21. They state, confusingly, that death 'may not' have been intended in the third category.
[41] *Ibid.*
[42] *Ibid.*

225

8100 (1350 + 6750) cases of increasing the dosage of palliative drugs; secondly, the 8750 (4000 + 4750) cases of withholding or withdrawing treatment without request and, finally, the 5800 (1508 + 4292) cases withholding or withdrawing treatment on request. Adding these 23,650 cases to the 2700 produces a total of 26,350 cases in which the Survey states that doctors intended, by act or omission, to shorten life. This raises the incidence of euthanasia from around 2% to over 20% of all deaths in Holland.

It could be argued that the 23,650 cases are not 'euthanasia' because they are not cases of intentional killing at the patient's request. There are, however, two counter-arguments. First, some of them clearly *are*. In relation, for example, to the 1350 cases in which it was the explicit purpose of the doctor to shorten life by increasing the dosage of palliative drugs, the survey discloses that 'In all these cases the patient had at some time indicated something about terminating life and an explicit request had been made in two thirds of the cases'. Indeed, the authors comment: 'This situation is therefore rather similar to euthanasia'.[43]

It is unclear, therefore, why the Commission does not regard these as cases of 'euthanasia'; they seem to fall squarely within its definition. It is equally unclear why the 5800 cases in which doctors withdrew or withheld treatment on request with intent to shorten life are not included.[44] Interestingly, a member of the Commission (who in fact wrote the report) has subsequently agreed with the proposition that those cases where doctors had, with the explicit purpose of shortening the patient's life and at the patient's explicit request, either administered palliative drugs or withdrawn treatment, could properly be categorised as 'euthanasia'.[45]

The second counter-argument is that the true scale of euthanasia can only properly be gauged when the Commission's abnormally narrow definition of euthanasia is replaced by the standard definition of 'the intentional killing of a patient as part of his medical care', whether or not at his request.[46] If this more realistic definition is applied, then the Survey's own presentation of the data suggests that there were a further 23,650 euthanasia deaths.

However, there remains a further question about the proper interpretation of the Survey's definitions, and thus of its figures. In particular, is it appropriate to include the 15,792 cases in which hastening death was only

[43] *Ibid.*, 72.

[44] By no means all of these patients were terminal. Life was shortened by one to four weeks in 16%, by one to six months in 43% and even longer in 13%. *Ibid.*, 82, *Table* 8.6. Moreover, three of the four reasons most frequently given by the patient for requesting withdrawal – 'loss of dignity' (31 %); 'tiredness of life' (28%) and 'dependence' (24%) *ibid.*, 82, *Table* 8.4 – appear (unlike the remaining reason – 'burden of treatment' (43%)) quite consistent with a suicidal intent. However, as the respondent doctors were not given the opportunity of stating that they withheld or withdrew treatment merely foreseeing that life would be shortened, the figures indicating that doctors intended to shorten life in *all* cases should be treated with some caution, and their categorisation here as cases of euthanasiast omissions is subject to that *caveat*.

[45] Interview by author with Mr. A Kors, Ministry of Justice, The Hague, 29 November 1991.

[46] *Euthanasia and Clinical Practice: The Report of a Working Party* (The Linacre Centre, 1982) 2(present volume, p.11). See also *Stedman's Medical Dictionary* (25th ed., 1990) 544 ('The intentional putting to death of a person with an incurable or painful disease'); *Dictionary of Medical Ethics* (A S Duncan, G R Dunstan, R B Welbourn eds.; 1981)164 (' ..."mercy killing", the administration of a drug deliberately and specifically to accelerate death in order to terminate suffering'.)

'partly' the doctor's intention? These cases were distinguished in the Survey from those where the doctor merely foresaw the acceleration of death (where he proceeded 'Taking into account the probability that life would be shortened'[47]). If the doctor's purpose in these cases was, albeit partly, to hasten death, then it seems quite appropriate to regard them as instances of euthanasia. By analogy, if racial discrimination is the intentional (purposeful) treating of one person less favourably than another on racial grounds and, say, an employer takes advantage of the need to make redundancies in order to get rid of his black workers, he may be said to have acted partly with a view to doing just that, even though his primary purpose is to save his company by reducing the wages' bill.

On the other hand, it is arguable that these are not necessarily cases in which the doctor's purpose was to hasten death. Notwithstanding the researchers' treatment of these as cases of purposeful killing, their explanation of this category and in particular their apparent understanding of the concept of 'purpose' in fact leave the matter unclear. The implication in their explanation that death in these cases was 'desired' does indeed suggest that the doctor intended to shorten life, but the reference to death as a 'not unwelcome' consequence suggests that death, while not regretted, may not, in some of these cases, have been any part of the doctor's purpose or goal.

Although it may well be that the doctor's intention in most if not all of these cases was to shorten life (a conclusion which would be consistent with the finding that no fewer than 88% of Dutch doctors had performed euthanasia or would be willing to do so[48]) the possibility that it was not cannot be ruled out. These cases are, therefore, regarded in this paper as cases of intentional shortening of life subject to this *caveat*. However, the force of the following critique of Dutch euthanasia in no way depends on their inclusion.

For even if they are discounted, the total number of life-shortening acts and omissions where the doctor's *primary* intention (more graphically but less precisely called 'explicit purpose' by the Survey) was to kill, and which are therefore indubitably euthanasiast, is 10,558. That figure is almost four times higher than the number of cases categorised as 'euthanasia' and assisted suicide by the Commission and amounts to over 8% of all deaths in Holland.

3. Criteria for euthanasia

How many of the 10,558 (or, if partly intended life-shortening is included, 26,350) euthanasiast acts and omissions satisfied the guidelines laid down by the courts and the KNMG? More specifically, in how many cases was there a 'free and voluntary' request which was 'well-considered, durable and persistent'?; in how many was there 'intolerable' suffering for which euthanasia was a 'last resort'?; and in how many cases did the doctor consult with a colleague

[47] Survey, 73, *Table* 7.2; *ibid.*, 90, *Table* 8.15.
[48] *Ibid.*, 40, *Table* 5.3.

and report the case to the legal authorities, whether prosecutor, police or local medical examiner?[49]

(i) an 'entirely free and voluntary' request which was 'well-considered, durable and persistent'

Doctors stated that in the '2700' cases of 'euthanasia' and assisted suicide there was an 'explicit request' in 96%; which was 'wholly made by the patient' in 99% of all cases and 'repeated' in 94%; and that in 100% of cases the patient had a 'good insight' into his disease and its prognosis. Oddly, no specific question was put about the voluntariness of the request and there is no evidence of any mechanism to ensure that the request was voluntary.[50] Moreover, the request was purely oral in 60% of cases[51] and, when made to a GP in cases where a nurse was in attendance on the patient, the GP more often than not failed to consult her.[52]

There is no way of gauging the accuracy of the doctors' statements, which are uncorroborated, about the patients' requests. Even if they are true, however, the survey data shows that in the 10,558 cases in which it was the doctor's primary purpose to hasten death, there was in the majority (52%) no explicit request from the patient. (Similarly, in a majority (58%) of the 26,350 cases in which it was the doctor's primary or secondary intention to shorten life, the doctor shortened life without the patient's explicit request.)

(a) 'life-terminating acts without the patient's explicit request'

In the light of the three studies, the Survey concludes:

On an annual basis there are, in The Netherlands, some thousand cases (0.8% of all deaths) for which physicians prescribe, supply or administer a drug with the explicit purpose of hastening the end of life without an explicit request of the patient.[53]

In over half these cases, the decision was discussed with the patient or the patient had previously indicated his wish for the hastening of death but 'In several hundred cases there was no discussion with the patient and there also was no known wish from the patient for hastening the end of life'. In virtually all cases, state the authors, seriously ill and terminal patients were involved who obviously were suffering a great deal and were no longer able to express their wishes, though there was a 'small number' of cases in which

---

[49] For a summary of the guidelines see *op. cit.* n1, *supra*, [52–61]. 98% of doctors stated that they were aware of the 'rules of due care' formulated by the KNMG, the Health Council and the Government. When asked what they were, 89% mentioned consultation but only 66% the need for a seriously considered request; 42% a voluntary request; 37% 'unacceptable' suffering, and 18% a long-standing desire to die. Survey, 95–96, *Table 9.1*. When shown 14 guidelines, however, and asked to rank them in importance, 98% mentioned voluntariness and only 67% consultation. *Ibid., Table 9.2*.

[50] *Ibid.*, 50, *Table 5.15*.

[51] *Ibid.*, 43.

[52] *Ibid.*,108, *Table 10.3*. (By contrast, 96% of specialists and nursing home doctors consulted nursing staff. *ibid.*) Further, two thirds of GPs said they felt it was up to the doctor in certain circumstances to raise the topic of euthanasia. *Ibid.*, 101.

[53] *Ibid.*, 182.

the decision could have been discussed with the patient.[54] The fact that doctors administered a lethal drug without an express request in 1,000 cases – almost half as many as they did on request – is startling. So too is the Commission's reaction to this statistic. The Commission observes that the ('few dozen') cases in which the doctor killed a competent patient without request 'must be prevented in future', and that one means would be 'strict compliance with the scrupulous care' required for euthanasia 'including the requirement that all facts of the case are put down in writ[i]ng'. However, the Commission defends the other cases of unrequested killing, stating that 'active intervention' by the doctor was usually 'inevitable' because of the patient's 'death agony'. That is why, it explains, it regards these cases as 'care for the dying'.[55]

The Report continues that the absence of a request 'only serves to make the decision process more difficult' than when there is a request. It adds:

The ultimate justification for the intervention is in both cases the patient's unbearable suffering. So, medically speaking, there is little difference between these situations and euthanasia, because in both cases patients are involved who suffer terribly. The absence of a special [sic] request for the termination of life stems partly from the circumstance that the party in question is not (any longer) able to express his will because he is already in the terminal stage, and partly because the demand for an explicit request is not in order when the treatment of pain and symptoms is intensified. The degrading condition the patient is in confronts the doctor with a case of force majeure. According to the Commission, the intervention by the doctor can easily be regarded as an action that is justified by necessity, just like euthanasia.[56]

The classification of killing without request as 'care for the dying' could be criticised as tendentious euphemism. It is, moreover, inconsistent even with established Dutch terminology. A leading authority on the definition and legal status of 'euthanasia' in Holland is HJJ Leenen, Emeritus Professor of Health Law at the University of Amsterdam (and, incidentally, a leading supporter of the legalisation of euthanasia). He has written:

In The Netherlands euthanasia is defined as the deliberate termination of the life of a person on his request, by another person. Central in this definition is the request of the patient. Without such a request the termination of a life would be murder.[57]

Leaving aside the Commission's resort to euphemism in its defence of killing without request, the reasons it gives in that defence are questionable. It asserts that the patient's 'unbearable suffering' is the ultimate justification for killing in these cases, but fails to explain the basis of this supposed justification. In view of the importance which has long been attached by many Dutch proponents of euthanasia to the need for a request by the patient, it is remarkable that the Commission, rather than setting out a reasoned ethical case to substantiate its opinion that killing without request

[54] Ibid.
[55] Outline, 3.
[56] Ibid.
[57] 'Legal Aspects of Euthanasia, Assistance to Suicide and Terminating the Medical Treatment of Incompetent Patients', 2. Unpublished paper delivered at a closed conference on euthanasia at the Institute of Bioethics, Maastricht, 2–4 December 1990.

can be justified, should simply assert that a request is no longer essential in all cases.

The Commission asserts that most of the 1,000 cases were incompetent patients in their 'death agony'. This assertion should, however, be considered in the light of the physician interviews which indicated that 14% of the patients were totally competent and a further 11% partly competent;[58] that 21% had a life expectancy of one to four weeks and 7% of one to six months (the survey classed patients as 'dying' if their life had been shortened only by 'hours or days', not by 'weeks or months'),[59] and that doctors did not list 'agony' as a reason for killing these patients. The reasons given by doctors were the absence of any prospect of improvement (60%); the futility of all medical therapy (39%); avoidance of 'needless prolongation' (33%); the relatives' inability to cope (32%); and 'low quality of life' (31%). Pain or suffering was mentioned by only 30%.[60] And, even in relation to this 30%, if they were essentially cases of increasing pain or symptom treatment to shorten life, why did the doctors not classify them under that heading?[61]

In short, the Commission's defence of these 1,000 cases would appear to be based on a shaky factual foundation and its attempted ethical justification amounts to little more than a bare assertion that killing without request, a practice in breach of one of the cardinal criteria for permissible euthanasia, is morally acceptable. On the basis of this assertion, it proceeds to recommend that doctors should report such cases in the same way as they report cases of voluntary euthanasia.[62]

The Government has accepted the Commission's recommendation that euthanasia without request should be reported. It is currently incorporating the reporting procedure into the statute regulating the disposal of the dead and is doing so in a way which makes it clear that the procedure applies whether the patient requested euthanasia or not.[63]

(b) other cases of intentional life-shortening without explicit request

In addition to the 1,000 cases, there were many others in which the patient made no explicit request that his life be shortened.

---

[58] 75% of the patients were 'totally unable to assess the situation and take a decision adequately'. However, 14% were totally, and 11% partly ('not totally') able to do so. Survey, 61, *Table* 6.4 The authors describe a person 'not totally able' as 'partially able to assess the situation and on this basis adequately take a decision'. *Ibid.*, 23. According to the death certificate study, 36% were competent. Loes Pijnenborg *et al.*, 'Life-terminating acts without explicit request of patient' (1993) 341 *Lancet* 1196, 1197 *Table* II.

[59] Survey, 66, *Table* 6.10. According to the Survey's (tentative) definition of 'dying' (*ibid.*, 24), therefore, in only 29% of the 2,700 cases of euthanasia and assisted suicide was the patient dying. *Ibid.*, 49, *Table* 5.13.

[60] *Ibid.*, 64, *Table* 6.7. Surprisingly, no question was asked about the doctor's intention which, as the authors note, 'complicates the interpretation of the results'. *Ibid.*, 57.

[61] Henk Jochemsen, 'Euthanasia in The Netherlands' *Journal of Medical Ethics* (forthcoming).

[62] Outline, 6. The Commission excepted from this recommendation cases where 'the vital functions have already and irreversibly begun to fail' on the ground that in such cases a natural death would have ensued anyway. *Ibid.* The Government has rejected this exception: see Gevers, *op cit* n63, *infra*, 140.

[63] J K M Gevers, 'Legislation on euthanasia: recent developments in the Netherlands' (1992) 18 *Journal of Medical Ethics* 138, 139–40.

In 59% (or 4,779) of the 8,100 cases in which doctors are said to have intended to hasten death by pain-killing drugs, the patient had 'never indicated anything about terminating life', and there had been no explicit request in a further 9% (or 729)[64], making a total of 5,508 cases in which there had been no explicit request.[65]

Additionally, there are the 8,750 cases in which treatment is said to have been withheld or withdrawn without explicit request and intentionally to shorten life.[66] The Commission would have it that these were cases of omitting to provide futile treatment. It states: 'After all, a doctor has the right to refrain from (further) treatment, if that treatment would be pointless according to objective medical standards. The commission would define a treatment without any medical use as therapeutical interference that gives no hope whatsoever for any positive effect upon the patient. To the application of this kind of futile medicine, no one is entitled. It is undisputed that the medical decision whether a particular action is useful or not, belongs to normal medical practice'.[67]

But this is misleading. First, the Survey did not use the concept of futile treatment in relation to withdrawal of treatment as the authors felt its meaning was open to 'variable' interpretation.[68] Secondly, it is clear from the preamble to the relevant questions that they were not asking about the withdrawal of futile treatment, that is, treatment which was unlikely or incapable of achieving its normal therapeutic purpose, but rather about the withdrawal of treatment which was preserving 'futile' lives, that is, lives which were not thought to be worth preserving:

In most instances this [decision to withhold or withdraw treatment] concerns situations in which the treating physician does not expect or does not observe sufficient success. However, there are situations in which a considerable life-prolonging effect can be expected from a certain treatment while the decision can nevertheless be made to withhold such treatment or to withdraw it. This implies that under such circumstances considerable prolongation of life is considered undesirable or even futile. "Considerable" is taken to mean more than one month.[69]

That the question was concerned with 'futile' lives rather than ineffectual treatment is confirmed by the authors' explanation of this series of questions:

Briefly, two types of situations are discussed here. On the one hand therapies are involved which will probably meet with little or no success. Such treatment can be withdrawn or withheld for this reason. On the other hand there are cases in which therapies which can have

---

[64] Survey, 76, *Table* 7.9.
[65] In 17% of cases, the patient had indicated something about life termination but the 'request was not strongly explicit'. *Ibid.* If these cases are included, the number of cases of life shortening without explicit request becomes 6,885. In only 15% of cases, therefore, was there a 'strongly explicit' request. *Ibid.*
[66] See text at n31, *supra*. In 18% of cases the patient had 'indicated something at some time about terminating life' and in a further 13% there had been some discussion with the patient. Survey, 88, *Table* 8.11.
[67] Outline, 3–4.
[68] Survey, 24.
[69] *Ibid.*, 84–85.

a considerable (more than one month) life-prolonging effect but in which prolongation of life is undesirable or pointless and treatment is withdrawn or withheld for this reason.[70]

They add that doctors were asked to discuss 'only the second type' of situation.[71]

Thirdly, it is clear that the question was so understood by the respondents, 35% of whom replied that their (primary or secondary) intention was to hasten death, not to withdraw a futile treatment.[72]

It is stiking that the lives of so many patients were shortened without explicit request. Hardly less striking is the fact that by no means all of the patients killed without request were incompetent. It will be recalled that of the 1,000 actively killed without request, 14% were (according to the physician interviews) totally competent and a further 11% partly competent. Van der Wal has aptly commented that in these cases the right to self-determination was 'seriously undermined'.[73] And of the 8,100 patients whose deaths are said to have been intentionally accelerated by palliative drugs, 60% (or 2,867) of those who had never indicated anything about life termination were competent.[74] Finally, the patient was totally competent in 22%, and partly competent in a further 21%, of all the cases where treatment was withheld or withdrawn without request.[75]

The Commission concludes that the Survey 'disproves the assertion often expressed, that non-voluntary active termination of life occurs more frequently in the Netherlands than voluntary termination'.[76] However, if intentional termination by omission is included, as it should be if an accurate overall picture is to be presented, the Survey indicates that non-voluntary euthanasia is in fact more frequent than voluntary euthanasia. As the above Table illustrates, the Survey discloses that in 1990 doctors intentionally sought to shorten more lives without than with the patient's explicit request. It was their primary aim to kill 10,558 patients, 5,450 (52%) of whom had not explicitly asked to have their lives shortened. If one includes cases in which the patient's death is referred to as part of what the doctor aimed to achieve, then the total number of intentional killings by doctors may not be far short of 26,350, in 15,258 of which (58%) the patient had not explicitly asked for death to be hastened when it was.

(ii) 'intolerable suffering with no prospect of improvement' with euthanasia as a 'last resort'

(a) 'intolerable suffering'

The Survey throws considerable doubt on whether euthanasia was confined to patients who were 'suffering unbearably' and for whom it was a 'last

---

[70] Ibid., 85.

[71] Ibid.

[72] See text at n.31, supra.

[73] Gerrit van der Wal, 'Unrequested termination of life: is it permissible?' (1993) 7 Bioethics 330, 337.

[74] Survey, 77.

[75] Ibid., 88. The Survey does not appear to provide separate figures for those whose lives were intentionally shortened.

[76] Outline, 3; Report, 33.

resort'.[77] For example, doctors were asked in interview which reason(s) patients most often gave for requesting euthanasia. Their replies to this question (and to that about the most important reasons for killing without request[78]) show that in most cases, 57%, it was 'loss of dignity'; in 46% 'not dying in a dignified way'; in 33% 'dependence' and in 23% 'tiredness of life'. Only 46% mentioned 'pain'.[79]

In relation to the withholding or withdrawal of treatment without explicit request and with intent to hasten death, the basis for the decision appears to have been simply a belief that, in the words of the preamble to the question put, 'considerable prolongation of life' was considered 'undesirable or even futile'.[80]

That Dutch doctors regard 'unbearable suffering' as an essential criterion is, moreover, hardly confirmed by the agreement of two thirds of those interviewed with the proposition that 'Everyone is entitled to decide over their own life and death'.[81]

(b) a 'last resort'

Nor does it appear that euthanasia was invariably a 'last resort'. Doctors said that treatment alternatives remained in one in five cases (21%) but that, in almost all of these cases, they were refused.[82] One in three GPs who decided that there were no alternatives had not sought advice from a colleague.[83] When asked to rank the guidelines in order of importance, only 64% of respondents said absence of treatment alternatives was '(very) important'.[84] Moreover, even in the four out of five cases in which the doctors said there were no treatment alternatives, this appears to mean 'alternatives to the current treatment' rather than 'alternatives to euthanasia'. This is suggested by the question asked ('Were alternatives available to the treatment given? Here I consider other therapeutic possibilities or possibilities to alleviate pain and/or symptoms',[85]) and by the doctors' response to another question about the aim of the treatment at the time when the decision to

---

[77] The Commission states that Dutch doctors regard the 'intolerable suffering of the patient and/or his natural desire for a quiet death' as the only grounds on which to perform euthanasia. *Ibid.*, 32. The reference to these grounds in the alternative, without disapproval, is revealing: it confirms that neither doctors nor the Commission regard both as essential for euthanasia to be permissible.

[78] See text at n.60, *supra*.

[79] Survey, 45, *Table 5.8*.

[80] *Ibid.*, 85. For example, the evidence in relation to the 8,750 cases in which doctors stated that they withheld or withdrew treatment without request with intent to shorten life does not indicate that all the patients were suffering unbearably and that euthanasia was a last resort. For one thing, 58% were incompetent, so how was the doctor able to assess the extent of the patients' suffering (if any), particularly as the patients' conditions varied? Survey, 88, *Table 8.12*.

[81] *Ibid.*, 102, *Table 9.7*.

[82] *Ibid.*, 45, *Table 5.7*.

[83] *Ibid.*, 43. Even in those cases where the doctors (two thirds of GPs and 80% of specialists) did consult, there is nothing to suggest that the colleague consulted was a specialist in palliative medicine.

[84] *Ibid.*, 96, *Table 9.2*.

[85] *Ibid.*, 43.

233

carry out euthanasia or assisted suicide was made. 77% replied it was palliative, 10% life prolonging, and 2% curative; only 14% said there was no treatment.[86] In other words, just because there might have been no treatment alternatives to the existing treatment does not mean that the existing treatment was not an alternative to euthanasia.

But even *if* the palliative treatment given in 77% of cases was not preventing intolerable suffering and was so ineffectual that euthanasia was thought to be the only alternative, does not this (and the fact that in 46% of cases pain was one of the reasons most frequently given by patients as a reason for wanting euthanasia) raise questions about the quality of the palliative care that the patients were receiving? It will be recalled that a report on palliative care published in 1987 by the Dutch Health Council concluded that a majority of cancer patients in pain suffered unnecessarily because of health professionals' lack of expertise.[87] Similarly, recently-published research into pain management at the Netherlands Cancer Institute, Amsterdam, contains the 'critical and worrisome overall finding ... that pain management was judged to be inadequate in slightly more than 50% of evaluated cases'.[88]

Interestingly, 40% of the Dutch doctors interviewed in the van der Maas survey expressed agreement with the proposition that 'Adequate alleviation of pain and/or symptoms and personal care of the dying patient make euthanasia unnecessary'.[89] Yet the Commission concludes that its total of 2,700 cases of 'euthanasia' and assisted suicide shows that 'euthanasia' is not being used as an alternative to good palliative medicine or terminal care.[90] This observation is quite unsupported by the data which reveals not 2,700 but over 10,500 unambiguously euthanasiast acts and omissions. It also sits uneasily with the Commission's later observation about the inadequacy of such care in Holland:

The research report shows that the medical decision process with regard to the end of life demands more and more expertise in a number of different areas. First of all medical and technical know-how, especially in the field of the treatment of pain, of prognosis and of alternative options for the treatment of disorders that cause insufferable pain.[91]

It adds:

Especially doctors, but nurses as well, will have to be trained in terminal care .... Optimal

---

[86] *Ibid.*, 45, *Table* 5.6. Why 14% were receiving no treatment is unexplained.

[87] *Op. cit.* n1, *supra*, 65. The British Medical Association Working Party on Euthanasia commented that palliative care in Holland is not as advanced as in Britain. *Euthanasia* (London: BMA, 1988) 49.

[88] Karin L. Dorrepaal *et al.*, 'Pain experience and pain management among hospitalized cancer patients' (1989) 63 *Cancer* 593, 598. Evidently, only 27% of Dutch GPs are trained to treat cancer pain and 40% are unaware of the sometimes severe pain suffered by their cancer patients. K L Dorrepaal, *Pijn bij patienten met kanker* (1989), cited by Z. Zylicz, 'Euthanasia' (1991) 338 *Lancet* 1150 (letter). Dr. Pieter Admiraal, one of Holland's leading practitioners of euthanasia, has written that 'in most cases, pain can be adequately controlled without the normal psychological functions of the patient being adversely affected'. 'Justifiable Euthanasia' (1988) 3 *Issues in Law & Medicine* 361, 362.

[89] Survey, 102, *Table* 9.7.

[90] Outline, 2; Report, 31.

[91] Outline, 7.

care for someone who is dying implies that the doctor has knowledge of adequate treatments for pain, of alternatives for the treatment of complaints about unbearable pain and that he is aware of the moment when he must allow the process of dying to run its natural course. Doctors still lack sufficient knowledge of this care . . . In a country that is rated among the best in the world when it comes to birth care, knowledge with regard to care for the dying should not be lacking.[92]

If there is such a lack of knowledge, does this not confirm and help to explain the Survey evidence which indicates that euthanasia is being used as an alternative to appropriate palliative care?[93]

(iii) performed by a doctor who has consulted an independent colleague and reported the case to the legal authorities

(a) consultation

The KNMG's proposed scheme of consultation with two colleagues, one of whom is independent, has never been put into effect. Doctors stated that they had consulted a colleague in 84% of cases of euthanasia and assisted suicide.[94] The Survey does not explain the form, substance or outcome of the consultations. Again, in the 1,000 killings without request – cases where it might be assumed that consultation assumed especial importance – only a minority (48%) of doctors consulted a colleague.[95] Moreover, 40% of GPs stated that they did not think that consultation was very important.[96]

(b) reporting

Only a minority of cases of 'euthanasia' were duly reported to the legal authorities. In almost three out of four cases (72%) doctors (three out of four GPs and two out of three specialists) certified that death was due to 'natural causes'.[97] By so doing, they not only failed to comply with one of the guidelines whose importance has been continually stressed by the KNMG, but they also committed the criminal offence of falsifying a death certificate.

[92] *Ibid.*
[93] An expert committee of the World Health Organisation has concluded: 'now that a practicable alternative to death in pain exists, there should be concentrated efforts to implement programmes of palliative care, rather than a yielding to pressure for legal euthanasia'. *Cancer Pain Relief and Palliative Care* (WHO Technical Report Series No. 804, Geneva, 1990).
[94] *Ibid.*, 47, *Table* 5.9.
[95] *Ibid.*, 64, *Table* 6.8 The reason given for not doing so in 68% of cases was that the doctor felt no need for consultation because the situation was clear. *Ibid.*, 65.
      Before withholding or withdrawing a treatment without request, doctors consulted a colleague in 54% of cases. *Ibid.*, 89, *Table* 8.13. (When there was a request the figure was 43%. *Ibid.*, 82, *Table* 8.5.) Before administering palliative drugs in such doses as might shorten life, doctors consulted in 47% of cases. *Ibid.*, 73, *Table* 7.4.
[96] *Ibid.*, 96, *Table* 9.2.
[97] *Ibid.*, 49, *Table* 5.14.

Doctors gave as their three most important reasons for falsifying the certificate the 'fuss' of a legal investigation (55%); a desire to protect relatives from a judicial enquiry (52%); and a fear of prosecution (25%).[98]

Similarly, virtually all of the 1,000 killings without request were certified as natural deaths. The most important reasons given by the doctors were the 'fuss' of a legal investigation (47%); the (remarkable) opinion that the death was in fact natural (43%); and the desire to safeguard the relatives from a judicial enquiry (28%).[99]

Interestingly, only 64% of doctors thought that each case of euthanasia should somehow be examined, and the most favoured form of scrutiny was by other doctors.[100]

Conclusions

My previous article maintained that the slippery slope argument in both its logical and practical forms applied to the Dutch experience of euthanasia. The Survey and the Report serve amply to reinforce that contention.

The examination of the guidelines in my earlier article suggested that they were vague, loose and incapable of preventing abuse.[101] This is vividly confirmed by the Survey, which shows that three of the most crucial guidelines – requiring a request which is free and voluntary; well-informed; and durable and persistent – have been widely disregarded. Doctors have killed with impunity. And on a scale previously only guessed at: the Survey discloses that it was the primary purpose of doctors to shorten the lives of over 10,000 patients in 1990, the majority without the patient's explicit request.

How the Remmelink Commission can so confidently conclude, in the light of the evidence unearthed by the Survey, that the 'medical actions and decision process concerning the end of life are of high quality'[102] is puzzling. The Commission's assessment is based solely on the doctors' uncorroborated replies, replies which disclose, surely far more reliably, widespread breach of the guidelines. In particular, the scale of intentional life-shortening without explicit request and of illegal certification of death by natural causes must cast grave doubt both on the Commission's conclusion that decision-making is of 'high quality' and on van der Maas's opinion that the Survey shows that doctors are 'prepared to account for their decisions'.[103] Even if all

---

[98] *Ibid.*, 48. The authors add that 23 doctors actually stated that they had regarded the death as natural.

[99] *Ibid.*, 65. Deaths hastened by withholding or withdrawing a treatment without request were almost all certified as natural deaths. *Ibid.*, 89. So too were all deaths hastened by the administration of palliative drugs, in over 90% of cases because the doctor felt the death was natural, but in 9% because he felt that reporting an unnatural death would be 'troublesome'. *Ibid.*, 74.

[100] *Ibid.*, 97, *Table* 9.3. See also *ibid.*, 98. It merits mention that in a small number of cases, the lethal drug was administered by someone other than the doctor, nurse or patient. See ibid., 140, *Table* 13.10; 143; 193.

[101] *Op.cit.*n.1, *supra*, 70. See this volume pp.209–10.

[102] Outline, 6. Remarkably, van der Maas also regards them as of 'good quality'. Survey, 199.

[103] Survey, 205.

cases had been reported, this would still, of course, have been no guarantee of propriety. Indeed, had they all been reported, it is doubtful whether prosecutors would have had the resources to subject them even to the limited check which reports currently receive.

As the 1,000 cases of unrequested killings graphically illustrate, the existing system cannot realistically hope to detect the doctor who ignores the guidelines since it essentially relies on him to expose his own wrongdoing. And the Remmelink Report's narrow categories of 'euthanasia' and 'intentional killing without request' may suggest to those who have not considered it before a neat way of side-stepping the reporting procedure. A doctor could kill not by a lethal drug, which he would be required to report, but by an overdose of morphine or by withdrawing treatment, which he could claim with at least some show of legitimacy (in the unlikely event of being challenged) to be 'normal medical practice'. It seems clear that the reporting procedure will continue to provide a wholly inadequate mechanism for regulating euthanasia and that the reports filed will continue to provide no more accurate a picture of the reality of euthanasia than they have done hitherto. Reports of killing without request promise to be particularly unrepresentative: how many doctors are likely to report a practice which has not (yet) been declared lawful by the courts?[104]

The Report uses the finding that doctors refused some 4,000 serious requests[105] to argue that 'euthanasia' is not used excessively and as an alternative to good palliative care.[106] Leaving aside the evident shortcomings in Dutch terminal care, this is simply illogical, particularly when viewed against the 10,500 occasions on which it was the doctor's primary purpose to shorten life.

That fact suggests rather the pertinence of the slippery slope argument in its 'logical' form, that acceptance of voluntary euthanasia implicitly involves condonation of (at least) non-voluntary euthanasia. The relevance of the argument is indeed quite strongly suggested by the fact that doctors had as their primary aim the shortening of the lives of some 5,500 patients without their explicit request (and are represented in the Survey as having had as their subordinate aim the shortening of the lives of upwards of a further 10,000 without their explicit request). The relevance is sufficiently striking even if one focuses simply on the 1,000 cases involving the administration of a lethal drug. Nor were these patients killed by a minority of maverick doctors: a majority of doctors admitted that they either had killed without request or would be prepared to do so.[107]

In any event, it is now clear that the legal and medical authorities in Holland no longer regard the patient's request as a *sine qua non* of permissible euthanasia. The Remmelink Commission seeks openly to defend the

---

[104] *Op. cit.* n.63, *supra*, 140.
[105] Survey, 52.
[106] Outline, 2.
[107] *Ibid.*, 58, *Table* 6.1.

vast majority of the thousand killings without request[108] and the Dutch Parliament is currently adopting Remmelink's recommendation that the reporting procedure for euthanasia should clearly allow for such cases.[109]

Similarly, the KNMG has condoned the killing, in certain circumstances, of incompetent patients including babies, patients in persistent coma and, most recently, patients with severe dementia.[110] It is surely only a matter of time before such 'responsible' medical opinion receives judicial approval. Indeed, this may not even be necessary: the Chief Prosecutors have already declined to prosecute in a number of cases of killing without request.

One such case involved a patient in a permanent coma after a heart attack. The local Chief Prosecutor, mindful of the Remmelink Commission's recommendation that such cases should be dealt with in the same way as killing on request, decided against prosecution; after questions had been raised in Parliament, his decision was affirmed at a meeting of all the Chief Prosecutors in February 1992.[111]

Another case concerned a dying 71 year-old man in a 'sub-comatose state and under sedation, who was no longer able to communicate'. He had not asked for his life to be shortened. At a meeting in November 1992 the Chief Prosecutors decided against prosecution since 'the action taken ... amounted to virtually the same as suspending ineffectual medical treatment', even though they regarded the case as 'potentially extending the boundaries of current practice'.[112]

The widespread readiness to kill without any request contrasts starkly with the refusal of many serious requests for euthanasia, and serves further to underline the dispensable role of patient autonomy in the reality, if not the rhetoric, of the Dutch experience. As ten Have and Welie shrewdly point out, acceptance of euthanasia is not resulting in greater patient autonomy

---

[108] A member of the Commission informed me that these killings came as a 'terrible shock' to its members, who had hoped that they did not exist. Interview, Mr. A Kors, 29 November 1991. This makes the Commission's defence of the bulk of these killings all the more puzzling.

[109] The Government has indicated that a different form may be introduced for reporting euthanasia without request and that additional requirements of 'careful practice' may be introduced for such cases. Jochemsen, *op. cit.* n61, *supra*.

[110] See *op. cit.* n.1, *supra*, 75. (This volume pp.214–15.) Henk Jochemsen, 'Life-Prolonging and Life-Terminating Treatment of Severely Handicapped Newborn Babies ...' (1992) 8 *Issues in Law & Medicine* 167; *Doen of laten*? (Nederlandse Vereniging voor Kindergeneeskude,1992)13; 'Dutch doctors support life termination in dementia' (1993) 306 *British Medical Journal* 1364.

[111] Personal communication, Staff Office of the Public Prosecutor, The Hague, 12 February 1993.

[112] A third case involved the killing of a 4 year-old handicapped child who was dying. Charges were dropped 'in view of the specific and unusual circumstances of the case, despite the fact that the patient had not expressly requested intervention'. *Ibid.*

One of the few cases in which a prosecution was launched recently came to trial. It concerned a 50 year-old woman suffering from severe depression who repeatedly asked her psychiatrist to help her die. The psychiatrist, who assisted her to commit suicide, was prosecuted but acquitted. The court found that the woman had been suffering unbearably: one son had committed suicide, the other had died of lung cancer and she had been repeatedly beaten over 25 years by her alcoholic husband. 'What the cause of her suffering was – illness or otherwise – is not important' stated the District Court at Assen. The prosecution intends to appeal. *Reuter*, 21 April 1993. See also Jochemsen, *op. cit.* n61, *supra*, n21.

but in doctors 'acquiring even more power over the life and death of their patients'.[113]

In 1990 Professor Leenen observed that there is an 'almost total lack of control on the administration of euthanasia'.[114] The Report and the Survey serve only to confirm the accuracy of that observation.[115] The Commission sought to paint a reassuring picture of the euthanasia landscape revealed by the Survey. As ten Have and Welie aptly observe:

> The Committee clearly tried to remove any social anxieties about the practice of euthanasia. Similar practices are brought under dissimilar headings to keep the numbers low. And at crucial places, particularly with the 1,000 non-voluntary euthanasia cases, the Committee uses fallacious rhetoric to emphasize that there is nothing to worry about.[116]

The picture painted by the Commission is an illusion. The hard evidence of the Survey indicates that, within a remarkably short time, the Dutch have proceeded down the slippery slope from voluntary to non-voluntary euthanasia. This is partly because the underlying justification for euthanasia in Holland is not now, if it ever has been, patient self-determination, but rather acceptance of the principle that certain lives are not worth living and that it is right to terminate them, and partly because of the inability of the vague and loose guidelines to ensure that euthanasia is only performed in accordance with the criteria laid down by the courts and the KNMG.

Whether the killing of competent patients without request, or against their will, will become as established a feature of the Dutch euthanasia landscape as nonvoluntary killing has become remains to be seen, but the extent to which some doctors have already proved themselves willing to shorten the lives of even competent patients without request suggests that a further slide cannot be ruled out.

In sum, the validity of the slippery slope argument in relation to euthanasia has been forcefully brought home by the Dutch experience. But this should come as no surprise. Some twenty years ago a perspicacious warning about the dangers of venturing onto the slope was sounded by one of the members of the House of Lords Select Committee on Medical Ethics:

> Legislation to permit euthanasia would in the long run bring about profound changes in social attitudes towards death, illness, old age and the role of the medical profession. The Abortion Act has shown what happens. Whatever the rights and wrongs concerning the present practice of abortion, there is no doubt about two consequences of the 1967 Act:
>
> (a) The safeguards and assurances given when the Bill was passed have to a considerable extent been ignored.
> (b) Abortion has now become a live option for *anybody* who is pregnant. This does not imply

---

[113] Henk A M J ten Have and Jos V M Welie, 'Euthanasia: Normal Medical Practice?' (1992) 22(2) *Hastings Center Report* 34, 38. See also Jos V M Welie, 'The Medical Exception: Physicians, Euthanasia and the Dutch Criminal Law' (1992) 17 *Journal of Medicine and Philosophy* 419, 435.

[114] *Op. cit.* n1, *supra*, 78. (This volume p.217.)

[115] The author of the Remmelink Report agreed that there was no control over cases which had not been reported and that, even in relation to the reported cases, the prosecutor did not know whether the doctor was telling the truth. He maintained that euthanasia occurred even if the law prohibited it, as was the case outside Holland, and that it was preferable to try to control it. Interview, Mr. A Kors, 29 November 1991.

[116] *Op. cit.* n.112, *supra*, 36.

that everyone who is facing an unwanted pregnancy automatically attempts to procure an abortion. But because abortion is now on the agenda, the climate of opinion in which such a pregnancy must be faced has radically altered.

One could expect similarly far-reaching and potentially more dangerous consequences from legalized euthanasia.[117]

This article maintains that the experience of The Netherlands illustrates the far-reaching and dangerous consequences of tolerating euthanasia and confirms the force of the slippery slope arguments against so doing. But these arguments, while underlining the difficulties of framing and enforcing safeguards against euthanasia without request and while indicating that the case for voluntary euthanasia rests on the principle that certain lives are not worth living and that it is morally acceptable to terminate them, cannot by themselves refute the case for euthanasia. For why should this principle not be accepted? That is a question which is answered elsewhere in this volume.

---

[117] Rt.Rev. J S Habgood, 'Euthanasia – A Christian View' [1974] 3 *Journal of the Royal Society of Health* 124, 126.

Contributors

John Finnis is a Fellow of University College, Oxford and Professor of Law and Legal Philosophy in the University. He is a Fellow of The British Academy and Vice-Chairman of the Board of Governors of The Linacre Centre. Among his important contributions to jurisprudence and moral philosophy are *Natural Law and Natural Rights* (Oxford 1980), *Fundamentals of Ethics* (Oxford 1983) and *Moral Absolutes* (CUA Press 1991).

Luke Gormally has been Director of The Linacre Centre for Health Care Ethics since 1981, and previously held a research post at the Centre. He has been a member of The Catholic Bishops' Joint Committee on Bioethical Issues for the past ten years. His publications include a recently edited volume on *The Dependent Elderly. Autonomy, Justice and Quality of Care* (Cambridge University Press 1992).

John Keown is a Fellow of The Queens' College, Cambridge, and a Lecturer in The Faculty of Law in the University specialising in medical law and ethics. He was previously a Director of The Centre for Health Care Law at The University of Leicester. He is a Governor of The Linacre Centre. His publications include *Abortion, Doctors and the Law* (Cambridge University Press 1988). Since 1989 he has devoted considerable time to research into the practice and regulation of euthanasia in Holland.

Index

abortion, 39, 42, 49, 56, 120–122, 155, 239–240
absolute prohibition, an, 39–43, 48–49, 56, 127–128, 180, 189 n.16
actions (acts): deliberate, 47, 48, 126–127, 154; ethically impossible, 47; ethically necessary, 47; illegal, 39; murderous, 39; and omission, 21, 27, 44, 46–48, 66, 75, 95, 126–127, 141, 169, 183–184; *see also* omission; positive, 46–47, 66, 156, 168–169, 183–184, 185–186; unlawful, 39; voluntary, 47; wrongful, 39
advance directives, 26, 145–149, 152–153, 157–158, 167–176; *see also* proxy
Airedale N.H.S. Trust v Bland *see* Bland case
Alkmaar case, 194–198, 203, 210, 213 n.119
allowing to die, 9, 16, 17–22, 27, 47–48, 80–81, 86, 94, 105–106, 126–127
amenity, 43
American Academy of Pediatrics, 16
animals, 29 n.53, 31, 35, 40, 42, 95, 125 n.13
answerability, 40
aphasia, 27, 97
Arthur case, 7–8, 104–107, 185 n.13
atheroarteriosclerosis, 27, 97
authority: civil, 39–40; religious, 39
autonomy, 61, 68, 129–135, 145–147, 164–165, 168–169, 171–172, 215, 231–232, 239

basal pneumonia, 93, 97
best interests *see* patient
Bible, 56
bilateral anophthalamia, 18, 97
Bland case, 118 n.1, 119 n.2, 125, 127 n.15, 129 n.19, 137 n.6, 141 n.8, 142 n.9, n.10, 143, 145 n.2, 148, 150–151, 153 n.1, 155–158, 168, 170, 171, 173 n.8, 174 n.12, 176 n.18
Bolam principle, 150–151
brain death, 27–28, 94, 125 n.13, 181–182
British Medical Association, 67 n.1;

Discussion Paper on Treatment of Patients in Persistent Vegetative State (1992), 127 n. 15; *Handbook of Medical Ethics* (1980), 67 n.1; *Report on Euthanasia* (1988), 125 n.13, 127 n.15, 177–192, 202, 234 n.87
British Paediatric Association, 67 n.1
bromide, 25, 97
bronchitis, 78
burdensome treatment *see* treatment

capital punishment, 37, 56, 119 n.2
care: comfort, 75, 77, 90–91, 134–135, 159–160, 175, 234–235; cost of, 21, 32–33, 147–148, 175–176; of elderly, 15, 25–27, 82, 91–93; of handicapped, 15, 19–21, 22–23, 81, 88–89; hospice, 24, 31, 90, 155, 159–160; intensive, 15, 27–28, 82, 93; kinds of, 73–97; medical, 11, 12, 15, 51, 68, 75, 78, 84, 91, 138–143; of newborn, 15–22, 84–88, 104–107, 187; 'nursing only', 18, 104–106; ordinary, 15, 85, 88, 138–139, 141–143, 147–148, 176; *see also* duty of care; feeding; team, 81–83; terminal, 15, 23–25, 50, 78–80, 82, 90–91, 138–139, 143, 155, 159–160, 162, 205, 229–230, 234–235
character of doctors *see* doctors
chemotherapy, 69, 78, 97
chloral hydrate, 18, 25, 97
Christian: belief, 51–55; Church, 51; faith, 54; morals, 56; teaching, 51–58, 135; tradition, 42, 51–58, 118–119, 135–136
Church Fathers, 53
clinical practice: British, 11, 16, 17, 23, 24, 25, 26, 27, 67 n.1, 183, 187; Dutch, 161–164, 204–210, 219–240; North American, 11, 16–17, 24, 26–27, 29 n.52
clinical team, 73, 81–83
colostomy, 70, 97
common good, 39
common morality, 12, 46, 156

243

competent *see* patient

consciousness, 43; *see also* Persistent Vegetative State

consent to treatment *see* treatment

consequentialism *see* utilitarianism

courts *see* law

creation, 51, 118

Criminal Justice Act 1967, 38 n.1

'custodial management', 21, 95

cystic fibrosis, 80

death: as benefit, 11, 16, 19, 42, 78, 80, 84, 95, 128, 153–154, 186; through dehydration and starvation, 18–19, 85, 104–107, 175–176, 187; diagnosis of, 27–28, 94, 125 n.13, 181–182; with dignity, 28, 42, 55, 93, 195, 203, 233; as end or as means, 49, 126, 168; hastening, 9, 17, 21, 23, 24, 25, 27 n.48, 46 n.8, 57, 64, 67, 75, 95, 141, 144, 162, 194, 209, 220, 223–227; inevitability of, 43, 65, 76, 90–94, 135; by omission, 15, 21, 27, 46–48, 64–65, 88, 95, 126–127; probability of, 28, 39; responsibility for, 37–38; unintended, 46, 127, 169–170, 184–185, 211, 225; voluntary, 35

Decalogue, 51, 52

diabetes, 62, 137, 152

doctors, character of, 154–155, 187–188, 189 n.16, 190, 192

'double effect', principle of, 48–50, 57

Down's syndrome, 16, 17, 18, 30, 32, 86, 95, 97, 104–107

drugs, cytotoxic, 92, 97; hypnotic, 19, 98; pain killing, 19, 48, 50, 56–57, 78–79, 85, 92, 222, 223, 225–226; psychotropic, 80, 99

dualism, 124–125

duodenal atresia, 16, 30, 70, 95, 98

Dutch Medical Association (KNMG), 163, 164, 198, 201, 202, 214, 215, 217, 220, 225, 227, 228 n.49, 238, 239; *Guidelines for Euthanasia*, 199–200, 203–204; *Report on Euthanasia* (1984), 160–162, 198–201, 205, 206, 214, 225, 235

duties of patients and doctors, 57, 61–71, 81, 92, 134–149, 176, 179–192, 211–212

duty of care, 141–144, 156–158, 164, 168

Dworkin, Ronald, 121–125, 132 n.20, 145 n.3, 146 n.4, 172 n.7, 174 n.12

euthanasia: active, 9, 18, 21, 25, 27 n.48, 223, 225, 232; advocacy of, 18 n.10, 22, 23, 27, 30–33, 42, 120, 128–129, 155, 213–216; in America, 16, 17, 18, 26–27, 173, 174; and Christian moral teaching, 55–58, 118–119, 135–136; definition of, 10–11, 203, 219, 222, 223, 225–227; and eugenics, 11 n.1, 23; in Germany in 1920s and 30s, 32, 164 n.25; of handicapped, 22–23, 89, 163, 209, 214–215; by instalments, 22, 23–24, 79; involuntary, 160, 194, 202, 203, 205, 208, 209, 213, 214, 216, 229, 239; justifications for, 9–10, 35, 120–124, 128–129, 187–190; and 'Lebensraum', 11 n.1; legalisation of, 9, 21 n.32, 25, 30–31, 45, 152–158, 163–165, 169–176, 177–190, 216–218; *see also* law; as 'mercy killing', 23, 31, 128–129, 154–155, 159–160, 162, 188–189, 195–197, 200, 211–212, 232–235; morality of, 37–58, 128–133; in the Netherlands, 160–164, 180, 193–240; non-voluntary, 11, 15, 21, 26 n.43, 28, 30 n.55, 31, 95, 128, 132–133, 152, 153, 154, 155, 162, 163, 164, 187, 194, 202, 207–210, 213, 214–217, 223–226; by omission, 21 n.32, 80, 95, 207, 209, 223, 226; *see also* omission; in paediatrics, 15–22, 35, 82, 84–88, 95, 104–107, 163, 187, 209, 214, 238; passive, 9, 18, 21, 26–27, 46–47, 223–226; policy of, 83; of terminally ill, 23–24, 90–91, 152, 173–174, 200, 228–230, 233–235; voluntary, 9, 28, 30–32, 35, 42–43, 45, 95, 128–132, 154–155, 160–165, 193–240; Voluntary Euthanasia Society, 30, 137 n.6, 152, 171, 173–175

evolution (human), 30

Exit, 9, 26 n.43, 30–32; *see also* Voluntary Euthanasia Society

exoneration, 37, 38, 39

extraordinary means, 26 n.43, 57, 62–63; *see also* ordinary means

extrophy of the bladder, 17, 98

family stress, 21 n.33, 31, 106, 203, 204, 208, 230

febrile infections, 27

feeding, 18, 46, 78, 89, 93, 95, 104–107, 141, 142 n.11, 153, 175–176, 185 n.13, 187; enteral, 26, 27, 89, 141–143, 147–148, 175–176

felony, 38 n.1

Finnis, John, 115 n.1, 125 n.12, 145 n.1, 155 n.3, 169 n.5, 211 n.113, 241

Foot, Philippa, 128 n.16, n.17

foresight, 38–39, 127–128, 155, 169, 211

freedom: and religious sense, 45; and self-determination, 42–43; *see also* autonomy

futile treatment *see* treatment

Gelfand, Gregory, 173 n.10, 174 n.11, 175 n.14, n.15, n.16

generosity, 55
Gillett, Grant, 120 n.3, 177 n.3, 182 n.9
Glover, Jonathan, 28 n.50, 48 n.12
glucose and water feed, 18
God: God's commands, 51–53; God's
    creation, 51, 53, 55, 56, 118; God's
    friendship, 54; God's gifts, 43, 51, 55, 57;
    God's likeness, 43, 56, 118; God's love,
    57; God's presence, 54–55; God's will,
    43, 53, 54, 95
Gomez, Carlos F., 161 n.7, 163 n.19, 217
Gormally, Luke, 115 n.1, 145 n.1, 241
government: and attack on people's lives,
    39–40, 122; first task of, 40, 122; and
    justice, 40, 122; and laws, 39–40
Grisez, Germain, 175 n.16
guilt: for death, 37, 48, 90; of doing evil,
    46–47; of murder, 37, 45

Habgood, J.S., 163 n.24, 239–240
handicapped patient, 21, 22–23, 28–29, 32,
    75, 84, 88–89, 141–143, 163, 183–184,
    187, 209, 214–215
Hare, R.M., 28 n.50, 188
hi-jackers (example of), 37–38
homicide: impermissible deliberate, 38, 119,
    127; laws, 29, 30, 95, 120, 122–123, 150,
    156, 157, 168–171, 193–194, 210–213; see
    also law; murder
hospice, 24, 25, 31, 90, 154, 155, 159–160,
human being, 41; see also person
human capacities, 118–126, 181–184, 185;
    point of, 119, 124; radical, 118–119, 124;
    short-term psychological, 120–124, 125–
    126, 181–184, 185
human dignity, 9, 12, 20, 22, 30, 31, 83, 97,
    119–120, 123–124, 125–126, 132–133; see
    also person; life
human flourishing, 124, 126, 130–131, 134,
    136, 138, 174
human heart, 43
human rights see rights
hydrocephalus, 17, 86, 88, 98

illness: acute, 76, 88; serious, 57, 138;
    terminal, 50, 61–62, 64, 65–66, 76–80,
    90–91, 138, 152, 173–174, 191–192, 228–
    230
incompetent see patient
innocence, 40, 50
innocent victim, 38, 39–40, 49, 52, 119
intention, 37, 38, 39, 46, 47, 65, 126–128,
    155–157, 168–171, 184–185
intentional killing see killing
Israel, 51, 52, 53

Jesus (Christ), 51, 52, 53, 54, 56, 95

Judaism, 52, 53
judgements: on burdensome treatment,
    63–64, 68–69, 96, 140–141; lucid and
    mature, 61; practical, 46; quality of life,
    19, 20–21, 33, 43–45, 46, 81, 140, 182–
    183, 185, 186, 187; value of life, 20–22,
    42, 43, 44, 78, 80, 82–83, 95, 120–122,
    138–139
justice, 40, 41, 43, 45, 83, 95, 119–120,
    122–124, 150, 151, 164

Kass, Leon R., 134 n.1
Keown, John, 115 n.1, 160 n.2, n.3, n.4,
    161 n.5, n.6, 162 n.16, 163 n.23, 169 n.5,
    241
kill(ing), 9, 17 n.9, 18, 19, 28, 37, 38, 39, 40,
    126–133; direct, 48–49, 170; divine
    command and, 51–53; of innocent
    people, 38, 39, 40, 119; intentional, 24,
    35, 37, 38, 39, 40, 48–49, 126–128, 135,
    141, 144, 155–158, 162–164, 168–171,
    184–185, 222–227; legitimate, 37, 52, 119,
    127–128; as mercy, 42–43, 44, 128–129,
    154–155, 188–189; by omission, 18, 21
    n.32, 27 n.48, 46–47, 95, 126–127, 141,
    143, 155–158, 162, 163, 164, 168–171,
    184–185, 186; see also omission; planned,
    38; as private decision, 40, 82; in self-
    defence, 38; as side-effect of other action,
    38–39, 48–50, 127–128, 184–185, 225;
    vengeful, 38
KNMG see Dutch Medical Association
Kuhse, Helga, 135 n.3, 191 n.21

law: American state, 26 n.43, 167, 169, 173,
    174, 175, 176; and courts, 104–105, 150–
    151, 155–157, 160–161, 174, 185 n.13,
    194–198, 201, 202, 203, 210–213; Dutch,
    160–163, 193–240; English, 38 n.1, 39,
    104–107, 150–158, 167, 168, 169, 170,
    171, 173, 174, 176, 185 n.13, 211 n.113;
    guilty intent and, 38, 155–158, 168–171,
    184–185, 211 n.113; homicide, 29, 30, 95,
    120, 122–123, 150, 156, 157, 168–171,
    193–194, 210–213; moral, 39, 48; and
    defence of necessity, 39, 160, 194–198,
    210, 213 n.119, 229; obedience to, 40; of
    God, 56; of human nature, 53; Victorian
    state, 167, 169, 170, 171, 173, 175
letting die see allowing to die
'letting nature take its course', 9
life (human): 'biological', 41, 121, 122, 124,
    125, 183; conception of, 30, 124–125;
    dignity of, 9, 12, 22, 30, 31, 41, 83, 97,
    119–126; disposable, 21, 57; as a gift
    from God, 43, 51, 56, 118–119; as a

245

good, 51, 55, 174, 175, 176; mystery of, 35, 43, 51, 95; prolongation of, 10, 26 n.43, 46, 48, 64, 65, 66, 67, 75, 78, 79, 80–81, 91, 95, 96, 134–135, 138, 139, 173–176, 185–187, 190–192, 231, 232; quality of, 9, 11, 19, 20, 21, 22, 32, 33, 43–44, 81, 88, 89, 140, 182–183, 185, 186, 187, 215, 230; rejection of, 65–66; religious valuation of, 45, 95, 118–119, 122 n.8; respect for, 43, 48, 53, 56, 95, 212, 213; reverence for, 83, 84; sanctity of, 9, 12, 56, 57, 95, 118–119, 121, 122, 129, 132, 133, 150, 190; shortening of, 44, 57, 79, 95; *see also* death, hastening; termination of, 26, 43, 44, 45, 53, 81, 94, 126–128; valuation of, 43–45, 82–83, 95, 106, 120–122, 128–129, 137, 139, 150, 151, 178, 179, 180, 212; value of, 20, 21, 28, 29, 32, 33, 43, 44, 45, 52 n.3, 86, 95, 96, 124–126, 128–129, 131, 132, 133, 135, 176, 178, 179, 180–184; worthless, 23, 32, 33, 42, 45, 78, 81, 95, 106–107, 120, 128–129, 131–132, 139, 163, 164, 170, 174, 178–179, 215–216, 231–232; worthwhile, 9, 20, 43–45, 84, 95, 139, 140, 174; wrongful, 19
living will *see* advance directives

malice, 38 n.1
magnet (example of), 41
management: custodial, 21, 95; no uniformly applicable positive rule of, 71, 93; of newborn, 15–22, 69–70, 84–88, 105–106, 187; policies of, 18–19; principles for good, 75–83
manslaughter, 39, 50, 168, 171
May, William, 175 n.16
McCormick, Richard, 174 n.13
meconium ileus, 80, 85, 98
medical ethics, 42, 45, 106, 160, 164, 195, 196, 210, 211
medical negligence *see* Bolam principle; duty of care
medical practice (an axiom of), 50, 79
medicine (ends of), 75, 134–135, 138–139, 164, 174, 192
meekness, 54
mercy, 42
Model Penal Code, 39
moral: law, 39, 48; pluralism, 30, 45–46; truth, 45
morphine, 18, 23, 79, 98
Moses, 54
mucoviscidosis, 80, 98
murder: absolute prohibition on, 40, 42, 48, 49, 56, 128; a class of acts, 37, 119;

definition of, 37–39, 157 n.6, 194, 229; and divine command, 51–53, 56; elements of, 37–39; as injustice to murdered, 40, 120, 150; and intentional killing, 37–39, 48–49, 126–128, 157, 168; intrinsically wrongful, 35, 40; mental element in, 38, 39, 157 n.6; by omission, 46–47, 95, 106, 126–127, 141, 168, 185 n.13; and the penumbra area, 50; self-murder, 52; verdict of, 38 n.1, 211
myeloblastic monocytic leukaemia, 69, 98
myocardial infarction, 26, 98–99

narcotic, 57, 99
Natural Death Act (California) 1976, 26 n.43
necessity *see* law
New Testament, 51, 56
nutrition and hydration *see* feeding

obligation: legal, 61, 168; moral, 61; *see also* duties; duty of care
obligation to undergo treatment *see* treatment
oesophagael atresia, 85, 99
Old Testament, 56
omission, 15, 17, 21, 25, 26, 44, 46–48, 66, 75, 80, 89, 95, 96; of life-saving measures, 47–48, 126–127, 141, 144, 155, 156, 157, 168, 169, 185
ordinary means, 57, 62–64, 78, 135; *see also* extraordinary means; care

palliative care *see* care
Pallis, Christopher, 181 n.7
parents' rights *see* rights
Parkinson's disease, 78, 191
patient: age of, 25, 27, 92; best interests of, 145, 146, 149, 151, 158, 172; 'brain dead', 94; burdens on, 44, 51, 63, 64, 75, 84, 93, 139–140, 147, 149, 186; classes of, 75–81, 84–94; competent, 12, 60–66, 84, 95, 96, 135–138, 232; dying, 23–25, 57, 66, 75–80, 93–94, 96, 143, 200, 229–230; incapacitating condition of, 81; incompetent, 33, 67–70, 84–88, 96, 140–143, 145–149, 152, 153, 167, 172, 174–176, 217; refusal of treatment by competent, 61–66, 135–138, 170–172, 186, 191–192; rights and duties of, 61–71, 135–149, 168–169, 172, 176, 190–192; selection of, 18; terminally ill, 23–25, 76–80, 152, 173–174, 191–192
peritonitis, 93
Persistent Vegetative State, 138, 141–143, 150, 157, 182, 183, 184; *see also* Bland case

person (human), 22–23, 29, 31, 41, 43–44, 55, 123–126, 181–184; concept of, 41, 123–126, 181–184; created for their own sake, 56, 57, 118; dignity of, 41–45, 55, 58, 91, 97, 119–120, 123–126, 132; as individual, 41; 'possessive individualist' conceptions of, 29; mystery of, 54
personhood, 29, 41
Pius X11, 56–58, 135
pneumonia, 62, 64, 65, 86, 191
Poor Law Hospitals, 25
pot-holer (example of), 49
power of attorney, 167; *see also* proxy
principles of good practice, 75–83, 134–144
prolongation of life *see* life
proxy, 26 n.43, 140–141, 145–147, 149, 152, 167, 170, 171, 172

quality of life *see* life; judgements

Rachels, James, 48 n.12, 129 n.18
rational: agent, 37, 38; nature, 41, 119, 124; *see also* human capacities
refusal of treatment *see* right; suicidal; treatment
Regina v Arthur *see* Arthur case
religious: attitude, 43, 45; valuation of life, 45, 95, 118–119, 122 n.8
Remmelink Commission (and Remmelink Report), 161, 162 n.13, 163, 164, 207, 209, 219, 220, 221, 222, 224, 225, 226, 227, 229, 230, 231, 232, 233 n.77, 234, 236, 237, 238, 239; *see also* Van der Maas Survey
respect for life *see* life
responsibility, 17, 28–29, 37–38, 42, 46–47, 61, 67, 68, 73, 75, 81, 82, 136, 141; clinical 75, 136, 141, 144; for death 37–38, 46, 126–127; notions of, 37–38; utilitarian views of, 28–29, 184–185
resurrection, 55
reverence for life *see* life
right(s): to die, 30, 213; doctor's and patient's, 57, 61–71, 145–148, 168–176; human, 22, 29, 45, 119–120; to life, 29, 40, 45; not to be murdered, 40, 45, 120, 151; of newborn, 29 n.53, 69–70; parents', 67; to refuse treatment, 61, 145–148, 167–176
Roman Catechism (1566), 56
Roman Catholic: Church, 55, 57, 115; teaching, 55–58, 62, 115, 135, 170
Royal Dutch Medical Association *see* Dutch Medical Association
rubella syndrome, 18, 99

Saint Paul, 52, 53

sanctity of life *see* life
Scripture (Sacred), 52
sedation and starvation (policy of), 18–19, 22, 85, 88, 187
Singer, Peter, 120 n.3, 135 n.3
Social Darwinism, 30
spina bifida, 15, 17, 18, 19, 20, 21 n.34, 32, 86, 87, 88, 95, 99
spirit, 35, 41, 42, 44, 45, 55, 95
State (competence of), 39; *see also* government
stewardship of life (man's), 53–55
substituted judgement *see* proxy
suffering, 9, 26, 27, 29 n.53, 31, 42, 43, 54, 55, 79, 80, 85, 89, 90, 91, 134, 154, 159, 160, 162, 163, 188, 189, 195, 196, 197, 199, 200, 203, 205, 211, 212, 213, 232–235
suicide, 35, 42–43, 45, 56, 61, 64–66, 137–138; ethics of, 35, 137–138, 145, 152, 153, 158, 160, 162, 168–171, 180, 194, 223, 224, 225; by omission, 68, 191; as self-murder, 52
suicidal: decision, 64; intent, 65, 147, 152–153, 169–171; refusal of treatment, 44, 61, 64–66, 137–138, 147, 148, 152–153, 168–171, 186, 191, 226 n.44
surgery, 16, 17, 18, 48, 49, 50, 70, 77, 85, 86, 88, 92

termination of life *see* life; death, hastening
tradition: Christian, 51–58, 118–119, 135–136; Judaeo-Christian, 35, 39, 52; legal, 67, 119–120, 156; moral, 67, 120, 156; religious, 35, 52, 120
transplantation (organ), 27, 48–49, 94
treatment: benefits of, 63–64, 67–71, 75, 81, 84, 92, 96; burdensome, 26, 44, 45–46, 51, 61–62, 63–64, 67–71, 77, 84, 95, 138, 139–141, 147, 149, 170, 186; consent to, 16, 61–66, 67, 135–140; efficaciousness of, 63; futile, 26, 31, 48, 51, 63, 66, 69, 70, 81, 94, 96, 138–139, 140, 142, 170, 231, 232; of handicapped, 88–89; kinds of, 75–94; life saving, 47–48, 57, 62, 75–81, 85–86, 95, 96, 137, 139, 142, 152–153; life-support, 76, 94, 142 n.11; life sustaining, 57, 61–62, 76, 78, 85, 93–94, 137, 138, 139, 142 n.11, 152–153, 173–174; minimal, 70; of newborn, 69–70, 84–88; non-treatment, 22, 27; obligation to undergo, 12, 61–66, 135–140; over-treatment, 26, 93–94; policies of, 9, 19, 25; refusal of, 26, 61–66, 69, 81, 95, 96, 135–140, 145–148, 167–176, 186, 191–192; selection of, 19, 20, 46; side-

effects of, 44; standard of, 67, 71; surgical, 70, 77; *see also* surgery; in terminal phase, 75–80, 90–91, 138; uniformity in, 71; withholding of, 16–17, 19–20, 25, 46 n.8, 52 n.3, 69–71, 81, 85, 94, 134–141, 144, 162, 163, 164, 167–175, 185–187, 223, 226, 231, 232
tube feeding *see* feeding, enteral

Utilitarianism (and consequentialism), 28–29, 40, 46, 184–185

Van der Maas Survey, 161–163, 207, 219–240
Vatican Council 11, 56, 57

valuation of life *see* life
value, 28–29, 43, 44, 124, 128, 129
value of life *see* life; judgements
voluntary behaviour, 47
virtue, 54

war, 41, 56, 119 n.2
Warnock, Mary, 121, 122, 123, 124, 135 n.3
will, 43, 65
withholding of treatment *see* treatment
worthless life *see* life
worthwhile life *see* life
wrongful life *see* life